Eat to Your Heart's Content!

Also By Dr David Dighton

Heart Sense
The 100 Calorie Heart Diet

Eat to Your Heart's Content!

The Diet and Lifestyle For a Healthy Heart

Dr David H. Dighton

HeartShield

First Published 2005

Copyright © D. H. Dighton

Published in Great Britain by Heartshield Ltd,
115, High Road, Loughton, Essex, IG10 4HJ UK
www.heartshield.org

British Library Cataloguing in Publication Data

A CIP catalogue record for this title is available from
the British Library

ISBN 0-9551072-0-2

Typeset by SX Composing DTP, Rayleigh, Essex
Printed and bound in Great Britain by
Mackays of Chatham plc, Chatham, Kent

CONTENTS

PART 1
HUNTING A KILLER
Chapter 1: The Silent Killer 3

What is our problem? Know your enemy . . . possibly your No 1 enemy. Inside arteries. How old are your arteries? Disabling arteries. Angina. Artery 'furring' and eggs. Is it all in our genes? To screen or not to screen? Artery 'furring', something old, something new. Remodelling. Plaque rupture. Detecting collateral damage. Limiting the damage. Repairing 'furred' arteries.

In the developed world, it is a fact that cardiovascular disease (strokes and heart attacks), not cancer, is our biggest killer. Other facts are that we are getting fatter and heart disease is reducing, but why? What are we getting right? What are we still getting wrong?

Artery 'furring' and High Blood Pressure, are they going to get you?

Chapter 2: Early Warning Signs 26

Survival strategies. Getting tested. The medical examination. Symptoms to be taken seriously. Chest pain – is it angina? Arm pain. Have you had a heart attack? Blackouts. Palpitations. Breathlessness. Claudication – pain in the calves when walking. Ankle swelling. Family history. The physical examination. Do you have high blood pressure? The tests or Investigations. Blood tests, ECG's, exercise ECG's, ultrasound pictures of arteries, IVUS, X-rays, EBCT scanning. Coronary arteriography. In the pipeline – new tests.

A summary of your needs. Further testing. Ruling out diabetes. Extra tests.

Looking for Trouble – Before it looks for *you*! A guide to the methods we use to detect early artery and heart disease.

PART 2
FEEDING THE ARTERIES

WHAT'S GOOD, WHAT'S BAD, AND WHAT'S JUST PLAIN UGLY.

Low fat diets. Atkins and beyond. Cholesterol in food – worried? Cholesterol and saturated fat in food. If anti-oxidants are good, are oxidants (copper and iron) bad. How bad are some foods for our arteries? The 'furring' factor. The AGI or Atherogenic Index. Healthy food for our arteries. Fats in food. Arginine and lysine.

The food we eat and its relationship to the 'furring' of arteries and high blood pressure.

What is good for our arteries. The clinical trial. Foods that might prevent heart attacks. Vitamins. Vitamins E and C. The B vitamins. Amino-acids. Minerals: magnesium, manganese, selenium, and zinc. Dietary fat and fatty acids. Dietary fibre. Phytosterols. Soya protein and isoflavones. Wine and alcohol. Garlic. Knowing what is good for our arteries. The API or Atheroprotective Index of foods.

Food to stop our arteries 'furring'.
Is any food good enough to stop our arteries 'furring'?

Chapter 5: The Cardiac Value of Food   109

'Heart' food! Recommended amounts of the good stuff. How big is a portion? Overall Cardiac Value (CVo). Cardiac Value scores and their meaning. The cardiac value of food groups. Have we progressed beyond our best? Dietary revolutions. Individual chemical cardiac value scores.

The Good / Bad Ratio: what food is good for the heart?

Chapter 6: The Cardiac Value of Different Diets   128

The value of different diets. The ideal cardiac protection diet. The Polymeal Diet. The 'Teen' diet. Gourmet diets. A very low calorie diet for dieting. The Atkins Diet. The vegetarian diet.

Is any diet really better than any other? The different diets we eat: the gourmet diet, the vegetarian diet, and the food our teenagers eat: how much better or worse are they? The Atkin's Diet – is it bad for your heart?

Chapter 7: Food Choice for Patients –
A Simple 100 Unit System.   147

Foods for those with high blood pressure and for those who want to lose weight. Diabetes and carbohydrate units.

Diabetics, the overweight, and those with high blood pressure – choose your foods using a simple point system. Have less than 100 units of some foods, and more than 100 units of others – and help your heart and circulation.

PART 3
ARE WE JUST WHAT WE EAT?
OTHER KILLER CAUSES - OTHER KILLER CURES

Chapter 8: Other 'Baddies'   155

The non-food baddies list. So you want to trust to luck? The smoking gun. Stop smoking! Giving up the habit. Influencing destiny? Ignorance as a culture. Inequality – is that the way it is? Knowledge and survival. Energy balance and stress. Disaster and stress. The stress of poverty. A personality issue. The energy secret. Smoking, Stress, and the Flat Battery Syndrome.

Chapter 9: Other 'Goodies'   182

Exercise. Some guidelines for exercise. Evidence for the benefits of exercise. Alcohol. The French Paradox. How much booze? Fatty liver and cirrhosis. Sleep and relaxation. What is stress? Joe and Bill – cured by love? Medicated or natural sleep? Blood cholesterol – the lower the better? Great mistakes? 'statin' drugs. Aspirin. Sleep and love, drugs and Rock n' Roll!

PART 4
CONCLUSIONS
Chapter 10: Is it true – No Food is Good Enough?   213

Introduction. Errors in Cardiac Value scores. Heart disease is really nothing new. The electric light bulb as a cause of heart disease? Is it a Social Disease? Anyone for Pie and Mash? Genes NOT Jeans. Nature and Nurture. Is 'natural' best? What are we actually eating? The Big Fight: 'The Goodies' versus 'The Baddies'. Low and High Blood Pressure. Food and other combo's. The Mediterranean Diet. The Polymeal Diet. Designer food. Science, the truth, and statistics. Who is at risk? Fat or thin? Fashionable numbers. Eating and other behaviour. Wealth, social status, and heart disease. Vitamins and supplements. Doing our homework.

Chapter 11: Where do we go from here? 246

Getting enough micronutrients. Further research. Some questions yet to be answered. Is artery scanning essential? What to do: Your personal check-list for preventing and modifying heart disease. Consider these questions.

Chapter 12: Further Topics 256

Truth and statistics (for those not interested in statistics). Further cardiovascular topics. Atheroma or plaque. Atherosclerosis. Footballs and golf-balls. What level of HDL should you have. The Anti-oxidant Theory. Cardiovascular disease. The circulation – what does it do? High blood pressure or hypertension. What is a normal blood pressure? The problem of high blood pressure.

APPENDICES

LIST OF FIGURES

LIST OF TABLES

ACKNOWLEDGEMENTS

From those who seem to know nothing,
there is much to be remembered.
From those who seem to know everything,
there is much to be forgotten.

This book is dedicated to
all those inquisitive patients of mine at
The Loughton Clinic,
and
The Cardiac Centre Loughton,
who asked . . .

'What *is* good for my heart and arteries?'

Once I thought I knew, and
they also thought I knew:
we were both wrong!
Then I started to do some research.

Now I know, just how much I didn't know;
just how much I still don't know,
and,
just how much more there is to be discovered.

* * * * *

None of the research work into heart and arterial disease undertaken at the Cardiac Centre Loughton could have been undertaken without my technician Noreen Connolly. Noreen is a treasure, and I value her as such.

My thanks to my daughter Anna for editing the text and for getting the book onto the bookshelves; to Tania Chicken, Kate Bridgman,

Andrew Elmes and Barbara Bird for reading and commenting on the earlier versions of this book. Thanks also to Jamie Nicholls for his computer skills in processing the photographs ready for inclusion.

I sought some expert advice about vitamins and supplements. Two men with long experience in the field gave me excellent professional advice. The first was Dilip Patel of Pharmadass, a large producer of vitamins and supplements, and the second was Tom Chapman of Essential Nutrition, of Brough near Hull in the UK. I would like to offer them both my thanks.

My thanks go to Mr Morton Stokes of Meat Markets, Seven Sisters Rd., London N7, for allowing me to take photographs of his meat, to Paul Christdoulou of Ocean Wave Fisheries, 60 Seven Sisters Rd., London N7, for allowing my take photographs of his fish, and to Michael of Michael's Fruiterers, 56, Seven Sisters Rd., London N7, for allowing me to take photographs of his fruit and vegetables.

My sincere thanks must go to my close friend Ken (Kenny Nicholls). I didn't ask his permission to use the words he might have used in the text – good friends don't have to!

My thanks in anticipation to anyone prepared to make constructive comments aimed at improving future editions. Please e-mail me at:
drdighton@loughtonclinic.co.uk

A proportion of the proceeds from this book in the UK will contribute to my own non-profit making research fund: The Heart and Artery Trust (H.A.R.T.). Charitable status for the fund will be sought later.

A proportion of the proceeds from this book in the UK will be donated to the British Heart Foundation. It was this foundation that funded my work at St George's Hospital, London, in the early 1970's and it has always been my wish to add to its funding in any small way that I can.

The British Heart Foundation has not been asked to approve of the views expressed in this book and in making them a beneficiary of its sale in no way implies that they condone its contents. The views expressed here are solely my own.

PREFACE

You may have seen the
British Heart Foundation advert:
fatty gunge oozing out of artery tubes,
or dripping from cigarettes as they are smoked.
You may have felt disgusted.
You may have been unmoved.
The fact remains that this 'furring' process
(the very same fatty gunge in the adverts) will contribute to most
middle-aged deaths in the western world.

This book is dedicated to explain all the ways we might prevent artery 'furring' while keeping blood pressure, weight, and diabetes under control.

If the right chemicals can stop the 'furring' in our arteries, help us prevent heart attacks, and avoid strokes, can food adequately supply them?

Food contains good things, and food contains bad things, but can we get enough of the 'goodies', without getting too many of the 'baddies'?

While food is neither 'all good', nor 'all bad', the ratio of good to bad could be of vital importance. Could it be that the beneficial chemical effects of the 'goodies' in food, out-weigh the adverse effects of the 'baddies'? Could it be that no food is good enough – that all food is relatively bad, and simply not good enough chemically to help us reduce heart disease? Along with smoking cessation, exercise, freedom from stress, weight and blood cholesterol reduction, could more intelligent food manufacture, and supplements of various sorts, improve our chances of survival?

UNLESS YOU ARE STARVING, FOOD IS MANY THINGS, BUT IT IS NOT A MEDICINE.

Without food we cannot live, but can it stop us from dying of cardiovascular disease? If food were a modern medicine, would some of it be allowed onto the market?

We harshly criticize drugs, even having tested them to the limit, and remain apprehensive of their possible side-effects. So how is it that we eat anything labelled: *'natural', 'organic', 'balanced', 'healthy', and 'good for us'* with enthusiasm, but give no further thought to it? Despite what is known of the importance to our future of smoking, exercise, stress, personality, attitude, lifestyle and genetic influence, we scarcely question the truth of the mantra: 'you are what you eat'!

Most food experts know little about cardiac medicine, and many cardiologists know little about food. Many nutritionists publish authoritative lists of what is 'healthy' and 'unhealthy' about food, but where is their evidence? If you are happy and comfortable with your opinions, presumptions, and beliefs about food, then simply eat, drink, and be merry! 'After all, you have to die of something don't you?'

Food once evolved through natural selection; now man has intervened with genetic modification. Food was not designed for human longevity, but could food science make it so? What we once ate, we now regard as 'uninteresting'. Most of us select food because it satiates our appetite, looks and tastes good and is culturally acceptable, regardless of whether it is good or bad for us.

Healthy food we now define as low fat, high roughage, low salt, and low calorie. We are not used to considering that the presence of many beneficial chemicals in food could be even more important to heart disease prevention.

Why do food companies continue to add so much sugar, salt, and saturated fat to their products? Why, apart from maintaining sales, would they wish to ignore the medical problems that these foods might bring?

Enough of questions: what about some answers?

HOW TO USE THIS BOOK

I have written this book challenged by trying to translate a new bit of food and medical science into a form understandable and usable by the general reader. It is important that some success is achieved because heart disease is now endemic, and knowledge about what is good and bad for our hearts and arteries, could help save us from heart attacks and strokes.

Go straight to the chapters on the food 'baddies', the food 'goodies', and the Cardiac Value of different foods and diets, if your only question is: 'What should I eat?'

For those with a wider interest but little time, there is a brief summary at the beginning of every chapter. You should explore the text if you want to know more. Some case histories and technical points that provide more detail are placed in boxes for those interested.

Because few understand the killer disease process that affects our arteries, in the chapter, 'The Silent Killer', I have given a brief overview of the process that kills most of us – atherosclerosis, or the 'furring' of arteries with cholesterol. In the chapter on 'Looking for Trouble – before it looks for you', I make the point that reconnaissance is a most valuable strategy for survival. First test your heart to see if you have a problem, and then decide what to do. I have briefly covered the tests, what they involve, and what they tell us about the heart, as well as indicating which ones you should have.

Under chapters entitled 'The Food Goodies' and 'The Food Baddies', I have dealt only with food. I have invented a way of weighing up just how good food is for the heart. It is simple – a ratio of what is good, to what is bad, in each foodstuff. I have called this the *Cardiac Value of food*, and you cannot afford to ignore this chapter if you have any predisposition to this killer disease within your arteries.

Those interested in lists of the food values that relate to heart and artery health (cardiac value, protective value, and adverse value), will find them in Tables in the various Appendices at the end of the book. Some of the Tables are listed alphabetically, others are in order of value – high to low Cardiac Value for instance. The Tables represent either calculation by portion size (as patients prefer), or calculation per 100 grams of food (as nutritionists prefer). If you come across an unfamiliar medical or technical word, try looking for an explanation in the Glossary of words. If you are interested in the original sources of information, refer to the Reading and References section.

I may be guilty of what some might judge to be unnecessary repetition. This has been largely deliberate because it will aid learning for those who will find this important subject unfamiliar territory.

Readers with a professional, technical and scientific background may wish to have the primary data and full working methods explained. For many reasons this information is not included here. This will be available later in an alternative monograph. Because my research is continuing I have also partly published the details in standard scientific format on the following websites:

www.cardiaccentres.co.uk and **www.heartshield.org**

Under 'What Ken says', I refer to the views of my friend Ken (Kenny Nicholls), since his views are likely to be closer to those of 'the man in the street', than mine. I have not quoted him but have written what I think he would say.

Ken is a diabetic who has had one heart, and two leg by-passes for 'furred' arteries. He is an accomplished person. Not only is he a singer songwriter and guitarist, but he knows most of what is worth knowing about plumbing, electrics, electronics, building computers, repairing outboard engines, cars, and guitars. However, when it comes to certain views about food and whether or not smoking has done him any harm, Ken and I differ. For decades now I have advised him on what is likely to be best for his ailing health but he still likes to smoke and eat chocolate biscuits, so I guess I have completely failed to influence him!

Is Ken not right when he says that he knows many very old and happy diabetic smokers? Would a new and 'healthier' lifestyle simply make him miserable, he asks. He says that he would rather have a few happy years left, than more miserable ones!

Perhaps he will read this book, and take some heed . . . but I wouldn't rely on it!

Introduction

As far as ill health and disease are concerned, I have never been inclined to believe that, 'we are what we eat', and after a lifetime in medicine, I definitely don't! There is a lot more to both ill health and disease than what we eat. But what exactly are we to believe, with the media telling us one thing, and experts telling us another? Just when you've decided on a particular food policy to follow, the chances are that some nutritionist guru will come along and overturn the whole idea.

Eggs are a good example. At one time, we were lucky to have them; at another, a little short of crazy if we did. If salmonella didn't zget you, the cholesterol would. Every week almost, a newspaper or journal article will appear, written by some famous chef or renowned food expert, inviting us to eat what is 'healthy'. The following week, another 'expert', will write something different. What *are* we to believe? With all this research into food going on, you would think that *someone* would know what is actually 'good' and 'bad' for us? More importantly, surely *someone* must know what is actually 'good' or 'bad' for the heart!

When it comes to food, I would guess that you have a very good idea of what is bad for you – and, you are likely to be correct. I'm also willing to bet that you have practically no idea about what is truly, proven to be, good for you. Even if you do know what is good, and what is bad, do you know 'how good', and 'how bad', each food is? For example, is milk better than cheese? Are nuts better than fish? What about the combination of foods we so readily take for granted? Could it be bad for you to mix dairy products with meat? You are about to find out!

Because food features in many of our human activities, it is not just a fuel for our bodies. For some, it can still be hard to come by, so getting it can itself be a cause for celebration. For the more fortunate, its role is centre-stage in our day or social calendar, as we celebrate birth, death, marriage and life. So why not just eat, drink, and be merry? After all, you have to die of something, so while you're here – enjoy yourself! Happiness is surely beneficial, and unhappiness must be a risk factor for heart disease? We will see.

I have never known much about food, and have never much cared about it either: the result of poor nutrition education at medical school, and a father who ate everything, and lived to 97! Unless we are dealing with the obese, a diabetic, or someone with high blood pressure and angina, doctors tend to have only a passing interest in what patients eat. For years I have dutifully trotted out the same old advice: 'what you need is a diet, low in animal fat, high in fibre, low in calories, rich in protein, with a moderate amount of carbo-hydrates'. Although it concerned my patients, my belief was that food, while pleasurable, was mostly irrelevant, and had very little to do with the life and death issues concerning a cardiologist.

For years, my patients have told me what they think is good for them. For years, I have listened to their theories about food, exercise, and innumerable preparations to be had in health food shops. I never have liked to ask them, "How they know that these things are good for us". Many patients are self-appointed 'experts' in their various fields of course, with strong beliefs in the benefits of all sorts of preparations, such as Echinacea, zinc, Royal Jelly, as well as many others. In fact, I have listened to as many time-honoured prescrip-tions for health and disease avoidance, as I have patients. At least they are interested enough in preventative strategies to take *some* action. This is credit-worthy survival strategy in itself, but to get it right, a bit of science is required.

So what did I know? Can I claim to have known any better? Not really. In fact, it wasn't until I started to do some serious research, that I began getting some scientific insight. I, too, am guilty of having handed out advice, based only on what I was taught, and on what I came to believe was correct, without really ever trying to verify it.

My initial interest was kindled by Vitamin E. One really good research study showed that it prevented heart trouble in a most difficult group: high-risk heart cases with proven coronary artery disease. For years, I told my patients to take it, until a more recent study showed that it was of little use. I asked myself, "What is Vitamin E?" I found I didn't really know, and what is more, few other doctors seemed to know either. All I remember from my medical school days was that rats needed it for fertility, and humans didn't actually need it at all!

Had I made a mistake in promoting Vitamin E to my patients? It was time to find out much, much more. What I discovered, led me to question all my beliefs about food,

> In the UK, 2.7 million people have heart disease. 268,000 people have heart attacks every year, 125,000 of which are fatal.

and its chemical components. I realized, that I needed to find evidence for what *is* actually good and bad for our heart and arteries. As cardiovascular disease kills over half the middle-aged population of the western world, I was not likely to be wasting my time. I became more interested in this subject, when I found it to be full of conflicting opinions and beliefs.

I decided to start with a real controversy: the place of vitamins in the prevention of heart disease. I needed to know if there was any evidence for thinking that vitamins could prevent heart disease. One thing was obvious from a little research: little belief exists within the medical profession for their usefulness. This disbelief was strong enough to have led to a clinical trial with a serious fault.

A trial was set up to compare the effects of 3 anti-oxidants (vitamins A and C with beta carotene) and a 'statin' drug on heart disease. The 'statin' drug prevented some of the complications the vitamin cocktail did not. Instead of using one anti-oxidant at a time, they mixed three together in a cocktail. The fact that the cocktail was shown not to work has at least two explanations. The first is that the cocktail was truly ineffective (likely), the second is that the effect of one vitamin on the others might have reduced any beneficial effects (unlikely, but an effect called confounding). This results in a real problem with interpretation and risked discrediting the trial. Perhaps there were those who did not believe in the anti-oxidants in the first place – they could hardly have been expected to believe that there was any risk in mixing them together. In contrast, they did use the 'statin' drug alone, with no possibility of confounding.

The food, supplement, and vitamin industries are huge. They also make huge claims for their products, many of which are completely refuted, or misunderstood, by the medical profession. Could there be some truth in the somewhat mystical beliefs of the health-food, vitamin, and supplement industries?

When lots of money is being made, as in the food and supplement industries, vested interests will abound and suspicions of bias are bound to stimulate interest. Let me state immediately therefore, that none of my research has had a sponsor, and none has yet been sought.

A close look at the subject soon showed that the science-based knowledge of food, vitamins, and supplements has a long history, but one that was often obscure, and did not cross the boundaries between disciplines such as nutrition and cardiology. Most of our common knowledge is negative, that is, we all seem to know what *not* to eat. We know, for instance, about the dangers of calories and obesity, saturated fat excess and blood cholesterol, salt and blood pressure, sugar and diabetes, but we have little scientific knowledge about what it is that might be positively good for us. We think of healthy foods as those without too much fat, salt, and too many calories for the weight-conscious.

What I needed was facts, not opinions. Where food and the heart are concerned, there are many opinions, but few proven facts. For instance, who knows if an English tomato has a different chemical composition to an Italian one? Are red wines all the same? Does Chilean Shiraz wine contain more beneficial substances than its Australian equivalent? Do the contents vary from one hillside to the next? I don't know. (Perhaps a subject for another book?) A few years travelling the world, wine-tasting and doing some chemical analysis, and I might make scientific sense of it all, if I survive that is!

Let me say right from the start what I mean by scientific sense. A theory is the starting point for all scientific enquiry, and at the very least, it must make scientific sense. That is not to say that it will prove correct, but it must make scientific sense in that it explains the observed facts. One trouble is, that the observed facts can easily be misinterpreted. For instance, the Earth proved not to be flat, the sun does not revolve around the Earth, and atoms do not obey the same physical Laws as snooker balls and planets. Because they appeared to make sense, many very clever people held these views, but were proved wrong. Once a theory is accepted as 'sensible' and worth trying to prove, the true scientist wants to know the truth, and nothing but the truth. He wants his theory to become justified by experimental proof, and proof so stringent, that every attempt to refute it, fails. You don't have to be a scientist to have this attitude; successful lawyers and businessmen have it too. 'People are going to love this product!' an enthusiastic inventor might say, looking for funds to produce and sell it. 'Where's your proof?' the cool investor will ask. Not much difference in attitude there!

> In 1632, Galileo published one of the first books about science for a public audience. In his book: *Dialogus de Systemate Mundi* (A discussion on the systems of the Universe), he compares the two views: that the sun revolves around the earth, and his correct, but heretical view, that the earth revolves around the Sun.

To make scientific sense a theory must be based on knowledge that has been experimentally verified or made likely by some clear line of reasoning. Scientific disciplines do vary in how easy their theories are to investigate in a laboratory. Because they deal with more complexity and inherent diversity, the biological sciences have taken a lot longer to develop than the physical sciences like physics and chemistry. If physics is a 'hard' science, then food science is a 'soft' science. By that I mean – the atomic weight of gold is the same on Earth and Mars, but the amount of saturated fat in a pork pie varies between London and New York!

As with most scientific matters, some questions, although simple, are not that easy to answer: 'How do you know that?' 'What is the evidence for that?' And sometimes: 'How is it possible to know that?' All are valid questions with involved answers.

What is the aim of science? In 1959 James Mason played the role of a scientist in the film, 'Journey to the Centre of the Earth'. He had two relevant lines to deliver: 'Science is not a guessing game', and, 'the ultimate aim of science is to penetrate the unknown'.

One way to the truth is to examine the original evidence. This is not always easy to do because experimenters assume a lot of knowledge, use a lot of scientific jargon and technical words that have been strictly defined and accepted by the many workers in the field. Unfortunately, scientific knowledge is hierarchical, and, by its very nature, impossible to truly understand without doing a lot of homework.

What do I mean by hierarchical? You may remember at school, when you first did simple arithmetic. After that you may have progressed to simple algebra, but not before you had understood the arithmetic. Then you progressed to equations, then simultaneous equations, then to calculus, then to . . . Each stage up the ladder had to be built on knowledge from the level before, making it impossible to understand further levels without mastering all the foundation levels. Because a true understanding of science involves so many levels of understanding, it will always be a bit impenetrable. That's not to say that an attempt shouldn't be made. One hope is that I can succeed in explaining to you, what you should eat . . . and why.

> *Because heart disease is so rampant, and the aim is to conquer it, it is important that we all gain a better understanding. It is not good enough that only medical scientists understand it, the man in the street, the politician, and those in the food industry, could do with some understanding as well.*

In interpreting the scientific research of others, and trying to write about it for the public, I *will* be guilty of unavoidable over-simplification. I hope that I have done justice to the authors of the works I quote (see reference section). All of the food chemical based calculations are my own, using formulae that I have developed. If there are errors, they are mine alone.

My particular interest is the prevention of heart attacks, so I decided to concentrate on these, with high blood pressure and strokes included for completeness. Both heart attacks and strokes are both unfortunate catastrophes best avoided. Could the right vitamins and supplements and eating the best food, really be a way of avoiding them? My intention was to find out, and to pass on the results, to those who need them most – my patients, and the general public.

We all know that eating cholesterol is bad for us. Isn't it obvious? After all, it collects in arteries, so it must be bad! Why then do low-cholesterol diets, not prevent heart disease that much? The same cannot be said about saturated fat and trans-fat in food; they *are* bad for us.

My father ate dripping, fatty meat, and eggs for almost all of his 97 years, but he also ate Brazil nuts and walnuts every day, as well as herrings and seafood, twice every week. Perhaps these foods reversed the harmful effects of the saturated fat he ate? My conclusion is that they might have, although it is more likely that he had such a good constitution, no food would ever have harmed him. That's anecdotal evidence for you. One case, while important, provides insufficient evidence for the sort of proof needed before applying food principles to everyone.

During the Second World War food was rationed in the UK. Ration books allowed people to eat only 2 ounces (66 grams) of margarine or butter per week. Fish was available, but meat was a luxury. When meat was roasted, the dripping, then thought to be so nutritious, was eaten on toast. Overall, the quantities of food then available, were much smaller than today. At this time, heart attacks were said to have decreased, although how anyone could have known this, with a war going on, I really don't know. Heart attacks were not much mentioned in medical textbooks of the time, the bigger problem being rheumatic heart disease and its effects. Without detailed autopsies to rely on, death certificates that list the causes of death as 'heart failure', 'coronary artery disease' or 'cardiac infarction' (heart attack), would always be suspect.

None of this would matter much now, except that it has led to the firm conviction that cutting down fat in the diet reduces coronary heart disease. Many research trials have subsequently shown that severe dietary fat restriction does have a beneficial effect, but only between zero and 15%, depending on the trial quoted. What has not been emphasized much is that a few trials showed a slight increase in cancer cases.

In 1970, when I was working, at St George's Hospital, Hyde Park Corner in London (now the Lancaster Hotel – the lease on the hospital ran out I believe!), a brilliant pathologist (the late Professor Michael Davies), showed us his detailed pictures of the whole coronary artery tree. For the first time, we realized just how bad the disease of atherosclerosis (artery 'furring') could be, without our being able to detect it clinically; and just how much worse it was, after we had detected it. Not that you need severely 'furred' arteries to get a heart attack.

But what are arteries? What does the heart look like and where is it exactly in the body? If you are not sure of the answers here are diagrams (Figs 1 – 3) to illustrate the answers. If this is just too elementary for you, I apologise.

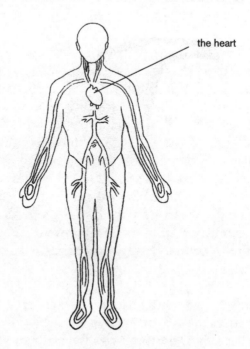

the heart

Fig 1: The position of the heart in the body.

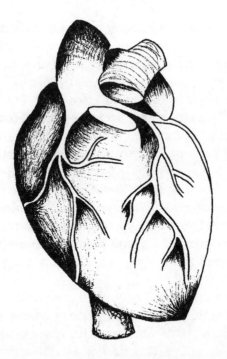

Fig 2: The front aspect of the heart showing the coronary arteries.

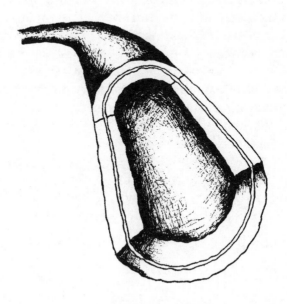

Fig 3: Cross-section of a normal artery.

When a coronary, or heart artery blocks completely, a heart attack may occur. If any heart muscle dies (infarction), we say that a heart attack or cardiac infarction has occurred. Heart attacks occur mostly from clotting on top of ruptured 'furring' – a bit like a slow growing boil or abscess, that comes to a head, and starts to ooze pus (cholesterol in the case of the artery). A clot forms to seal the hole, but in so doing, may extend to completely block the flow of blood in that artery. This is how heart attacks and some strokes happen.

I decided I needed much more basic information about food and its effects on our arteries, so I started to look at animal experiments. These date back further than I had imagined, to 1909 in fact. What they showed was fascinating, and entirely unexpected. Fats do affect arteries, about that there is no doubt; but antidotes exist to the fat that I never anticipated.

If there are antidotes or 'goodies', and 'baddies' such as fat, there might also be foods that are 'neutral', that is, foods that have no good or bad effects. In fact, I needed to find something completely neutral for comparative purposes – a sort of 'gold standard', of zero effect. All food contains complicated chemicals – even lettuce, so maybe even that isn't truly neutral. But what about tap, or spring water – is that neutral? Well, maybe not, since heart disease in the UK does vary between 10 – 15%, depending on the hardness of water in different regions – the harder the water, the lower the risk. The minerals and other substances dissolved in the water we drink clearly have some beneficial value. I decided it had to be water, with all the minerals and other chemicals removed. That was it, the 'neutral' gold standard – pure water.

What I decided to do next, was to take the known chemistry of foods and then develop some health-related scores –

- **one for how bad it is likely to be for our arteries,**

- **one for how good it might be for them,**

- **and the ultimate goal – one single score that would express the balance between the two – a good / bad ratio. With this score, and only this score to look at, any shopper would see instantly** just how good or bad any foodstuff would be for their arteries and heart, without reading all those important, but just too complicated details, on the back of food packets. Besides sugar, fat, and salt, there are of course many other chemicals that need to be taken into account such as fatty acids, zinc, selenium etc. (at least 17 others in fact). This single score – *the cardiac value of food,* as I have called it, draws them all together in one score for the first time.

With water as the neutral standard, anything good for the heart would have a score better than water, and anything bad for the heart, would have a score worse than water. Initially, my concern was just the 'furring' of arteries – after all, this is the single most important disease factor in cardiovascular disease. There are, however, two other very important factors included for completeness – a factor for diabetes (diabetics are more liable than normal people to develop 'furring'), and a factor for high blood pressure (the major cause of strokes). With these two added I could now call my single score: **the Overall Cardiac Value of food.**

There are of course many other factors as important as food, when it comes to preventing the 'furring' process, or improving our overall cardiac

> **The Overall Cardiac Value of food reflects three factors:**
> • the like tendency of any food to cause 'furring' of the arteries,
> • how bad the food is for diabetics, and,
> • how likely it is to raise blood pressure.

health. For this reason it is vitally important to consider the roles of smoking, exercise, weight and stress, so I decided to include these topics in this book, covered at a practical, rather than an 'in-depth' level.

Cardiovascular disease has a lot to do with the genes that control our metabolism. The understanding of these basic mechanisms is just emerging, and still the subject of much research. Ahead of us lies the individualisation of risk, which the mapping of genes will make possible for each individual. This could make disease liability known before any symptom emerges. Once the influence of each risk gene is understood, metabolic manipulation, using specific drugs and gene therapy, could become the means by which inherited diseases and predispositions are reversed. Once there, we should be able to prevent heart disease, while perhaps ignoring diet and the other risk factors. We will have to wait and see, but that is the prediction for the next two decades! It should come, but not all science-based guesses have proven correct. For instance, it was suggested, as an argument for its inception in the UK, that the NHS would eradicate ill health and lead to a diminishing need for health expenditure. How wrong can you be!

What then might kill us, if not heart disease? Perhaps heart disease is a good way to go – at the right time that is! So what should be the objective of cardiologists? I had to decide on a personal objective at least. Could eating the best food, and doing all the right things, result in a healthy heart for life? With a completely healthy heart, could we all live forever? Of course not! Mind you, anything that even vaguely intimates the possibility of immortality is greatly sought after, and for many of us, food and health seem to hold some promise. We have to be realistic though – we will all have to die of something, so until the geneticists can successfully fiddle with our longevity genes, and switch off all of our disease inducing genes, we might as well resign ourselves to do the best we can to avoid disease, and boost the quality of our lives. *To attain these objectives a healthy heart is going to be essential.*

So what was it to be, this objective of mine? In the end, I decided on a modest one – to try and add one extra day of life! Just imagine what you could do with that one extra day!

On second thoughts, is that such a modest objective?

PART 1

HUNTING
A
KILLER

For many of us,
a killer process threatens from within.
It slowly and silently narrows our lifelines;
sometimes cutting them off completely.
Ignore it and take what comes if you will, or,
mount an effective defence –
these are our only options.

To know your enemy,
you must be vigilant:
watch and listen, then test and learn.
Knowledge is the decisive weapon.
When you have learned enough – decide:
to attack, hold fast, or retreat.
The decision is yours.
Remember,
the clock is ticking.

CHAPTER 1

The Silent Killer

> ***In a Nutshell:*** *As we age our arteries progressively 'fur'*
> *a little (so-called plaque, atheroma, or atherosclerosis).*
> *When this 'furring' goes beyond the normal and is*
> *sufficient to narrow or block our arteries, serious*
> *medical conditions can result. Even small amounts of*
> *the wrong type of 'furring' (so called vulnerable plaque),*
> *can have grave consequences. The 'furring' of arteries*
> *can cause angina, heart attacks and some strokes – the*
> *commonest causes of middle-aged death in the western*
> *world, but not a subject much talked about.*
>
> *'Furring' is largely controlled by our genes but can be*
> *significantly modified by factors such as diet, exercise,*
> *alcohol, smoking, and 'statin' drugs.*

WHAT IS OUR PROBLEM?

The most sinister medical condition we have in the western world possesses two of the most dangerous characteristics of any adversary: advancement by stealth and suddenness of attack. This disease grows slowly within us over decades and then, as if out of the blue, strikes without warning. Nothing actually comes out of the blue of course it's just that we are only rarely aware of that inevitable build up which precedes every catastrophe.

Ask anyone in the street what they think is the commonest killer. Most will say 'cancer' of course, simply because it is so greatly feared. There is a condition, however, that competes with cancer for that sinister claim – 'the commonest cause of death in the western world'. In those prone to it, the cause grows silently within us, narrowing our arteries. Those who have the sinister form of this disease will suffer heart attacks or strokes. Those with the benign form will never know of its existence.

As a nation, we die more from heart attacks and strokes than from anything else. The strange thing is, heart attacks are becoming less common than they were in the 1960's, and that is a bit of a mystery in a world of ever increasing stress, excess, and obesity. So we must be getting something right – but what? The truth is, we are not sure, although there are a number of theories. We are certainly eating less saturated fat (butter, fatty meat, dripping etc), and more low-fat dairy produce. Some of us are even doing more regular exercise training, although many of us spend our lives doing no more exercise than is required to change TV channels! We get out of bed, get into the car, walk a short distance to our office desk, sit all day, then go back to bed again – having devoured many more calories than we need. Modern labour-saving devices, and the availability of prepared food, are making us lazy. Every shopping area is now a cafeteria – lots of food outlets, providing quick, calorie-laden meals, for less money than they would cost to prepare ourselves, and in a shorter time.

In the U.K. we are smoking less, eating better, and taking many more vitamins and supplements, most of which are thought to be ineffective by a sceptical medical profession. Perhaps we are also less stressed, although I've never heard anyone voice that opinion, mainly because it runs counter to our perception. Could these factors be reducing heart attack rates?

What is stress anyway? We cannot define it, yet we all know what it is and when we have it. To some, like Margaret Thatcher, an 18-hour super-charged day of interviews, challenges, and conflict, might not have been perceived as 'stressful'. To others, the anticipated arrival of their telephone bill can precipitate a state of frenzy. If stress is involved in the origins of heart disease, can we explain why it affects us all so differently?

Could global warming, over the same period, be somehow responsible for fewer heart attacks? Although this may sound a little ridiculous, it does raise an important issue. Because two separate trends are associated, it does not mean to say that one causes the other. Global warming has increased since 1968, while heart attacks have reduced, but does that mean that global warming is responsible? *Put another way: is association proof of causation?* Just because saturated fat consumption has reduced in the same period, it does not necessarily mean that this is causally linked to fewer coronary deaths. For other plausible reasons though, most medical experts (epidemiologists) do believe that the latter two are causally related.

What are the reasons for believing that saturated fat is bad for us? Well, it raises our blood cholesterol, and that is known to be associated with more heart attacks in a population. Also, animals fed fat, get 'furred' arteries – so the idea is quite plausible. Why then have many trials of a low fat diet failed to show much of a reduction in heart attacks? These trials compare the results of those on a reduced fat diet, to those who were not. Some twenty or so such trials, undertaken over the last 25 years, have only been on-going for a decade or so, which may not be long enough for them to give us a clear picture. Should we now give up our butter, eggs, and cheese, and stop eating suet puddings – or should we ask a few more questions?

KNOW YOUR ENEMY . . . POSSIBLY, YOUR NO 1 ENEMY!

Most of us worry about the wrong things. We worry about flying, but not about driving – yet flying is safer. We worry about cancer, but artery 'furring' is far more common, and sometimes just as lethal. This disease causes narrowing of our arteries with cholesterol, in a way similar to the build-up of 'furring' in our domestic water pipes. **The name of this killer disease is athero-sclerosis, and because it lends itself to an easy mental image, I have referred to it throughout this book as artery 'furring'.** While many of us have it for years without knowing, in others it can cause heart attacks, some strokes, a type of dementia, cold and painful legs, and sudden death. 'Furring' can be detected directly using various artery scanning and imaging techniques of the heart, neck and leg arteries, although few have been tested in this way so far. We can influence its progress greatly, so it is well worth detecting – if you think you can handle knowing that you have it!

A recent British Heart Foundation anti-smoking advertisement (Fig. 4) graphically portrayed atherosclerosis as a sticky, messy material, oozing out of a cigarette. The cigarette in the advertisement represents an artery tube, filled with 'fatty deposits'. (Grace International Miracle Ministries in East London are not claiming to have the cure, but I couldn't resist the photograph!)

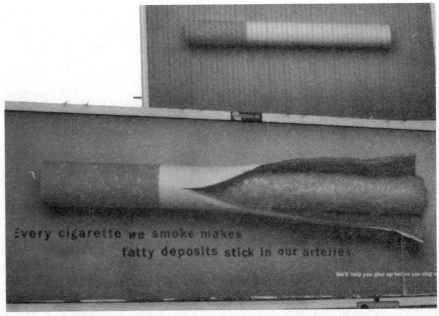

Fig 4: UK British Heart Foundation Anti-Smoking Advert (Jan 2004)

Arteries are our lifelines. Through these delicate muscular tubes, blood carrying oxygen, is pumped through an ever-branching network of blood vessels, to supply all of our organs. Our veins collect the used blood from the organs and return it to the heart and lungs where it is replenished with more oxygen. Without the right amount of blood and oxygen, delivered to them by our arteries, our organs could not work healthily. Without the right amount of blood, our heart, our brain, and our kidneys, could become fatally damaged. For these reasons we need our oxygen delivery pipes – our arteries, open and free, not clogged and narrowed with cholesterol.

> Five hundred years ago Leonardo da Vinci and his contemporaries conceived of the heart and circulation as a seed from which many branching roots extend.

Atherosclerosis would seem simple enough – it is the steady build - up of cholesterol in our arteries over many years. This causes a progressive narrowing that could eventually stop the flow of blood altogether. When the blood in an artery clots – the resulting thrombosis, as it is called, may suddenly and completely block the artery. When no oxygen then reaches the tissue, a part of that tissue may die. In the heart, this is referred to as a heart attack; in the brain, a stroke results, although strokes do have a commoner cause – bleeding into the brain, caused by high blood pressure.

In contrast to the British Heart Foundation advertisement image, actual atherosclerosis is a little different. Atherosclerosis is not a sticky mess that can ooze out of the artery, but rather a fatty, cheesy, or hard chalky material under the inner lining of the artery. The point of the advert was not to portray the actual 'furring' process, but to shock and horrify the public into an awareness of what smoking can do. An animated video clip was also shown on TV to support the billboard advertisement. The TV video advertisement showed smokers with fatty material dripping out of their cigarettes, spoiling their clothes. I wonder how many gave up smoking in response to it?

I did say that atherosclerosis was a simple process. Well it is, at a basic level, but the more it has been studied, the more difficult it has become to understand. It certainly is due to cholesterol build up. So a good first question might be, where does the cholesterol come from? I guess you know – from eggs and animal fat . . .correct? Well, only partly correct I'm afraid. **This disease is largely genetic – if it isn't in your family, you are much less likely to get it.** Your genes control your metabolism, and the metabolism of the inner artery lining can promote the build up of cholesterol.

Survival, if it is not to depend entirely on luck alone, requires inside knowledge. Every soldier (and heart disease is a battle we are fighting) knows that reconnaissance, or knowledge of an enemy, gives you an advantage.

When it comes to **atherosclerosis,** if you are over 30 years of age, and have never heard of it, now is the time to find out all you can. Atherosclerosis first forms streaks on the inside of arteries; it then goes on to form mounds of porridge-like cholesterol, mixed with crystals and chalk. The chalk is thought to arise as a result of long-term inflammation, not only in arteries, but also in joints and injured muscles. The chalky remnants of inflammation have been imaginatively referred to as 'the gravestones of past inflammation'. Let's take a look at some real live arteries, and look at actual atherosclerosis as it is imaged in the echo-soundings of the main arteries in the neck (called the carotid arteries).

The picture in Fig 5a is of one such mound, plaque, or lesion, representing one of the most advanced forms of atherosclerosis to be seen in arteries. This type of narrowing can be deadly. With this degree of narrowing in the neck, the patient is bound to have atherosclerosis or 'furring' elsewhere. **Without treatment, such people have a greatly increased chance of a heart attack or stroke.** This particular patient had a heart attack the day after we found his problem!

In Fig 5b, a smaller plaque of cholesterol is seen, and in Fig 6, a completely normal artery image is shown for comparison. You can see how easy it is to make the distinction between 'normal' and 'furred' arteries.

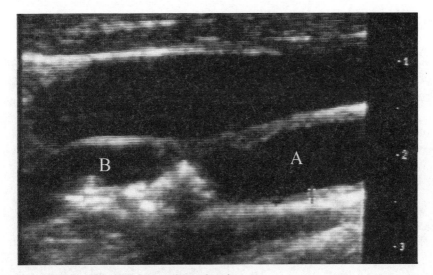

Fig 5a An ultrasound image of severe atherosclerosis:
* 'A' is where blood runs inside the neck (carotid) artery,
* Below 'B' is 'furring', not too dissimilar to an iceberg in shape, that is almost blocking the artery (so called Class 5 atheroma), composed mainly of chalk, mixed with cholesterol.

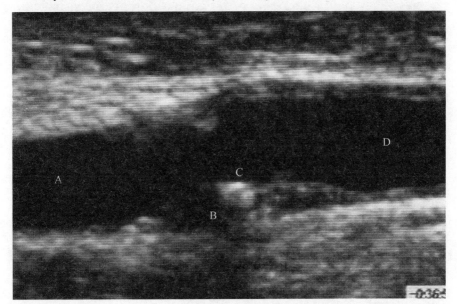

Fig 5b An ultrasound image of a moderately severe, mixed and vulnerable, lesion of atherosclerosis (Class 4):
* 'A' and 'D' are where blood runs inside the neck (carotid) artery,
* 'B' is fatty material within the 'furring' plaque. If this bit ruptures, blood will clot on top, and could completely block the artery (therefore we call it 'vulnerable plaque').
* 'C' is a safer 'chalky' area, much less likely to rupture.

Compare these to the echo-sounding of a normal artery:

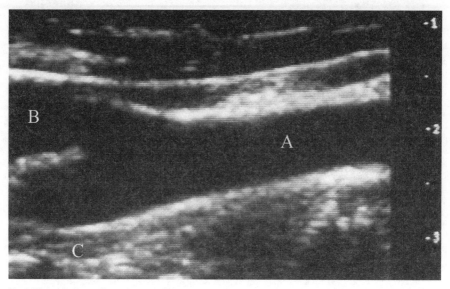

Fig 6 The echo-sounding of a normal artery:
- 'A' and 'B' are inside the neck or carotid artery, where the blood runs.
- 'C' is in the surrounding tissue.

To get these pictures we used my own echo-sounding machine at the Cardiac Centre, Loughton Clinic.

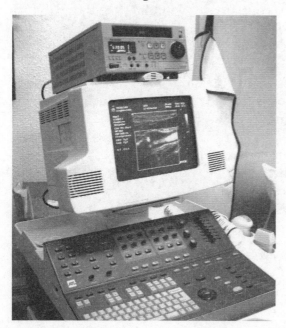

Fig 7 An Echocardiogram
Machine

HOW OLD ARE YOUR ARTERIES?

The inner lining of our arteries gets thicker with age. Age is so closely related to the thickness of the inner lining (the intima), that age predicts the likely thickness, and vice versa.

In Fig 5b, a thickened inner lining can be seen above and below the letter 'D', whereas in the normal artery (Fig 6), almost no inner lining is visible above and below the letter 'A'.

> ♡ *Technical Point: For the mathematicians among you, we can state that age is directly proportional to inner artery lining thickness – the plot or graph, of one against the other, is almost exactly a straight line (see Appendix 4).*

What is the significance of this thickening? In the average person, we would expect the inner artery lining thickness (the intimal thickness, or IMT for short – in your neck) to be 1 millimetre at 75 years old, but only half a millimetre at 15 years old. Suppose you are 40 years old and have an inner lining thickness of one millimetre. This isn't good news, because at 40, your arteries would be like those of a 75 year old. The implication is that you are aging inside, faster than you know. For me, this is quite a common finding, perhaps because I am dealing with a lot of heart disease patients. I less commonly see 70 year olds with the arteries of 40 year olds. This illustrates the point that **there can be a major difference between our actual chronological age, and our internal biological age.**

I would doubt that we can reach one hundred years of age, without young open arteries at the age of 60 – bad arteries, are bad news. What age are your arteries I wonder?

ARTERY 'FURRING' AND EGGS

To doctors, claudication and angina (see Chapter 2) are both familiar and serious conditions, known to result from the build up of cholesterol in our arteries. But where does this cholesterol come from?

Twenty years ago we thought we knew everything about cholesterol in arteries. It was simple – you eat eggs rich in cholesterol, this raises your blood cholesterol, which then deposits like snow, on the walls of our arteries. We know now that this is only partly true.

Feeding animals with fatty food can certainly cause cholesterol to build up in their arteries, but only to some extent. If you take 100 people with 'furred' arteries (visualised by echo-sounding), 60 of them will have a raised blood cholesterol, the remaining 40 will not. Let's look at it the other way round – if you take people aged between 40 and 55 years of age with a blood cholesterol of over 7 mmols/l, half of them have no evidence of the 'furring' process within their arteries (EBCT scanning results – see later). For those over seventy years of age with a raised cholesterol, 10% of men and 30% of women have no evidence of any 'furring'. **This suggests that a blood cholesterol level in the middle-aged is a no better test than tossing a coin, when it comes to detecting the presence of artery 'furring'. In the elderly however it is a better indicator, mainly because artery 'furring' is commoner, the older we get.**

The average blood cholesterol of a population can be used to predict the number of heart attacks that will occur in that group. For individuals however, blood cholesterol is far from an accurate predictor of future heart events. How can this be?

Imagine yourself in the middle of a large football crowd. If I told you that the average height of all those in the crowd was 5 feet 8 inches, what money would you place on the bet that the person standing behind you, was 5ft 8inches tall? If I were you, I wouldn't waste my money – not that I'm against gambling – life is one long series of gambles anyway. The fact is, that an 'average measure' is a group measure, and nothing to do with the measure of individuals, whether it be their physical height, or their level of blood cholesterol. For this reason **you might still have a heart attack risk, even if you do have a low blood cholesterol; and you may not be liable to a future heart attack, even if you do have a high blood cholesterol level.**

The principle is this: *it is invalid to deduce anything about individuals from a statistical average.* Equally, it is invalid to deduce averages from your knowledge of a few individuals. Like the man standing behind you at that football match, his 5 feet 10 inches, doesn't mean that the average of all those attending the match is 5 feet 10 inches.

Statistics can however bring us a statement like this: *because the average blood cholesterol in Glasgow is much higher than that in Bournemouth (that's a guess – I don't know that to be true), there are likely to be more heart attacks in Glasgow.* So where do Alistair McBride of Caledonian Road., Glasgow, and Mrs Betty Smith of Poole Road, Bournemouth, come into the picture – do their blood cholesterols predict their individual heart attack risk? The answer is: no they don't! Statistics simply cannot be used to predict individual liabilities – neither theirs, nor ours. Because statistics will be used to justify any treatment suggested for our blood cholesterol, we might as well be as clear as we can about its power and relevance to us as individuals.

Almost all of what is held to be true by the medical profession today is based on statistics, so it helps to know a little about the subject. Whether you are sceptical about statistics, or accept them uncritically, read the section on 'Truth and Statistics', at the end of the book, if you want to know my unorthodox view of them.

If we work on the assumption that total blood cholesterol is a bad predictor of artery 'furring' in individuals, perhaps the different types of cholesterol (or fractions as they are called) could reveal more. Cholesterol comes in at least two forms – so-called 'good' cholesterol (HDL, or high density lipoprotein), and 'bad' cholesterol (LDL, or low density lipoprotein). Microscopically, these represent large and small chemical collections (molecules) respectively.

Because the details will not be of interest to everyone, I have written more about these, and the anti-oxidants that are thought to influence them, in the further facts section at the end of this book.

With any medical test that claims to detect the 'furring' process, we must ask: 'will it reliably reveal the truth about our arteries?' As I have indicated, blood cholesterol level is far from being a reliable test. I have shown you echo pictures of arteries, so is that a better test? Well, it isn't necessarily the best test of all. In fact there is no 100% reliable test, but it is certainly safe (no X-rays), painless, and repeatable. Blood cholesterol tests detect 50% of middle-aged people with a 'furring' problem; artery ultrasound detects over 95% (in technical jargon we would say that its diagnostic accuracy positive, is better). You will later read about other tests, all of which have their advantages and disadvantages.

IS IT ALL IN OUR GENES?

Could it be that we inherit a type of metabolism that drives us to 'fur' our arteries, regardless of what we eat? There can be little doubt that this is true because many people, who do suffer the consequences of 'furred' arteries, have a family history of similar trouble. By the way, this also applies to high blood pressure, diabetes, stomach ulcers, hay fever, asthma, migraine, and many other conditions. You don't have to be a doctor for many years to realise that the tendency to inherit these conditions is really quite strong.

Can a person with no obvious inheritance, get 'furred' arteries by eating the wrong things? I don't think so. **Can someone who has inherited the problem, avoid it, by eating all the right things?** I didn't think so before the results of a typical Mediterranean diet were published – now I have to say 'probably' to the question. Ultimately, we will benefit directly from knowing our individual genetic profiles, but for now, we have only indirect ways of preventing artery 'furring' by employing diet, drugs, and lifestyle measures.

Genetic instructions define the good and bad features we are heir to. An exact copy is kept in every cell. If the whole set of our chromosomes (23 pairs) is like a book with twenty-three chapters, the genes would be the subject subheadings within each chapter. (Chromosomes are the lumps of DNA or genetic material, carried in the nucleus of each of our cells, that carry all of our inherited genetic instructions). The problem is, there are millions of coded instructions written throughout the book. The codes for an angina sufferer might for instance, be written on pages 5, 161, 345, and 897, with many subtle variations in different people. These different distributions of code are called genotypes. We now know, for instance, that there are many genotypes for muscular dystrophy, representing many different forms of the disease (phenotypes), yet to be recognised as separate medical conditions. Maybe the same applies to atherosclerosis ('furring')?

Our book of genes is written in an alphabet of only four letters (amino-acids actually), so the basic code is quite simple, while the number of possible combinations (equivalent to words) is infinite. Their combination is a bit of a lottery. Just occasionally they will combine in one individual to define someone of outstanding talent, or someone who has such a serious disease, they will die in childhood. One serious defect is called **hyper-homocysteinaemia**. This is important because it is a cause of artery 'furring' and heart attacks running in families and has nothing to do with blood cholesterol. It is due to a detectable enzyme defect – children carrying the gene, get rapid, and serious, 'furring' of their arteries, and have heart attacks even as teenagers.

Those with half of the defect (the recessive trait) have a raised **blood homocysteine** level, and 'fur' their arteries more than usual. Folic acid (and other B vitamins), found in green vegetables, liver, and some supplement tablets, will sometimes lower the blood level of homocysteine, and may lessen the risk. We will have to await the results of current trials, to see whether folic acid is better than chalk, in reducing heart attacks in general, and artery 'furring' in particular.

I have been measuring blood cholesterol and other fats for decades, but I have only in the last three years started to measure the blood homocysteine level routinely. Already I have come across a few families at risk, but one family in particular is worthy of mention.

A Case History: *Sonia came to me with her two sisters and brother. They had sadly lost two brothers and their father with heart attacks at a very young age. Their question was, could I tell them if they too were at risk? I measured their blood fat levels and found them to be normal. I scanned their neck arteries, to see if their arteries were 'furred', and also measured their blood homocysteine levels. To my surprise, three out of the four of them had a raised homocysteine level, and some 'furring' of their arteries. I started them on folic acid and now await their next test results to see if it has reduced their blood homocysteine. Whether that will be sufficient to protect them, I am not yet sure. Just because the homocysteine in the blood has been lowered, it does not necessarily mean that their tissue processes have been corrected. They will also need exercise, the best diet possible, weight reduction, advice about stress, and perhaps a 'statin' drug, until we can define exactly what level of intervention is good enough. (Cholesterol lowering 'statin' drugs are of undoubted value and are discussed later.)*

TO SCREEN OR NOT TO SCREEN?

A medical 'MOT', or health screen, can make people feel secure when all appears to be 'normal', but are they worth doing? Might they not give a false sense of security? Is there a risk of worrying people unnecessarily? Many doctors are sceptical about the benefits. Screening consumes a lot of time, effort, and money, and the resulting information can often be trivial. However, the medical information gained can be of real value to patients: they can come to know their actual state of health, and can decide to change their lifestyle and diet if necessary – based on objective risk assessment, not guesswork. Patients often see these examinations as a wise precaution. Occasionally, really important early diagnoses are made that lead on to early treatment, and a better chance of avoiding catastrophe.

All forms of medical screening have a tough challenge to face – demonstrating that they can improve outcome. Ten years on from the test, are those who were screened better off than those who were not screened?

Cervical smear testing and breast self-examination, have both been shown to reduce female mortality, so they are both 'good' tests. Lowering blood cholesterol in a population leads to fewer heart attacks, so measuring blood cholesterol is definitely worthwhile for groups. Ultrasound screening of neck arteries can detect those with a four to one chance of a serious cardiovascular event within four years, but it remains to be shown that such people, most of whom are without symptoms, can have their outlook improved. The onus is always on those who undertake the research, to prove the benefit of their tests and interventions. This can take a long time, but it is our duty to do it.

While we are finding the facts, and doing what we regard as 'our best' for patients, are we not creating unnecessary anxiety? Without question, the answer is 'yes', although, most of us would regard death as worse than anxiety. Nevertheless, the onus is on those engaged in medical screening, to make sure that any anxiety is kept to a minimum, and that the end results are worthwhile. Inducing anxiety, over something we can do nothing about, is cruel. People are sometimes better off not knowing, although not all would agree. Some prefer to know the worst, if only to be able to get their affairs in order. We are capable of helping people with 'furred' arteries, but it takes motivation and courage for them to get their arteries checked in the first place. In this way, they are at least given the opportunity – but it is only an opportunity – to take advantage of all the available interventions and treatments possible.

ARTERY 'FURRING' – SOMETHING OLD, SOMETHING NEW.

It's the number one killer, so let's take a closer look at the whole process of artery 'furring', from its early beginnings in childhood, to the blockages that cause heart attacks in adults. There is an amazing amount of detailed information now available about the biology and chemistry of the artery wall, so I have had to limit the discussion to key topics.

Leonardo da Vinci observed that, by comparison to a child's inner anatomy, an elderly man of 100, had 'very parched, shrunk and withered' blood vessels. Leonardo had been talking to him only hours before his death, when 'without any movement, or sign of anything amiss, he passed away from this life'. Could this be the first description of atherosclerosis or 'furring' in the major arteries? I suspect so. These remarkable observations do not rest on statistical proof, their truth rests on the accurate observation of one individual – still profound, four hundred years after they were written!

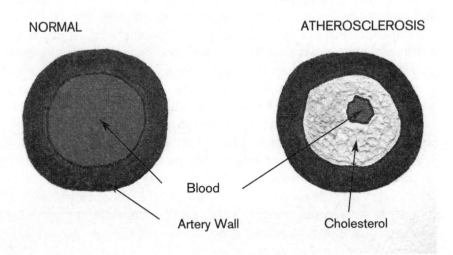

NORMAL

ATHEROSCLEROSIS

Blood

Artery Wall

Cholesterol

Fig 8 Cross section of a normal and a 'furred' artery. A normal artery (cross section), and one with severe cholesterol narrowing due to atherosclerosis. In a heart artery this degree of narrowing is likely to cause angina.

In those liable to it, cholesterol forms in the inner lining of arteries from an early age. It tends to accumulate at sites where arteries bend and where the flow is subject to turbulence. Unlike the drains in our houses, which will block if enough solid material is put down the kitchen sink, these artery pipes block themselves – that is, the pipes themselves grow the blockages. What is the reason for this, if it is not a lot to do with what we eat? In fact, the biggest factor is likely to be genetic, but there are theories for other factors:

Theory 1: that slight injury to the inner lining of the artery starts the process.

Theory 2: that the cholesterol formation is an adaptive process, intended to strengthen the artery tube where it needs to be reinforced.

Theory 3: if you don't use it, you lose it (it silts up).

Cholesterol first collects inside scavenger cells called **macrophages** (Greek for 'distant eaters'), just under the artery inner lining. These cells can travel a long way from other organs in the body to collect in the inner lining of an arteries, attracted to any site of soreness or inflammation, one of which may be that of the 'furring' process or atherosclerosis. They can also devour cholesterol at a distance from the main body of the cell by extending an arm or two (like an amoeba). These cells release chemicals that attract more macrophage cells, thus perpetuating the process. Some doctors think that microbes of various sorts are involved – Chlamydia pneumoniae and Mycoplasma pneumoniae are the ones in the news – so they have advocated the use of antibiotics to treat it. Others have logically suggested the use of anti-inflammatory drugs as a form of treatment. Both treatments are in the process of being evaluated.

The next step in the process is the further collection of cells and cholesterol, to form an inner crescent (Stage B in Fig 9). At the same time something quite extraordinary occurs. While the cholesterol 'crescent' is tending to narrow the artery, the whole artery expands (a process called **re-modelling**), in order to compensate. In this way, the lumen (through which the blood passes) of the artery remains open, despite the build-up of more cholesterol. The remodelling process eventually fails and the inner diameter finally starts to narrow, causing the blood flow to diminish. Eventually, insufficient blood flows for the demands of the tissue it supplies with oxygen (a process called **ischaemia**) – perhaps decades after the process first began. When sufficient oxygen fails to reach the heart tissue, angina (a tight feeling in the chest on exercise), makes its first appearance.

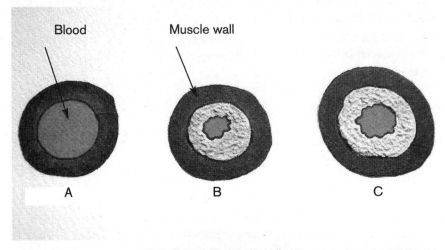

Fig 9: Remodelling of a 'furred' artery.
- 'A' represents a normal artery.
- In 'B' the artery is 'furring'.
- In 'C' the whole artery expands to allow more blood through.

As the process of atherosclerosis (artery 'furring') progresses, **crystals of oxidised cholesterol and calcium** may form within the artery wall, and things start to get more serious. The inner lining (intima) covering these crystals may rupture, bringing blood into contact with the cholesterol. This serious event may precipitate thrombosis, or **clotting within the artery**.

PLAQUE RUPTURE

This is one of the hottest topics in cardiology to day. Why do some patches of cholesterol in arteries rupture and spill out some of their contents, and why do others remain stable? Some of these patches are actively inflamed and, like a boil, will come to a head and rupture; others will never rupture – either because of their structure, or because they were once inflamed, but are now inactive, and no longer vulnerable to rupture.

Some plaques are vulnerable to rupture others are not. In general, the vulnerable ones are full of cholesterol and the non-vulnerable ones are made either of scar tissue (fibrous plaques) or are burned-out (the inflammation was in the past) and contain lots of calcium.

Because of the chemicals released, rupture of the plaque attracts clot, which can easily block the artery within minutes. *The plaques of cholesterol that lead to the most trouble can be quite small. It isn't their size that counts, but their biological activity.* Probes inserted to test their temperature have found them to be hotter than the surrounding inner artery lining.

> ☼ *Technical Point: Not all the plaques that rupture cause clotting and artery blockage. Many rupture and heal without any complications. The recently published research of Hong Myeong-Ki (2004), reveals some interesting findings. In those who had a recent heart attack, at least one ruptured plaque was seen in 70% of cases, whereas in those with angina and no recent heart attack, 31% had at least one rupture. This information was obtained by examining the interior of coronary arteries with a special ultrasound probe (so called intravascular ultrasound, or IVUS for short).*

- Two crucial questions that need to be answered are –
- can the type of 'furring' in the neck arteries predict the type of 'furring' to be found in other arteries,
- and can we tell from the neck arteries, how liable our other 'furring' plaques are to rupture?

When a clot forms, and an artery blocks in the heart, a heart attack (cardiac infarction) may occur. If a supply of blood can reach the tissue from some other nearby artery, the damage will be reduced (Fig. 10).

Occasionally, bits of clot will break off from the inside of a 'furred' artery, travel downstream, and lodge elsewhere. When this happens

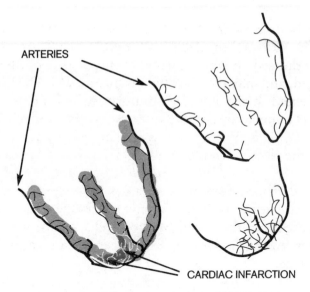

ARTERIES

CARDIAC INFARCTION

Fig 10 The coronary arteries and a heart attack.
When a heart, or coronary artery blocks with cholesterol and clots, heart tissue dies due to lack of blood supply. This is called a heart attack or cardiac infarction. If two arteries supply the area (bottom right), the area of damage will be small or non-existent because of the alternative blood supply available to the heart muscle. Top right: only one artery supplies the area of damage.

in the neck arteries, clot may come to lodge in the brain. This can cause death or damage to brain tissue and manifest itself as –

- a permanent stroke (cerebrovascular accident or CVA),

- a transient, but similar event – a transient ischaemic attack (TIA for short), or

- if enough heart or brain tissue is damaged all at once, sudden death may occur.

- If lots of very small clots fly off and lodge in the brain over a long period, dementia could result.

DETECTING COLLATERAL DAMAGE

The heart beats by virtue of its own electrical system, on less power than one AA battery (1/25 of that power to be exact). The ticking of the heart arises from specialized cells, located in one of the top chambers of the heart. From there, an electrical wave spreads from the top to the bottom of the heart, the passage of which can be recorded on the skin as an **electrocardiogram** (ECG for short). Disturbance of the way in which this wave travels occurs when the heart is damaged, and may then be obvious on an ECG. The ECG as a test was invented in the late 19th century, so it isn't the latest technology. It is quite an insensitive test, so even when the heart is damaged, the ECG may look normal. The plumbing may be abnormal, but the electrics can look all right!

Sometimes, the damaged area of the heart is limited to a few cells only; in which case, it can be detected only by finding some specific chemicals, released into the blood by those cells – these are called **cardiac enzymes**. An ECG is not usually sensitive enough to detect such slight damage.

In the brain, a transient loss of speech, sight, or power in an arm, leg, or one side of the face (T.I.A.), may indicate that something small, but sinister, has occurred. Such symptoms represent the tip of a very serious iceberg, and ignoring them can lead to regrets later on. Every patient with these symptoms should be investigated, because, they may be the only warning given of a more devastating stroke to come. Equivalent warnings of impending catastrophe do arise from the heart, but they are often ignored. Chest tightness, shortness of breath, and unaccustomed tiredness, are all symptoms worthy of further investigation.

Whether it is your heart or your brain that is involved, what you need to know is,

the condition of your arteries.

'Furred' or not, that is the question!

LIMITING THE DAMAGE – CLOT BUSTING

When I worked in Amsterdam in the early 1980's, my colleagues there (but especially Pim de Feyter, who is still hard at work in Holland researching coronary artery disease), were admitting patients with chest pain. Because Amsterdam is a relatively small and efficiently run city, we were able to get our patients into the cardiac department within one hour of the onset of chest pain – a feat still unknown in many other cities. We then investigated them (**cardiac catheterisation**), in order to get good pictures of their heart arteries (**coronary arteriography**). If a complete blockage was seen, a **'clot-busting' drug called streptokinase,** was injected directly into the artery with the clot. As we watched, the clot dissolved; blood would flow again, and heart tissue would be saved. The patient was seen to recover before our eyes. Any pain they had quickly disappeared; their pale skin became pink, their blood pressure rose, and they quickly felt better. If you did not know that this was the appliance of science, you could be forgiven for thinking that it was magic, or some divine intervention. Few techniques in medicine give such immediate relief, other than perhaps, delivering a baby, lancing a boil, and shocking the heart (defibrillation) at a cardiac arrest! Later on, others found that the same clot-busting drugs were just as effective when dripped into a vein, so the procedure has now become much simpler. Different drugs, with the same effect, are now given by paramedics in ambulances – a procedure that saves lives every day.

Success in the treatment of cardiac emergencies will always depend on the speed of medical response. Forty years ago the significance of this was not fully appreciated. With experience, junior doctors soon came to know that the quicker they treated a cardiac emergency, the more likely the patient was to survive. It seems strange now, but this was not obvious at the time. What followed in the late 1960's was that Dr J.F.Pantridge in Belfast pioneered the taking of a 'crash' team and their resuscitation equipment out of the hospital environment and into the patient's home.

When discoveries are first made by junior doctors acceptance by more experienced doctors can be slow. It's hard to teach old dogs new tricks! I'm now an old dog myself, so I have to be very careful when I think of barking at new ideas!

REPAIRING 'FURRED' ARTERIES

Cardiac catheterisation is not the most pleasant of procedures, but it can be life-saving, quick, and painless. It involves passing a small tube from an artery in the leg or arm, up the main artery until it reaches the heart. Once there, video pictures can be taken of the heart arteries. If we are able to catheterise a patient quickly, it is sometimes possible, not only to dissolve the clot, but also to open out the artery with a balloon (**angioplasty**). Thereafter, a **stent** can be inserted (a very small steel mesh cylinder), to keep it open. The cholesterol on the inside of an artery has the consistency of wet sand, so once it is pressed outward with a balloon, it tends to stay put! No big operation or general anaesthetic is required, just a local anaesthetic procedure to numb the skin around the groin.

The 'furring' in arteries has only rarely been seen to disappear on its own, although there are some reports of 'statin' drugs reducing it. Our first priority must therefore be to limit its growth from an early age using the best of diets, exercise, anti-smoking campaigns, drugs and several other interventions for which there is evidence of benefit.

Chelation therapy, aims at removing metals and artery 'furring' from the body – an attractive idea with little evidence that it is effective. It is currently the subject of a scientific trial, the results of which will be eagerly awaited.

CHAPTER 2

Early Warning Signs

Looking for trouble –
before it looks for you!

In a Nutshell: What are the early warning signs of heart disease? Breathlessness and chest tightness are both important. Medical examinations – are they any good? What uses have blood tests, heart tracings (ECG's), and exercise tests?

For doctors whose responsibility it is to give advice to a nation, the average blood cholesterol is a useful measure because it roughly predicts the number of heart attacks that will occur. For doctors dealing with individuals, the test is almost useless, because it cannot differentiate those who actually have artery 'furring' and coronary artery disease, from those of who do not.

Newer scanning techniques offer hope of detecting heart disease long before it proves to be a medical problem – so should we scan everyone aged 35 and older? Is this a sensible policy – find and defeat the enemy before it strikes? It sounds like a good idea, but, can we afford it? Can we afford not to? Will our accountancy – driven world try to deny us cardiac health prevention strategies? At the moment, our NHS and some UK medical insurers, prefer us to get sick first, then to ask for advice!

John Wayne often faced the problem. The question a wagon-train boss had to ask himself was: Do you first look for the Apaches, or do you settle down to fry your breakfast, and wait for the Apaches to look for you? What John Wayne chose to do defined his likelihood of survival. Arrows, heart attacks, and strokes are all quick ways to die, so if you simply want to chance your luck, or are too scared to deal with reality, read no further.

Life moves on, and the threats change. For many people in the world, car bombs, not bows and arrows, are now to be feared. With an ever-growing number of choices to make, life is no longer a simple choice between cooking breakfast and looking for trouble, although the question still remains: are fried breakfasts more dangerous than arrows?

Is there any point in waiting for heart trouble to happen? Why don't we try to detect it early? The surprising answer is, we can't all be bothered. Heart screening is expensive, and there are many doctors who don't much enjoy 'wasting their time on the worried well, or rich neurotics'. Doctors, after all, are trained to deal with real illness like pneumonia, ulcerative colitis, dementia, and Parkinson's disease! As a result, not all doctors are inclined to believe in the benefits of early detection. Those who do believe in it, rightly want to know whether it is worth doing – that is, whether it leads to a better outcome such as fewer heart attacks, fewer strokes, or added years of healthy life.

> The commonest early symptom of heart disease is increasing shortness of breath. Only 5% of us with heart disease will get chest pain as a first sign.

It's a doctor's job to be concerned if the results of testing lead to unnecessary worry. The concern is that finding some small, and perhaps harmless problem, might create enough worry to induce a heart attack. This is a real possibility – I have seen it happen. However, this must be balanced against the benefit for those who might have their lives redirected by early detection and intervention. This is not a choice you will ever be given, but which would you choose – unnecessary anxiety or unnecessary death?

Let's change perspective – 125,000 people die in the UK from heart disease every year; many die through a lack of early detection of their condition, and the preventative treatment that could ensue. In this country, facilities for effective early detection testing are not yet widely available. Even if there were, I wonder how many of those who might have been helped, would have wanted to be tested, before their heart attack or stroke? A few will be members of easily-defined groups: there's the 'nothing wrong with me' group; the fatalistic 'what will be, will be' group, and the resigned 'you've got to die of something, haven't you?' faction. Are they being honest, or are they just a little scared? The honest ones will be those who are truly happy to accept their fate, whatever it has in store for them. Others have greater priorities, and choose not to be tested, although some may have no knowledge of what testing is all about in the first place. While that is understandable, such ignorance may allow false security! Others, who do know all about it, may be inhibited by fear. The brave fear testing, but still go through with it. Although frustrating, none of this would matter much of course, if it were not for the fact that we are trying to deal with the commonest fatal disease of the western world, for which there are many effective preventative strategies.

> Those with a learning disability are 50 times more likely to die prematurely.

Once those who decide to get tested, do actually get tested, there are some technical issues to consider like: 'What tests are best?' Not all those who get tested, get the tests they need, or should have – that is, those tests capable of actually detecting early heart and artery disease. *Many of the tests we have put our faith in for so long, like ECG's and blood cholesterol, are actually pretty useless in detecting early disease.* If this conflicts with your belief remember that all of our beliefs can benefit from a good shake-up now and again, just to see if our faith remains justified. Firmly-held beliefs can be really hard to shake loose, even when the evidence against them is overwhelming.

Unfortunately, we have to face a fact: not all of those who have their artery disease detected early will survive, whatever we do for them. They will undoubtedly have a better chance of survival, but may still not benefit, even with the best treatment. Apart from the anxiety that may be induced, there are other reactions. Some are consoled by knowing what to do for the best, others are relieved by the finding of normal results. However, only the very best tests are worthy of providing such relief. False security might be forgivable if nothing can be done anyway, but it is unforgivable if it denies the patient the chance of beneficial intervention. For years, doctors have listened to chests with a stethoscope and pronounced to their patients: 'There's nothing wrong with your heart!' To day, no serious expert would ever condone such reassurance, based on that evidence at least.

There is more to being a doctor than being a scientist, but requiring all doctors to be scientists, even before they enter medical school, means that the art of medicine will lose some of its recognition. Gone are the days of complete faith and confidence in doctors – I wonder if the public have sensed the change in priority? A doctor's power has been partly transferred to machines. If the scan says you're all right – you're all right! That attitude, combined with an acute awareness of medico-legal issues, means that doctors are no longer as free to practise their art as they were, without referring to the results of blood tests, scans, and other impressive technological tests. The art of medicine must endure for the sake of our patients. Despite the interest and expertise expended on all the technical information acquired about a patient, we must always treat the person, never just their technical results.

Fear inhibits action, and fear of the unknown – that something awful might be discovered, will prevent many of us from getting tested. This may be so, even if an effective treatment is known to be available. A negative attitude, a lack of courage, and insufficient knowledge could thus affect our fate.

OK, so you have decided to get your heart checked.

There are several objectives to keep in mind.

Firstly, you will want to know

IF you already have heart or artery disease.

Secondly, you will want to know, if you have it in the early phases. You will want to know – how bad it is, and where it is. You will want to know – what can, or could, be done about it.

A little knowledge will allow you to know if you are being tested correctly. This testing is a science, and **no science is of any use at all unless it can predict the future –** *your* **future.**

Heart attacks and strokes, caused by 'furring', and clotting within our arteries, kill 60% of middle-aged people in the UK. Because effective preventative treatment is available, knowing which of these you might have, ten years before you suffer them, could be valuable. (High blood pressure is another cause of strokes, but is not a cause of heart attacks.)

Research has revealed some facts the would-be survivor needs to know about. Here is a summary:

(1) **The 'furring' in arteries (atheroma, atherosclerosis, or cholesterol in your arteries), can be visualised early,** by using ultrasound scanning of your neck (carotid) and leg arteries, and by other forms of direct scanning (EBCT, MRI, and PET – I will come to these later). If you have 'furring' in your neck (carotid) arteries, you are very likely to have it elsewhere. The more severe it is in the neck arteries, the more likely it is to be present elsewhere in your body.

(2) **Blood cholesterol testing detects only 60% of those with artery 'furring'.** Forty percent of patients who actually have artery 'furring', will be wrongly told that they are OK, because their blood cholesterol is 'normal'. There is no connection (correlation) between blood cholesterol level and the severity of artery 'furring' in the neck.

(3) **Heart attacks occur, when a clot forms on top of the 'furring' in a coronary or heart artery.** This can happen quickly, giving the impression that heart attacks 'come out of the blue'. Unfortunately the tendency to form clots is not that easy to detect with certainty.

(4) We do not need a lot of 'furring' in our arteries to initiate the clotting process. A small, but vulnerable plaque, can rupture without warning and result in the sudden and complete blockage of an artery. Just how common these vulnerable 'furred' areas are within our arteries, is as yet unknown.

THE MEDICAL EXAMINATION

What should you expect from your doctor, the specialist he may refer you to, and the tests they might do? It would be as well to know about the effectiveness of a doctor's examination and his test results. All interventions have their strengths and weaknesses, and it might help you to be acquainted with some of them.

It may surprise you to know that the most important part of any medical examination is the 'history taking', that is, accessing and analysing your present symptoms and what has happened to you in the past. This involves an ancient art – that of personal communication, a skill that cannot have changed much since Hippocrates advocated its sensitive use. It helps if you 'get on' with your doctor, and if sufficient time is made available. I am fortunate enough not to have to work in a system where managers are empowered to tell doctors how much time is 'sufficient' for their patients.

If you want to buy a shop, or run a successful business, the golden rule is:
'location', 'location', and 'location'.

If you want to do the best for your patients, as a doctor, the rule is:
'history', 'history', and 'history'.

Your medical history and any observations you may have, produce a catalogue of useful clues and 'red herrings', all of which may have to be investigated.

SYMPTOMS TO BE TAKEN SERIOUSLY

The main symptoms of serious heart disease are **tightness in the chest with exercise, and shortness of breath**. There are others, but they are less specific, such as tiredness, 'running out of steam', palpitation, leg pains, and ankle swelling.

Symptoms often occur late in the progression of heart and artery disease, although from the patient's perspective, this may not always appear to be the case. By 'late', I mean that the actual disease process may have been there for many years, before it is detected. As a result, an opportunity exists to detect the condition early, and to do something about it before symptoms do develop.

The consequences of heart and artery disease can be dramatic. Rarely, but significantly, your first symptom could be your last! Just occasionally, the first effect of a narrowed or blocked artery is electrical instability. One particular type, called ventricular fibrillation, can cause sudden death, unless a resuscitation team is on hand ('fibrillation' is a sort of quivering, at least that's what it looks like). This is one good reason to find trouble, before it finds you! Another type is called atrial fibrillation. This was in the news recently because Prime Minister Tony Blair suffered from it and had to be admitted to hospital for treatment. It is an irregular (sometimes very fast) heartbeat, arising from the top part of the heart (the atrium). This condition can occur due to narrowed arteries, but is just as likely to arise from an innocent form of scarring in the thin-walled, upper chambers of the heart, called the atria.

CHEST PAIN: IS IT ANGINA?

Severe chest pain is not often due to heart disease, but must never be taken for granted. **Chest wall pain – the commonest form of chest pain, can be severe, but is never serious. By contrast, chest tightness might not seem very dramatic, but it can be serious.** If it occurs regularly when exercising, then it is likely to be angina.

> **Angina:** A tight feeling in the chest, induced by exercise or emotion, and relieved by rest and calm. It does not usually develop until a coronary artery is narrowed by more than 85%.

Ken's Story: Ken was sitting in my car, parked outside the Wellington Hospital in London, when he received a rather upsetting mobile phone call from his daughter. His daughter and her fiancé had decided to get married, not in the UK, but on holiday in Goa... and they couldn't afford to pay for him to go. Because he had no money himself, he wasn't going to be at his daughter's wedding!

For a while before this, Ken had been unable to walk as fast as usual. 'I just run out of steam', he would say, 'I can't explain it in any other way'.

Sitting in my car, he had his first episode of chest tightness and breathlessness. That was his first attack of angina.

Angina is a symptom, not a disease. William Heberden, an English physician, was first described it in the eighteenth century. **Angina** arises from narrowed heart or coronary arteries, while claudication (pain in the calf muscles on walking), arises from narrowing in the leg arteries. Angina is experienced as tightness in the chest, brought on by exercise (sometimes also by emotion), and relieved by rest. The tightness in the chest, or calves (claudication), usually disappears within minutes of stopping. In both cases, the oxygen supply needed to power the heart or leg muscles, is restricted by the narrowed arteries: in other words, there is fuel starvation – a mismatch between the muscle demand for fuel (oxygen) during exercise, and its supply. Because this oxygen deficit gets worse and worse with more and more exercise, so do the symptoms of both angina and claudication (see Chapter 2).

What to do if you have chest pain or tightness?

An ECG at rest and on exercise, are both essential. Carotid (neck artery) ultrasound is useful to detect the presence of the 'furring' process in general. If both tests are normal, the chance of heart disease is small, but not completely ruled out.

Quite often, changes are seen on heart tracings that make little sense. There are certain changes that accurately indicate heart disease, and others that are confusing, because they look abnormal, but are in fact, variations of normal. If this should happen to you there are several important points to be borne in mind.

- When these indefinite ECG changes are seen, uncertainty about the correct diagnosis will arise.

- In this situation the result of an EBCT scan can be useful. If an EBCT scan is abnormal, arteriography may be needed to take a closer look at the coronary arteries.

- In cases where angina occurs on exercise, an EBCT scan is not required because a coronary arteriogram will be needed anyway to define the coronary artery anatomy.

- If abnormal, the coronary arteriogram could lead us to suggest a balloon angioplasty (now often done at the same time), if one or two narrowings are present. Bypass surgery may be required if there are many more than two narrowings.

One of the commonest causes of chest pain is inflammation of the cartilages connecting the ribs to the breast-bone (**costochondritis**). This hurts to press and is made worse by some movements, including breathing. Perhaps the first doctor to describe this was Carl Tiertze, (Tiertze's syndrome), a German physician/surgeon who lived in the middle years of the 19th century. Treatment isn't easy, or very effective. Press-up type exercises can help, as can anti-inflammatory drugs. One problem is that these cartilages are a bit like plastic inside – pliable, but with a minimal blood supply in comparison to most tissues. For this reason, few drugs affect them and stop the pain.

Another type of chest pain was first described in soldiers, on the brink of battle, in the American Civil War. Their fear induced left-sided chest discomfort which became known as 'Soldiers Heart'. Today, life stresses can induce the same pain. The symptom is nearly always associated with anxiety. Spasm of the coronary arteries, similar to cramp in the leg muscles, caused by the direct effects of adrenalin-like chemicals on the artery and chest wall muscles, is one possible explanation. 'Furred', or otherwise narrowed heart arteries, are a rare finding in such cases.

ARM PAIN

Heart pain can be felt, or referred to, the arm and the neck, rather than being experienced in the chest. If it is of cardiac origin (related to the heart), it usually occurs on exercise and associated with some chest tightness or discomfort. A 'slipped disc' in the neck is a common cause of arm pain, as are muscle and tendon injuries, induced by lifting heavy weights.

HAVE YOU HAD A HEART ATTACK?

A heart attack is said to have occurred when some heart muscle has been damaged as the result of a blocked coronary artery. **This will surprise you – 95% of all small heart attacks go unnoticed because they are not associated with chest pain.** It is

> If you have had a heart attack, your foremost aim should be to prevent another one!

possible that many victims of a small heart attack simply feel unwell, as if they had had a bout of flu, although this is difficult to prove after the event. Just occasionally, I have seen patients whose only symptom had been a flu-like illness, before the finding of an abnormal heart tracing. Don't run away with the idea that all bouts of 'flu' are heart attacks in disguise. If you are unusually breathless, have chest pain, or have a known heart disease risk, that is a different matter. If doctors had to check every 'flu' victim with an ECG, they wouldn't be doing much else!

Case History: John was in his shop, sitting at his desk, when he developed chest pain. He telephoned me to tell me about his symptoms. He didn't have pain, just a bad discomfort, as if an elephant was sitting on his chest. Nothing he did seemed to make it better. It sounded typical of heart pain, so I suggested that he went straight to the nearest NHS hospital. They released him after 5 days, with no better test of heart fitness, than two nurses walking with him up one flight of stairs and pronouncing: 'OK, you're alright to go home', followed by, 'We'll send for you!'

A few days after that, the coronary arteriogram I performed, showed that he had a 95% blockage in his main left coronary artery. Had this blocked completely he would have dropped dead! His life, without him knowing it, had long depended on what there was left of blood, flowing through that crucial artery. Next day he had a by-pass operation. Eight years on, he is still a bit overweight, but very fit, and still successfully running his businesses!

I later tested his neck arteries (I didn't then know how useful neck artery scanning would prove to be). These arteries were also 'furred'. I now test him annually to make sure that the 'statin' drug he takes, is doing its job. It is not good enough just to know that the drugs lower his blood cholesterol, I want to see for myself that they stop the progression of 'furring' in his arteries.

Once a heart attack has been confirmed, many cardiologists will do a coronary arteriogram to assess the coronary arteries. This is done to exclude serious blockages, which might otherwise remain undiagnosed and untreated. Repeated ultrasound assessments of the neck arteries are important because we can follow the progress of any artery 'furring' process in all such cases, without unnecessary X-rays. This could be done with EBCT scanning or angiograms, but the radiation and other risks, prohibit their use.

Thinking that there is a catastrophe lying in wait around every corner can lead to a psychiatric state of anxiety. What happened to John is unlikely to happen to you, but there are lessons to be learned. John must have had a lot of 'furring' in his arteries well before his heart attack. Could I have prevented his heart attack, had I known of the 'furring' years before? I don't know. Knowing all about his arteries, after his heart attack, has very likely saved his life. Knowing about them as we do now will hopefully prevent him having another attack. None of this can be guaranteed – nothing much in life is guaranteed, but his odds of surviving have certainly been improved. For me, such cases make the point that getting tested and treated early, is worthwhile, whatever the personal cost.

Those who make judgements on behalf of the poorer members of a nation, have to decide whether prevention is financially expedient. The cost will surely prohibit them, and will continue to inhibit them, while weapons are given more priority than health! Their decisions will contribute to health differences between the rich and the poor.

What to do if you have had a heart attack

An annual exercise test, carotid ultrasound, and blood tests, are appropriate for all those who have had a **heart attack**. This allows early detection of further problems, in those most at risk. We then have the opportunity to prevent the progression of artery 'furring'.

There are quite a few possible **complications of heart attacks.** If there is any suggestion of a murmur (valve problem), or heart failure, then an echocardiogram is essential. This test uses ultrasound to visualize the heart pumping chambers (the ventricles) and the valves. When a heart attack has damaged a lot of muscle, an abnormal pattern of contraction may be seen. **Heart failure (a weak heart)** is associated with an enlarged heart and poor contraction. Poor pumping action means less blood flow, so the hands, feet, and nose, may grow cold. When blood isn't being pumped out of the heart properly, it dams back in the lungs, causing breathlessness, and dams back in the limbs causing swollen feet. When this is mild, the patient will feel a bit breathless on walking; when severe, there will be shortness of breath on minimal exercise, and on lying down. Patients sometimes awake breathless from sleep, have to sit up, and feel that they need to open a window in order to get more air. These serious symptoms require urgent diagnosis and treatment.

BLACKOUTS (SYNCOPE)

There are two basic types of blackout: those that result from a brain disturbance, like epilepsy, and those that arise from the heart when it beats too slow or too fast. In 'faints', and heart rhythm disturbances, insufficient blood reaches the brain because the heart pumps ineffectively. In epilepsy, an electrical 'brain-storm' can result in various degrees of unconsciousness. Differentiating one from another can be difficult. Both the history and the observations of others can be of crucial importance.

Fainting is the commonest type of blackout and is only rarely of serious significance. It is common in early pregnancy, undiagnosed illnesses of all sorts, and stress. The heart is an engine, whose rate of action is controlled by an accelerator and a brake, both working at the same time. 'Faints' which are due to the combination of a slow heart rate and low blood pressure, result in the subject becoming pale and sweaty – a so-called 'cold sweat'. This is due to an overactive braking system, acting on the heart in response to pain, the sight of blood, or feeling ill. The best thing you can do, if you see this happening to someone, is to lay them down flat, in a cool environment – if possible with their feet up on a chair. If you then get them to use their calf muscles, you will encourage more blood to reach their brain. Don't sit them up and pour tea or whisky down their throat – that will encourage blood flow to their feet when it is needed in their brain! The result could be to maintain a semi-state of consciousness.

Rarer, and much more serious forms of syncope, are caused by heart muscle disease, and narrowed heart valves. An echocardiogram is done to exclude these.

What to do if you have frequent blackouts, or near-blackouts

The possibility of epilepsy as a cause of blackouts must always be taken seriously. This necessitates a brain tracing (EEG). An ECG at rest, a 24-hour heart beat recording, an ECG exercise test, and occasionally an echocardiogram are necessary. All may be required to differentiate one cause from another.

PALPITATIONS

Palpitations are a nuisance and in most cases, that is all they are.
They are only rarely associated with serious heart disease. They are
found mostly in stressed and anxious people, when adrenaline – like
substances, drive the heart to produce extra beats (called 'ectopics').
Stress management, and beta-blockers (drugs which block the effect
of adrenaline), can be useful, but so too is the increased confidence
and adrenaline resistance, achieved through athletic fitness.

An echocardiogram is needed to define heart valve function, and to
measure the heart chamber sizes, since stretching of the heart
chambers does sometimes lead to palpitation. While exercise often
suppresses innocent palpitations, it can make them worse, when
they have a more sinister origin. This means that we have to exclude
heart muscle disease, and heart muscle damage resulting from a
heart attack.

What to do if you have palpitations:

Because **palpitations** may be a sign of heart disease, testing with an
ECG at rest; on exercise, and over a 24 hour period, together with an
echocardiogram (echo sounding of the heart), will all be required to
define the cause. Electrical recordings from inside of the heart
(electrophysiological studies), are sometimes required for diagnosis.

BREATHLESSNESS

Breathlessness should never be ignored. It is due to less oxygen than
required, reaching the tissues. Breathlessness must be regarded as an
early sign of heart or lung disease, until proven otherwise.

Breathlessness is commonly due to being overweight, and the over-
breathing (hyper-ventilation) that may accompany anxiety and
panic. These are not indicative of heart disease, but are risk factors.
Much less commonly, breathlessness is an early symptom of heart
disease. In some cases, a change of heart rhythm to uncontrolled fast

beating, is the cause of the breathlessness. One particularly common form, in middle-aged and older people, is **atrial fibrillation**. This is an electrically chaotic rhythm, affecting the upper chambers (atria) of the heart. The irregular fast rhythm that results, can lead to

---

IMPORTANT WARNING SYMPTOMS

Have you noticed that you are losing strength, 'running out of steam', or more easily losing your breath? If the answer to either question is 'Yes' – GET TESTED

If lying flat makes you feel breathless – get tested URGENTLY

HEALTH WARNING

These symptoms can be a sign of serious heart disease (heart failure), or lung disease.

---

inefficient pumping of the heart and therefore to breathlessness.

When I was a young doctor, one of the common cardiac causes of breathlessness, was heart valve disease. This is because, in the 1930's, 1940's, and 1950's, children suffered from rheumatic fever. Twenty years after their fever, heart valve damage first became apparent. Thereafter, the condition almost disappeared from the western world, so few new cases emerged after 1980. Valve problems (narrowing and leakage), are potent causes of breathlessness, associated with heart murmurs. (Murmurs are noises

---

What to do

Patients with breathlessness must have a clinical examination, an ECG at rest (and perhaps on exercise), lung function studies, and perhaps a chest X-ray. An echocardiogram may become necessary, if heart valve problems are suspected, and a 24-hour ECG is essential, if heart rhythm problems are thought to be the cause.

---

detected by a stethoscope, caused by valve narrowing or leakage, and sometimes by holes in the heart).

CLAUDICATION – PAIN IN THE CALF MUSCLES WHEN WALKING.

This is a sign of 'furred' arteries in the legs. Walking causes a tightening in the calf muscles that subsides after a short rest. All (99.9%) of those with this condition are smokers. I have only once seen a non-smoker with the problem; and he was reported as a special case in the Lancet medical journal!

Leg pain can also be caused by vein thrombosis (clots), but if painful, this is more likely to be due to vein inflammation (thrombo-phlebitis), which is less dangerous. This is because free, painless clots in the veins, can dislodge, and travel to the lungs (pulmonary embolus), whereas painful inflamed clot, is stuck to the vein walls and doesn't usually travel. That's the thinking anyway!

What to do if you have leg pain on walking:

An exercise test, together with ultrasound testing of the arteries and veins in the legs, and lower abdomen, are the investigations required.

ANKLE SWELLING

Ankle swelling due to heart failure and kidney failure used to be called 'dropsy'. The commonest cause of ankle swelling now is immobility – sitting around for long periods for whatever reason.

The presence of ankle swelling often causes worry to people. True, it can be caused by heart failure, but it is far more commonly caused by inactivity, varicose veins (especially in hot weather), taking pills that cause either fluid retention (anti-inflammatory drugs), or an increase in blood flow to the legs (like the drug amlodipine). When it is due to these conditions, or chronic lung disease (emphysema), immobility may have played a major part.

Deep vein thrombosis is a potentially dangerous cause of ankle swelling seen after operations, leg injuries, and under some circumstances, associated with the contraceptive pill and stress. It only very rarely occurs as a result of travel, but remaining still over long distances and an inherited tendency to clot, will both contribute.

FAMILY HISTORY

Your family history can be an important indicator of future risk. Although it is true that heart attacks, and some strokes, do run in families, this can be misleading. Both the 'furring' process in arteries (atherosclerosis), and high blood pressure – are largely inherited. If you have one parent with such a problem, your personal risk of similar trouble, will be at least four to one. With both parents affected, it would be wise to assume that you will develop the same problems, until proven otherwise. This is not necessarily the case, but your need to be tested, should be put on high priority – especially if you are over the age of forty. My research data shows, that by the age of 55, the 'furring' process is usually well on its way, so don't leave it too late to get tested.

> **Research into family history:** My own research results into those who have proven coronary artery disease, show that a family history of heart disease, diabetes, and high blood pressure is much more common than in people of the same age, who do not have such evidence – in fact 2–3 times more common.

THE PHYSICAL EXAMINATION

The physical examination, and the special tests that may follow, are used to find evidence for a doctor's diagnostic suspicions. All of this takes time, and without this time, a good job cannot be done. So don't be rushed into having tests, without having your history taken, and your body examined. Short cuts give short measure!

DO YOU HAVE HIGH BLOOD PRESSURE?

Strokes are most often caused by high blood pressure, although they are also due directly to artery disease. The important questions are:

(1) Has high blood pressure affected your heart muscle and your smaller arteries in general? (this means it definitely needs treatment).

(2) Is your blood pressure high all of the time, or just when you are stressed?

How can we answer these questions? To start with, it is a good idea to learn to take your own blood pressure. Many companies make reliable machines, the best of which use the upper arm.

A 24-hour BP test is available. It entails wearing a machine that takes your heart tracing (ECG), and blood pressure, every half hour. In this way the repeated recording of your blood pressure can be achieved, even while you are asleep. 'Real' high blood pressure, is often raised during sleep.

The problem with high blood pressure is that it thickens both the muscular walls of the heart and the arteries in the body; at the same time it thins those in the brain (for more information see 'Further Facts' at the end of this book). By testing the thickness of the heart muscle with ultrasound (echocardiogram), we can tell whether blood pressure has had any adverse effect. This will help define the risk of a stroke, and the need for treatment.

Newer blood pressure treatments, with ACE inhibitors and 'sartan' drugs, are looked on favourably, because they are thought to stop the muscle thickening, and reduce the risk of complications. Such generalized claims, made by drug companies, that these drugs will achieve this, need proving in individual cases. Too much is at stake for assumption and guesswork. **Regardless of these reservations, the effective treatment of high blood pressure has been shown to be very worthwhile in preventing strokes and many other cardiovascular problems.**

> ## What to do if you are thought to have high blood pressure:
>
> Take your own blood pressure under differing circumstances – relaxed and calm, active and worried. Have a 24-hour blood pressure recording. Have your blood pressure tested on exercise. Have a baseline echocardiogram done, and thereafter, on an annual or bi-annual basis.

What other important aspects of the physical examination relate to the heart and circulation? What follows is the briefest of examination features, sufficient only to orientate you to what is happening when you are examined.

In the skin: cholesterol may collect around the eye (called **xanthelasma**), and even in the creases of the hand when severe. These will alert the physician to the possible presence of a very high blood cholesterol level. Although rare, this inherited condition may indicate a strong tendency to coronary artery disease within a family.

Diminished touch sensations in the feet are sometimes the result of diabetes. They can actually be present before diabetes becomes obvious. It can be detected by the diminished ability to feel the vibration of a tuning fork.

In the eye cholesterol may deposit around the iris (on the outer edge of the blue or brown ring that encloses the pupil). This is called **arcus senilis** because it is a ring that gets more prominent with age. My own research has found that arcus senilis is significantly associated with 'furring' in the neck arteries, and with the presence of coronary artery disease, but not with blood cholesterol levels.

At the back of the eye, evidence can sometimes be found for high blood pressure and diabetes. Opticians are often the first to discover these features.

The pulses: These can be felt in the neck, in the arms, in the abdomen, and in the legs and feet. If the feet are cold it is important to check all the leg arteries for reduced blood flow. This requires a sensitive touch because narrowed arteries may diminish the blood flow to the point where a pulse can hardly be felt. In the abdomen an enlarged artery (the abdominal aorta) may be an indication of an aneurysm – equivalent to a blow-out in an old-fashioned bicycle tyre. These conditions are associated with advancing age and high blood pressure.

The pulses at the wrist and in the neck are a study in themselves, allowing the discovery of the many abnormal rhythms as well as features of heart failure and various valve disorders.

The heart itself can be felt (palpated) and listened to (auscultated). These two techniques are very sensitive to the trained hand and ear and can yield much information. The heart can feel enlarged or normal in size. It is possible to detect the features of a weak heart as well as those of a heart made more muscular by prolonged high blood pressure. Listening to the heart can reveal abnormal sounds from each of the four valves as well as extra sounds associated with heart failure, athletic adaptation, and high blood pressure. With a lot of experience, a skilled cardiologist can predict the pressures and various blood flows within the heart, just from listening and feeling the heart. One such expert was my boss at St George's Hospital, Dr Aubrey Latham. He wrote the classic work on the subject. Nowadays, a doctor has only to request an echocardiogram to acquire the same information. The experience gained from listening to the heart for a lifetime, is no longer required. That's progress!

The nervous system must always be examined for signs of damage – strokes and transient ischaemic attacks, as well as the diminished sensitivity of the skin, previously mentioned in connection with diabetes.

Some patients are breathless at rest and will need their lungs examined. Some patients have blue lips and cold feet and can be in a very poor state if advanced heart failure is the cause. In such cases one can make a diagnosis from the end of the bed!

THE TESTS OR INVESTIGATIONS

- **Blood tests:** Many people have faith in blood tests! That faith can be misplaced, because the blood, while it flows through many organs like the heart and brain, may carry little or nothing away from these organs. The blood is however an organ in its own right, so testing it is good for examining the blood itself. Blood testing has many diagnostic uses, but we do it as often to exclude certain medical conditions, as we do to diagnose them.

The following test results could indicate the likelihood of coronary artery disease: a **high blood cholesterol** (with a raised LDL – or bad component); **a low HDL** (good component cholesterol), and **a raised homocysteine** level. I am sorry to disappoint all those believers in blood testing, but my own research into arteries shows that these are all pretty useless tests when it comes to detecting the presence of 'furring' in the arteries of individuals. Every day, I see people with 'furred' arteries and normal cholesterol levels, and others with normal arteries and a high cholesterol level. Although blood tests have gained universal acceptance, it could be argued that we should stop wasting our money on them, and test arteries themselves. In those with 'furred' arteries – blood tests are a useful guide to treatment. This view is an unconventional one at present, because both patients and doctors still want to treat blood cholesterol. The alternative strategy of using scanning techniques is generally not on offer, is too expensive, and there are too few experienced operators. I prefer to treat the arteries, not the blood cholesterol (which relates more to the liver function than artery disease). So why the focus on blood cholesterol?

Statistical studies have shown a definite benefit in treating populations with a high average blood cholesterol level. It has not yet been shown that treating arteries is of equivalent benefit to individuals so, until then, we are all duty bound to treat both actively. Unfortunately, only the very few know what is actually going on in their arteries, while most of us now can quote our blood cholesterol level – to at least one decimal place!

Blood clotting tests are not often done, but blood **fibrinogen and PAI 1,** are two among many, thought to be of some use. The greater the clotting tendency, the more likely is any form of thrombosis (blood clotting) – including a heart attack. Smokers are more likely than others to have a raised fibrinogen (blood clotting tendency) level and a higher associated risk of heart attack.

Blood tests are very good for detecting the chemicals released by damaged muscle cells during a heart attack. Blood **troponin levels and cardiac enzyme levels** are both used for this purpose. As mentioned before, it can be quite difficult to tell when a small heart attack has occurred, since only a few heart muscle cells may have been damaged. In doubtful cases, if these blood chemicals are not raised, the evidence will be against any heart damage having occurred.

- **ECG's:** An ECG (electrocardiogram, or electric heart tracing), is a recording of the electrical activity of the heart used in practice to detect problems with the coronary arteries and heart muscle. **How, you might wonder, can an electrical test be a good test of plumbing (the arteries), unless the plumbing has affected the electrics?** After heart attacks, and sometimes when severely narrowed coronary arteries exist, the electrocardiogram does show abnormalities. Despite its shortcomings, an ECG is always performed, as part of a routine heart check.

- **Exercise ECG tests** are to the heart, what 'road tests' are to the car. The hope is that the exercise, will reveal signs of trouble not present at rest. We also use the test to observe blood pressure on exercise. A useful, simple, and inexpensive test; it will detect 85%+ of all those with narrowed heart arteries. Because blood will find its way through, the arteries have to be more than 85% narrowed before the test can reveal an abnormality. For this reason, the test will be normal if your arteries are only 60% narrowed. The exercise test has its place in detection, but not in very early detection of heart disease.

There are several types of exercise testing apparatus. There is the moving walkway or treadmill, the bicycle (ergometer), and the very simple, but still effective, step test (stepping up and down, on one or two steps). All these tests are performed with an ECG machine attached to the patient, so that it can be viewed as it happens – now referred to as 'in real time'. (What, I wonder, is 'unreal time'?)

A treadmill test is the best type of exercise test, because it utilizes a standardized, reproducible protocol, the commonest of which is called the **Bruce Protocol.** This protocol divides exercise into periods of 3 minutes, from a slow beginning on a low upward slope, to very fast, on a high slope or gradient. Anyone who completes Stage 3 of the Bruce Protocol is of average fitness; Stage 4 is better than average, and Stage 5 is expected of those in training. Those who reach Stage 6 are athletic. Stages 7 and above, are the preserve of top athletes.

Because a treadmill test is reproducible, results can be compared wherever, and whenever, they are performed. The results are a measure of progress in exercise ability when done from time to time. This is especially useful information when arteries have been expanded using a balloon technique (angioplasty), or after a by-pass operation. Reproducibility makes the treadmill test superior to bicycle-based exercise tests. It is simply not possible to cycle at a constant rate, and then to repeat exactly the same thing at another time. Bicycle tests do, however, allow an initial diagnosis in those capable of cycling.

My boss at St George's Hospital (formerly at Hyde Park Corner London) in the early 1970's, Aubrey Leatham, was of the opinion that, if a patient could climb the flight of stairs to his rooms in Harley Street, there was little practically wrong with his heart! For him, this was almost a standardized test. By judging the rate of climb, and the condition of the patient at the end of it, much could be learned. He was always sceptical about the extra benefits of bicycle exercise testing (which was all we had at that time). Unfortunately, his test lacked that universal standard which would allow it to be performed, by any other doctor, at any other time, in exactly the same way. It did, however, provide Aubrey Leatham with what he wanted – an important rule of thumb, a comparable heart assessment of each of his patients.

Case History: Andrew and I used to play squash together, but he became somewhat fed-up with me winning all the time! He came to me with a very unusual form of chest and arm pain. Having examined him, I told him that I thought it very unlikely that he had heart trouble.

Noreen, my cardiac technician, having found his neck arteries to be quite 'furred' with cholesterol proceeded to exercise him. She had to stop him prematurely. What we saw, concerned us greatly. His ECG soon showed a change, indicative of a severe coronary artery narrowing. That was one Friday evening. I booked him into hospital, in order to take pictures of his heart arteries (cardiac catheterization), the following Wednesday. He didn't quite make it. Two days later he had a small heart attack! Ten days later he had been catheterised, his one almost blocked artery (98%) dilated with a balloon (angioplasty), and a tubular wire cylinder (stent) inserted, in order to keep it open.

He still can't beat me at squash!

- **Ultrasound examination of the neck arteries** is simple, painless, and quick. It can be repeated as often as necessary, because, unlike many alternative scans, X-rays are not involved. If atherosclerosis ('furring') is present in our neck arteries, it is 95% + likely to be present in our heart (coronary) arteries as well – and that is likely to be a conservative estimate. From my own research, I know that the more severe the neck 'furring' (atheroma), the more likely it is to be associated with coronary artery 'furring'. **Research suggests that those with this serious problem, left untreated, have a 4:1 chance of a heart attack or stroke, within four years.**

Introduced in the late 1960's, this painless technique uses high frequency sound (called ultrasound) to image the larger arteries, the heart, babies in the womb, and the gallbladder etc. It involves no more than placing a microphone-like probe on the skin. The probe produces ultra-sound waves, and then 'listens' for reflected echoes. Recent advances in image processing technology have greatly improved the quality of the resulting images.

Ultrasound from within the coronary arteries is possible – **intravascular ultrasound, or IVUS** for short. This detects the amount of actual 'furring' within the walls of coronary arteries. Results of these studies are worrying because they often show more 'furring' than a coronary arteriogram might suggest. This is very far from being a screening test and so I have not considered it further here.

- **Chest and other X-rays:** We are doing fewer and fewer chest X-rays for heart related conditions. We are no longer required to do them, unless the subject has prolonged coughing, unexplained shortness of breath, coughing of blood, or certain forms of known heart or lung disease. We used to do **chest X-rays** on all patients with suspected heart disease, but we are now concerned about the effects of unnecessary radiation.

- For those with lung disease, X-rays are still very useful.

> ♥️**Technical Point:** The relative danger of any X-ray test is assessed, by comparing it to the background radiation from the environment. In one year we are usually exposed naturally to 2.7 milliSieverts (mSvs) of radiation. A coronary angiogram would give you 2.1 mSvs.

Smokers often want a chest X-ray to rule out lung cancer. Ruling it out quickly consoles, but I regret to say that the early detection of lung cancer only rarely leads to a longer life. There are exceptions, of course, but they are rare in my limited experience of only 38 years! (A word of warning – it is inadvisable to make generalizations based on personal experience.)

EBCT (Electron-Beam Computerised Tomography) is an X-ray of the heart, which shows the presence of chalk (calcification) in the coronary arteries. A negative test is a very reliable way of ruling out narrowed heart arteries. A positive test is not quite so helpful. The reason is that lesions or plaques of cholesterol in arteries, detected because they contain chalk, are not always associated with artery narrowing. Nevertheless, a positive test means that narrowed coronary arteries are likely to be present. Because a coronary arteriogram may then be necessary to confirm such narrowings (stenoses), the thinking is – why not do an angiogram in the first place? The simple reason is that coronary arteriography is much more dangerous to perform, and involves a lot more radiation.

My policy is to do an EBCT scan when I wish to avoid doing an angiogram, in cases where there is a reasonable suspicion, but not very good evidence, that the patient has coronary artery disease. Such suspicion would be made stronger by a number of features: artery 'furring' in the neck arteries, if she/he is a diabetic or a smoker, if she/he has a strong family history of heart disease, and if a raised total blood cholesterol (especially a raised LDL and a low HDL), or a high blood homocysteine level are found.

An EBCT scan is simple and quick to do. While it is certainly of value in screening out normal subjects, its true place in cardiac investigation policy has yet to be fully agreed.

In passing, I must mention **perfusion scans.** These are radioactive tests that can show how well blood is reaching the heart muscle. They are used to further assess those with proven, or strongly suspected, heart disease. It can be surprising just how well some patients get blood through their severely narrowed arteries to supply their heart muscle with oxygen. This is because the small blood vessels that are hardly seen on angiograms are of crucial importance, especially when the main arteries are narrowed. Research into small blood vessel growth and disease has a long way to go, but it is underway.

- A **coronary arteriogram** (X-ray picture of the heart arteries) is done during **catheterization of the heart.** First to perform the procedure was Dr Mason Sones in 1958. It involves injecting dye into the arteries of the heart, through a tube inserted under local anaesthetic, into an arm or groin artery. Iodine-based dyes are injected into the pumping chambers and arteries, revealing their interior form, while being recorded as digital video X-rays.

It has its dangers, it is expensive, and involves a lot of X-rays. Essential, if angina or a heart attack have just been diagnosed, but not a test for routine early detection. This test is obligatory for those patients with evidence of heart disease, who need confirmation and further definition of their artery disease, before proceeding to an angioplasty (balloon opening of an artery or valve), or a by-pass operation (CABG, or Coronary Artery By-pass Grafting – CABG is pronounced 'CABBAGE' in the trade).

IN THE PIPELINE

Although it has been in existence for well over twenty-five years, the most exciting test in the pipeline for detecting 'furring' is called a **P.E.T scan (Positron Emission Tomography)**. Using radio-activated glucose, this test can spot the inflamed patches of 'furring' in arteries. When combined with an EBCT scan, the exact location of the 'furring' can be demonstrated.

Magnetic Resonance scanning is already in use, but not for the coronary arteries. Current scanners are not yet fast enough to capture pictures while the heart is beating.

A SUMMARY OF YOUR NEEDS

For those with no obvious risk, the minimum requirement is to rule out artery 'furring', high blood pressure, and diabetes. This must include a structured questionnaire to assess symptoms, past and family history, social, and treatment history. It should include measurement of height, weight, and abdominal girth; measurements of your blood pressure at rest and after exercise, as well as a urine test for sugar (glucose) and a blood test for cholesterol. All of these are valuable basic interventions that all doctors make available.

FURTHER TESTING

Artery Ultrasound: A painless ultrasound scan of your neck arteries will indicate whether or not you are a 'furrer'. **I am advocating this**

as a routine test for all those who wish to undergo cardiac screening, whether they have any relevant symptoms or not. This should be repeated every 3 – 5 years in those found to be normal, and every 1 – 2 years when any degree of 'furring', or atherosclerosis, has been detected.

The blood tests: Blood cholesterol and its subfractions (LDL, HDL, and lipoproteins –a and b), homocysteine, clotting factors, and an inflammation indicator called C-reactive protein (CRP), are used to assess future heart attack risk. Because the diagnostic accuracy of these tests in individuals is not that good, a patient could have all normal tests, yet still have a major problem with his arteries.

Ruling out diabetes, even in its earliest stages, is crucial. In the very early stages of diabetes there are no symptoms. Later on, the patient experiences an unusual thirst, the frequent need to pass urine, and tiredness, which they quickly get used to. Diabetes is diagnosed by finding a raised blood glucose level. Initially, a random blood glucose estimate will allow an earlier diagnosis than one taken after several hours of not eating. Fasting before a blood test could normalise the blood glucose level so that the diagnosis is missed. **If early diabetes, or the tendency to diabetes (pre-diabetes) is suspected, a glucose tolerance test must be done.** This involves testing the blood several times after drinking a glucose drink. Diabetes occurs because of a problem with insulin (too little, or too much of a defective sort). Because insulin is an important factor in the 'furring' process, testing for diabetes is an essential, when 'furred' arteries are suspected or discovered.

ECG's: An ECG at rest, and an ECG exercise test, are necessary in order to 'road-test' the heart. These are minimum requirements together with routine artery ultrasound, for anyone seeking valid assessment of their heart attack and stroke risk. An indefinite, or equivocal exercise test result, will need to be followed up by a further test, such as an EBCT scan, or perhaps a perfusion scan (MIBI or thallium scan), in order to be sure of what is going on. When definitely abnormal, an exercise test will need to be followed by a coronary angiogram, in order to exclude or diagnose, potentially dangerous coronary artery narrowings.

EXTRA TESTS

If the problem is high blood pressure, blackouts, heart failure, or heart valve problems, a 24 hour ECG, and an ultrasound of the heart itself (echocardiogram), are both required.

Key Point:

Whatever else these tests might do for you, they will provide a useful baseline for the future. It is from this base, that future diagnoses and management, are more easily made.

Experience shows that abnormalities quite often occur when they are least expected, so the principle must always be to test more, rather than less. This is why non-X-ray and non-invasive methods are so important.

Reconnaissance does save lives, but it can be difficult to cope with indefinite results. Cardiac screening is perhaps better suited to stoics, with a strong survival instinct, rather than to the faint-hearted. However, we cannot all be brave, and everybody benefits from the reassurance of 'normal findings'.

Consider emulating Noah – build the Ark before it starts to rain!

In the moments just after a medical catastrophe, your choices are limited. Before catastrophe strikes, the information gained from testing will provide time for reflection, and perhaps the dignity of choice as to what to do. The object is to improve the chances of survival, for those prepared to adapt. Many unwilling people, sent by someone else for testing, may have no wish to change in the first place – they could be wasting their time, and perhaps, someone else's money!

PART 2

FEEDING OUR ARTERIES: WHAT'S 'GOOD' . . . WHAT'S 'BAD' . . . & WHAT IS . . . JUST PLAIN UGLY!

CHAPTER 3

The Food 'Baddies'

In a Nutshell: Food is a great source of the 'baddies': saturated fat, cholesterol, and what are called trans-fats – these are the primary villains. They are more likely to 'fur' arteries when combined with animal-derived protein (from dairy produce, fish, and meat), and much less likely to cause a problem, when combined with plant protein.

Dairy products combined with fish and meat products, are likely to create the most dangerous type of food for our arteries. Lysine is the component of animal protein that multiplies the problem. One beneficial component of plant protein is arginine. Nuts contain quite a lot of saturated fat, but they are rendered less dangerous by their high arginine and low lysine content. Dairy products combined with meat (as in a cheeseburger), contain saturated fat, and lots of lysine mixed together, so this combination is likely to 'fur' our arteries. The Atkins Diet works well for weight loss but it allows the mixture of lots of lysine (animal protein) with lots of fat, so it would be bad for the heart and arteries if eaten in any period other than the very short term.

By measuring the 'baddies' in food (fat and lysine), it is possible to grade food for just how bad it is likely to be for our arteries. Foods can be scored on a scale from those that are most bad, to those that are least bad. This score, the Atherogenic Index or AGI, allows you to directly compare the artery 'furring' potential of one food with another.

We have all come to assume that too much fat and cholesterol in our food is bad for us. Because deaths from heart disease and the general consumption of fat have both reduced by 30% since the 1960's, some food scientists believe that the two are linked – that a lower fat intake has led to fewer heart attacks. The idea has gained such universal acceptance, that we now refer to low-fat food as 'healthy food'. But is that entirely true?

By contrast, angina, due to 'furring' of the coronary arteries increased in men between 1978 and 2000, despite a reduction in saturated fat consumption during the period (Lampe, F.C. BMJ.May 2005). Could it be that heart attacks are prevented by dietary fat reduction, but the 'furring' of arteries remains unaffected?

There is little doubt that animals, fed a mixture of fat and protein, will 'fur' their arteries more than with fat alone, but is the same true for humans?

Since evidence is gathered thick and fast these days, you have to be prepared to junk a few of your old ideas, and even change your mind completely. This partly explains the observation that the medical profession tells you one thing one year, and something different the next. What follows may not be very palatable, because you may have to consider different views about 'good' and 'bad' diets. You might even have to change your views about cholesterol.

Is it true that fat is that bad for our arteries? All we have to do to prove it, is compare two groups of people over many years, one group eating as much fat as they like, the other following a rigid low fat diet. The question is, which group will get the heart attacks? This sort of trial has been done many times, in fact almost thirty times in the last thirty years, and the results are not quite what you would expect, if you are one of those (probably the majority), convinced that fat restriction is the keystone strategy for heart attack prevention. **A review of 27 fat restriction diet studies, showed 2% fewer deaths overall; 9% fewer heart related deaths, and 16% fewer heart attacks and strokes.**

These results show that dietary fat restriction is valuable but not the whole answer. Perhaps the studies were not carried on for long enough? Also, what about the presence of chemicals, known to be good for the heart, such as arginine, fish, and other oils? Might not supplementation with these chemicals prove more successful? There are, in fact, many important factors in food that make it positively 'healthy', while at the same time, fats and lysine make it 'unhealthy'. Perhaps we need an idea of the balance between the good and the bad substances, if we are to get any complete answer to the question: what foods are actually best for our heart and circulation? A measure of this balance I have called **the Cardiac Value of food**, and I will come on to this crucial subject in a later chapter, after describing to you how we might measure all of the 'baddies' and all of the 'goodies' in the food we eat.

You might ask: why bother to measure things? Surely it's obvious what is good and bad? Without measuring we are in danger of fooling ourselves. After measuring, we can make better judgements and even compare one food to another. Sure, there will be errors and measured guesses, but we can take errors into account, and our guesses will at least be the best possible. Belief without verified evidence just isn't good enough when it comes to health – it could lead to all sorts of wrong food choices. There are, of course, more serious consequences of decisions based on unverified belief! Need I do more than mention 'weapons of mass destruction'?

One of the original reasons for thinking that a low fat diet is good for the heart, resulted from the serious misinterpretation of one clinical trial done in a large Scandinavian psychiatric hospital. For years, one half of the hospital patients were subjected to non-smoking, a low fat diet, and exercise; the other half were not. After many years, the results showed a big difference in favour of those who had eaten the low fat diet. The researchers concluded that it was the diet that had reduced the number of heart attacks, not the smoking cessation or the exercise – two factors now known (but perhaps not then known) to be of great preventative significance (both can reduce heart attacks by about 50%). The result was clear enough; it was just that the interpretation was biased in favour of diet.

Research into what does 'fur' arteries was first published in 1909, so this is not a new subject. Having read much of this old research, it seems to me that much of what was learned in the past has either been ignored or forgotten. There is nothing new in that. Scientists now rarely quote old experiments. There is a very strong trend these days to quote as reliable, only research published within the last few years, and to apologise for quoting anything older. When they are quoted, old research results are mentioned merely to add historical perspective, not to add weight to the argument. This is a pity, since I doubt that the best eyes, ears, and brains have changed much in the last couple of million years!

Leonardo da Vinci knew nothing of statistics and computers yet discovered more of importance than has any other scientist. I wonder whether he would have been taken seriously these days? I doubt it, if all he had to offer were his personal observations. 'Things have moved on', I hear someone say. One thing that will never move on is this – the further away we get from primary observation, the more likely we are to be indulging in fantasy.

Taken together the animal experiments of the past lead to two overall conclusions:

(1) **The arteries of animals can be made to 'fur', or 'thicken', in at least three separate ways, depending on the type of feed they are given.**

(2) **The early 'furring' process of animals can be partly prevented by a number of additions to their feed: substances such as fish oil, arginine and magnesium, as well as many other chemicals.**

The very first researchers fed animals different feeds, and found that cholesterol, alone, did not 'fur' their arteries, as much as it did when mixed with meat. More recently, in the 1930's, it was shown that the combination of milk protein with fats, had 2 – 3 times more potential to 'fur' arteries, than when vegetable protein (from soy for instance) was mixed with meat. This is an interesting fact that has been largely overlooked, in favour of something simpler – the idea that fat alone, is bad for the heart and arteries.

ATKINS AND BEYOND

The Atkins diet works well for weight loss, mainly because its high protein content somehow modifies our appetite and makes us take in fewer calories. When I asked my old school pal, Mike Stock, an expert on nutrition, what he thought of this, he said it was simple –'you just can't eat a lot of protein!' Other more complicated mechanisms are now being investigated. The world lost a great scientist, and I lost an old school buddy, when Mike died a few years ago.

The Atkins diet allows you to eat lots of protein, together with lots of fat. This makes the Atkins diet potentially bad for arteries, because lysine and saturated fat together, cause more 'furring' than fat alone. However, few people will be on an uncompromised Atkins diet for long, so perhaps the Atkins diet would only be bad for our arteries if it was followed religiously for decades. It is a very effective diet for weight loss and that alone can hold enormous benefits. What do I do myself ? I modify the Atkins diet by avoiding fat and alcohol whenever possible, at the same time as eating a high protein, low carbohydrate diet, combined with increased exercise.

I have given you two conclusions from some old experiments, here is a third, which summarises some of what has been mentioned before:

(3) fats, such as saturated fat (solid fat, like butter and dripping that solidifies on the plate), trans-fats (those produced by baking, and processing fats), and cholesterol, are the 'baddies', but the type of protein eaten with them, is crucial to the degree of 'furring' that will develop.

Proteins are made up of building blocks called amino-acids. These components of protein are good for arteries, when derived from nut and vegetable sources (the amino-acid arginine in particular), or shellfish sources (taurine); and bad by comparison, when derived from animal sources – dairy produce, meat, and fish (the amino-acid lysine for instance). This will prove to be an over-simplification, but it serves to make the point that it is not only fat that is bad for our arteries.

To summarize so far: the 'baddies' are definitely the saturated or solid fats, the trans-fats, (such as those in compound cooking oil), and what little cholesterol there is in food. What we don't know is just 'how bad' each of these is, on its own. Furthermore, the presence of the amino-acid lysine makes the effect of these fats worse; the presence of the amino-acids arginine and taurine lessen the 'bad' (atherogenic) effect on the arteries.

CHOLESTEROL IN FOOD – NO WORRIES?

This fact might surprise you – there is very little cholesterol in any food. When someone says 'there's a lot of cholesterol in seafood', they are usually implying that it is bad for you. They are making two mistakes. Firstly they haven't worked out just how much cholesterol there is in seafood (only a little), and secondly, cholesterol itself is not that bad for you, although saturated fat is.

In Table 1 is an abbreviated list of foods, ranked from high to low, in cholesterol content. Note the content of prawns and a triple meat cheeseburger. Both are almost at the top of the list and are commonly thought to contain a lot of cholesterol, but the analysis shows that a 50 gram portion of prawn (1½ ounce) contains very little cholesterol. It contains 0.14 grams (1/214 of an ounce) of cholesterol, only half of which is absorbed in the bowel (1/428 of an ounce)! True, a 12 ounce (400 grams) cheeseburger portion contains slightly less cholesterol (0.13 grams), but look at the difference in the saturated fat. The portion of prawn contains 500mgs of saturated fat (half of a gram, or one 60th of an ounce), whereas the cheeseburger contains 24,800 milligrams (24.8 grams), or ⅔ of an ounce, of this most dangerous fat.

Table 1

CHOLESTEROL & SATURATED FAT IN FOOD

Note: I gram = approximately one thirtieth of an ounce.
Weight of portion = average portion size per meal.

FOOD	WEIGHT of Portion Grams	CHOLESTEROL Grams	SATURATED FAT Grams
KIDNEY (BEEF)	85	0.39	0.90
LIVER (CHICKEN)	85	0.30	1.60
PANCREAS	85	0.22	5.00
HEART (BEEF)	85	0.22	2.50
LIVER (BEEF)	85	0.20	1.36
EGG (YOLK)	17	0.19	1.60
HAMBURGER	250	0.19	10.00
CHICKEN BREAST (ROASTED)	196	0.18	4.30
LOBSTER	145	0.16	2.40
LIVER (PIG)	54	0.16	1.35
PRAWN	50	0.14	0.50
CHEESEBURGER (triple meat)	400	0.13	24.80
OCTOPUS	85	0.12	0.64
EEL	136	0.11	3.60
TURKEY (DARK MEAT)	85	0.10	2.60
COD	180	0.10	0.30
DUCK (ROASTED)	85	0.10	8.20
CHICKEN (DARK MEAT)	114	0.09	4.20
SOLE	127	0.09	0.50
SALMON (PINK/BAKED)	150	0.09	0.85
WHELK	85	0.09	0
LAMB (LEG ROASTED)	85	0.09	7.00
PORK (LEG ROASTED)	85	0.09	5.50
CRAB (STEAMED)	118	0.09	0.30
OIL (COD LIVER)	14	0.08	3.20
BEEF (RUMP) COOKED	100	0.08	7.77
TUNA	150	0.08	0.40
OYSTERS	70	0.07	1.10
SHRIMP	50	0.07	0.23
TURKEY (BREAST ROASTED)	85	0.06	1.80
HALIBUT	150	0.06	0.61
HERRING	143	0.06	3.70
HADDOCK	150	0.06	0.30
SWORDFISH	106	0.06	1.50
SAUSAGES (PORK)	100	0.06	4.90

ANCHOVY (in oil)	85	0.05	1.10
MUSSEL	85	0.05	0.70
MACKEREL	88	0.05	3.70
CAMEMBERT	62	0.05	9.50
SARDINES (in oil)	50	0.03	0.83
CHEDDAR	28	0.03	5.90
ICE CREAM	66	0.02	4.50
BUTTER	5	0.01	2.50
CHOCOLATE: MILK	44	0.01	8.05
CHOCOLATE: WHITE	44	0.01	8.10

Recent news is of a hamburger, so large, you would need both hands to hold it. One portion delivers 1400 Kcals and an undeclared amount of saturated fat – useful provision for anyone planning to walk from London to Siberia! Enormous variation exists between individuals but an average active adult will use 1500 Kcals per day to fuel bodily activities.

The message is: stop worrying about the cholesterol content of food and start worrying about its saturated fat content.

Want to know how much fat there is in food? The complete saturated fat and trans-fat lists, for the foods that I have studied, are given in Appendix 5, and in abridged form at the end of this chapter.

IF ANTI-OXIDANTS ARE GOOD, ARE OXIDANTS BAD?

Oxygen rusts iron. Oxygen, while essential to life, also helps 'fur' our arteries by converting cholesterol (LDL to be specific) into the irritant form – oxidized LDL (cholesterol), that can induce inflammation. Anti-oxidants stop the rusting of iron and also stop the 'furring' of arteries, or at least that is what we are told.

There are other possible contenders for the title of food 'baddy'. Copper and iron in excess could be a problem, but only rudimentary information is available about their influence on the 'furring' process. The idea is that, **if anti-oxidants are good, 'oxidants' should be 'bad'. Both copper and iron carry oxygen around in the body and**

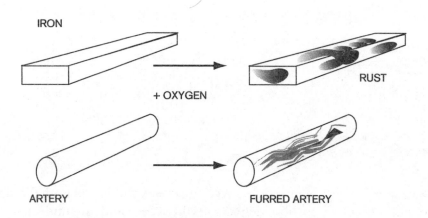

IRON

+ OXYGEN

RUST

ARTERY

FURRED ARTERY

Fig 11 Oxygen causes iron to turn to rust, and the cholesterol in our arteries, to turn to oxidised cholesterol.

act as 'oxidants'. How significant they are to the 'furring' process is not yet defined, but there is enough information to say that their oxidant effect could be part of the problem.

It could be that food with the greatest content of iron and copper, taken in excess of daily requirements, could have a deleterious effect on our arteries. It is therefore worth noting the top iron and copper containing foods. *It is very important to state that both iron and copper are essential to health, so beware, this could be a Goldilocks situation: too much and too little, could both be a bad thing.* It would be best to have only one recommended daily nutritional intake every day, unless you are advised on medical grounds, to take more. Those with iron deficiency anemia for instance, may need iron, in which case they will be replacing their diminished reserves, but they should not take more than they need. Once anemia is corrected and the iron reserves are replaced, it is important for the patient not to continue taking iron supplements.

Top Sources

Copper: veal and beef liver, oysters, cashew nuts, brazil nuts, king crab, hazelnuts, almonds, soy-nuts, walnuts, molasses, pumpkin seeds, pistachios and peanuts.

Iron: Clams, oysters, chicken, turkey, and beef liver, kidney, pistachios, molasses, ground beef, lamb, seaweed, unsweetened chocolate.

HOW BAD ARE SOME FOOD TYPES FOR OUR ARTERIES?

Table 2

TYPE OF FOOD	AVERAGE 'BAD' SCORE
Prepared Food	14.74
Meat	11.30
Confection	8.33
Fish	5.16
Dairy	5.02
Nuts and Seeds	4.45
Offal	4.12
Oils	3.42
Shellfish	2.49
Pulses	1.84
Breakfast Cereals	1.28
Vegetables	1.07
Fruit	1.06
Alcohol	1.00
WATER	1.00

If we total the amounts of fat and lysine in food and do some arithmetic, we can calculate a 'bad' score, or **atherogenic index (AGI)**, for each food.

Table 2 gives the average score for each of various food groups – the higher the score, the more likely the food is to 'fur' our arteries. Pure water is the neutral 'gold standard' – it definitely does not 'fur' arteries, and scores '1'. From Table 2, you can see that dairy produce is 5 times more likely to 'fur' our arteries than vegetables, and prepared foods like hamburgers, are five times more likely than shellfish to do the same.

This data allows us to compare one food group with another, based on food chemistry, not guesswork. Instead of stating that meat is worse for you than breakfast cereal, we can say that meat is nine times worse for you than breakfast cereal. Although food science is made inexact by large variations in food chemistry, this sort of calculation, based on what little science there is, does allow a better class of guesswork. The figures I have given are calculated from the actual chemistry of food, so it is interesting that the results follow what we might otherwise have guessed. Many will say: "I could have told you that meat was worse for you than fruit!" True, but they would not be able to say, how much worse meat is for our arteries than fruit.

I did mention in the introduction that most people would have a pretty good idea of what is bad for them. Knowing what is bad in food, is only half of the matter, since the 'good' things in food could be more important. *Two important questions are: 'how much fat do you need to eat to 'fur' your arteries, and can small amounts of the antidotes (the 'goodies') overcome the 'furring' effects of fat?'* Unfortunately, we just don't know the answers to these crucial questions at the moment.

One of the many problems with food is that its chemistry can be very variable. Is a banana from Nigeria, the same chemically as one from Antigua? They must be fairly similar, I guess, if only because they are both bananas, but they cannot be exactly the same, because the soil in which they were grown will have been different, and it is from the soil that some important food chemicals are derived. While this is an important source of error, the difference between really different foods – a lemon and a piece of steak for example, is so vast, that the small differences between the same foods, shrink to relative insignificance. Another source of error is that food laboratories may use different methods of analysis. Both are errors that need to be considered when we come to judge the reliability of our estimates of 'how good', and 'how bad', different foods are for our heart and arteries.

THE 'FURRING' FACTOR

The first thing I thought to do was to add up the three different types of fat in food, and call the result, the 'furring factor'. Another way is to include lysine in the calculation. Remember that in animals, the amino-acid lysine, taken with fat, can 'fur' the arteries up to two and a half times more than fat alone. My guess is, that this is less true for cholesterol, which does relatively little harm on its own, but is especially true for saturated fat, which is dangerous with whatever it is mixed. My guess also, is that lysine is as bad for humans, as it is for animals.

The word 'saturated', is a chemical term meaning no vacancies for guest atoms – all of the attachment sites are occupied or saturated. By the same token, 'unsaturated' fats are those with spaces to spare for those atoms that might wish to attach themselves. They can absorb other, perhaps dangerous chemicals, and neutralize them into a harmless form. Trans-fats are the product of cooking and heating fats to a very high temperature. They are found in biscuits, baked products, and confectionary. Like saturated fats, they are thought to be particularly bad for us.

Atherogenesis is the name we give to the 'furring' process, so the figure I calculated had to be given an appropriate name. **I chose 'AtheroGenic Index' or AGI, to express the idea of how likely food is to generate 'furring' (in other words: the *genesis of atheroma*). One way to remember it is that a lot of fat forming in your arteries could result in a lot of AG!**

Let's take some tasty examples – wine and cheese for instance. Without any reference to fat content, Camembert cheese has a high lysine/arginine ratio (making it relatively bad); red wine has a very low ratio (lots more arginine than lysine), making it good for our arteries (forget your liver for the moment!) So what happens when we drink wine with our cheese? Wine is an antidote to the 'furring' effect of cheese, but you would need a lot of wine to overcome the bad effects of lysine in cheese.

In working out AGI scores, I wanted as many food groups as possible to be represented, such as meat, fish, cereals, and fruit etc. I also wanted to be sure to include some of the foods with the highest concentrations of each beneficial chemical, such as selenium, zinc, omega-3 oils etc. I calculated the AGI ('baddy') formula for all of these foods, and sorted them into a list, from worst to best. The quoted chemical contents of food vary from one reference book to another and I found that the books I referred to, quoted figures that were +70%, to −50%, of the average for each constituent. So any quoted figure could actually be 70% more, or 50% less, than I originally thought. When you come to compare the 'furring index', or AGI for each food, this error, caused by natural variation, must be borne in mind.

You can directly compare AGI scores. If hamburgers score 64.8, then they are 21.6 times worse for you than sesame seeds, which score 3.0.

Technical Point about Lysine: If there is more lysine than arginine in the food, the fat present will cause much more artery furring. Much more arginine than lysine can exist − for instance, in red wine, there is 221 times as much arginine as lysine; one reason, at least, why it might be good for our arteries. At the end of this chapter I have given a list of the Arginine to Lysine ratios (Table 7). The higher the score, the less 'furring' potential any fat content will have. Why not just use this score then? It is a valuable consideration, but it takes no account of the other bad stuff − the actual fat content itself, or the anti-furring effect of any beneficial chemicals like selenium, zinc, omega 3 oils etc, all of which contribute to the end result.

How to Interpret the AGI Score:

There are two scores: the score per portion (Table 3), and the score per 100grams of each food (Table 4).

Table 3: This list strictly refers to the average edible portions of each food, so the AGI number allows us to say, from a practical point of view, how much more 'furring' potential one portion of any particular food has than another.

Table 4: Nutritionists prefer to quote their nutritional information in terms of 100g of food, so this is given as well. We obviously do not eat as much milk chocolate (AGI 100g = 24), as we do chicken breast (AGI 100g = 6). So if chocolate has 4 times the 'furring' potential of chicken breast (i.e. the AGI score for chocolate is 4 times greater than that of chicken breast), then you can eat 100 grams of chicken breast, or 25 grams of chocolate, and suffer the same 'furring' effect.

Table 3

Atherogenic Index (AGI)

Analysis per portion. Top ten foods only. Descending order of AGI.
(NB: One ounce = approximately 30 grams)

(For the full lists, go to Appendix 5, where the same Table numbers have been retained for ease of reference.)

Food	Portion Size (in grams)	AGI Score
CHEESEBURGER (triple meat)	400	64.81
HAMBURGER	250	20.89
CAMEMBERT	62	17.27
BEEF (RUMP) COOKED	100	16.08
LAMB (LEG ROASTED)	85	14.70
CHICKEN BREAST (ROASTED)	196	14.38
COCONUT	23	13.38
DUCK (ROASTED)	85	12.78
OIL (PALM)	14	12.40
PORK (LEG ROASTED)	85	11.23

Table 4

Atherogenic Index (AGI):

Top ten foods. 100g of food, in descending order.

Food	AGI Score
OIL (PALM)	82.44
PARMESAN	65.40
COCONUT	56.17
BUTTER	55.79
CHEDDAR	48.20
CAMEMBERT	33.25
OIL (COD LIVER)	24.43
CHOCOLATE: MILK	23.76
MAGARINE	21.70
OIL (WHEATGERM)	19.58

The two lists are clearly different in order of AGI, or 'bad' potential. This is because Table 3 assumes a portion size – after all, nobody eats the same amount of honey as steak, so quoting figures only for 100grams of food is not practicable for us consumers. However if you want to know the *concentration* of 'bad' chemicals in food, then the 100g list (Table 4), is the one for you.

For the full lists, go to Appendix 5, where the same Table numbers have been retained for ease of reference.

Using these lists, **it is possible to state that the worst foods by portion are: burgers, Camembert cheese, beef and lamb, whereas by concentration, they are palm oil, Parmesan cheese, coconut, butter, Camembert cheese, cod liver oil, and milk chocolate.** Because we do not eat much of any of these items, their effect is not perhaps as bad as the list might suggest. For instance, although Parmesan is second in the concentration list (Table 4), it is 57th in the portion list. Coconut, on the other hand, is 7th in the portion list, and 3rd in the concentration list – bad either way.

The AGI score gives an indication only of the 'bad' components in food – it takes no account of any possible 'good' components it might have.

Because the AGI score reflects how bad food is likely to be for us, it must be taken into account (in one form or another), in any definition of 'healthy' food, but so must the presence of the 'goodies'. Without both, no definition of healthy food is complete.

The lower the AGI score, the more 'healthy' the food is for our arteries. When the 'good' components are taken into account as well, this will offer a new way of classifying food, according to both its 'good', and its 'bad' chemical components.

Healthy food for our arteries

Healthy food for our arteries is food with little or no fat, more arginine than lysine, and lots of positively beneficial chemicals.

For the health of the heart and circulation we also have to include factors which keep down blood pressure, control body weight, and help control diabetes, since these all have a major influence on heart disease.

Let's broaden the definition to include these factors.

Healthy food for the Heart and Circulation

Healthy food for our heart and arteries will have to have: –

little or no fat, more arginine than lysine, be low in salt (sodium), high in potassium, have a limited amount of carbohydrate, limited calories, and lots of protective chemicals.

In the next chapter we will consider the protective chemicals, or 'goodies', and create a separate score for them. The 'goodies' act as antidotes to the 'baddies', so we cannot consider one without the other.

Table 5

Saturated Fat & Cholesterol in Food

Top 20 for Saturated Fat content

Ranked in descending order of saturated fat content
Note: I gram = approx. one thirtieth of an ounce.
One milligram (mg) = one thousandth of one gram
100 MILLIGRAMS = ONE THREE HUNDREDTHS OF AN OUNCE

FOOD	WEIGHT of Portion grams	CHOLESTEROL milligrams	SATURATED FAT milligrams
CHEESEBURGER (triple meat)	400	128	24800
HAMBURGER	250	188	10000
CAMEMBERT	62	45	9500
DUCK (ROASTED)	85	98	8200
CHOCOLATE:WHITE	44	10	8096
CHOCOLATE: MILK	44	10	8052
BEEF (RUMP) COOKED	100	76	7765
LAMB (LEG ROASTED)	85	85	7000

CHEDDAR	28	27	5900
PORK (LEG ROASTED)	85	85	5500
PANCREAS	85	223	5000
SAUSAGES (PORK)	100	55	4900
ICE CREAM	66	16	4500
CHICKEN BREAST (ROASTED)	196	184	4300
CHICKEN (DARK MEAT)	114	93	4200
HERRING	143	61	3700
MACKEREL	88	48	3700
EEL	136	107	3600
OIL (COD LIVER)	14	80	3200
TURKEY (DARK MEAT)	85	102	2600
HEART (BEEF)	85	221	2500
BUTTER	5	11	2500

Table 6

Trans-Fat & Cholesterol in Food
(top 20 for trans-fat content)

Ranked in descending order of trans-fat content
Note: I gram = one thirtieth of an ounce.
One milligram = one thousandth of one gram
100 MILLIGRAMS = ONE THREE HUNDREDTHS OF AN OUNCE

FOOD	WEIGHT of Portion grams	CHOLESTEROL milligrams	TRANS-FAT milligrams
HAMBURGER	250	188	1400
CHEESEBURGER (triple meat)	400	128	1200
LAMB (LEG ROASTED)	85	85	595
ICE CREAM	66	16	528
SAUSAGES (PORK)	100	55	410
CHEDDAR	28	27	392
MAGARINE	5	0	335
PEANUT BUTTER	32	0	300
BEEF (RUMP) COOKED	100	76	200
CHOCOLATE:WHITE	44	10	176
CHOCOLATE: MILK	44	10	176
BUTTER	5	11	150
CHICKEN (DARK MEAT)	114	93	114
DUCK (ROASTED)	85	98	85
TURKEY (DARK MEAT)	85	102	85
KIDNEY (BEEF)	85	391	85
PARMESAN	6	5	66

SARDINES (in oil)	50	33	50
CHOCOLATE: PLAIN	44	3	44
CRISPS (POTATO)	30	0	30

Table 7

Arginine (A) to Lysine (L) Ratio (A/L) of Foods
(ie plant to animal amino-acid ratios – abridged version)
The higher the score – the better for your arteries

More arginine than lysine	A/L Ratio
RED WINE	221.50
WHITE WINE	139.00
SHRIMP	10.00
PINE NUTS	5.25
HAZELNUTS	5.20
BRAZIL NUTS	5.05
WALNUTS	5.00
SESAME SEEDS	4.64
ORANGE JUICE	4.00
ALMONDS	3.77
Lysine content = Arginine content	
CRAB (STEAMED)	1.00
ASPARAGUS	1.00
BANANA	1.00
BROCCOLI	1.00
CABBAGE	1.00
CARROTS	1.00
CAULIFLOWER	1.00
CORN	1.00
STRAWBERRY	1.00
More Lysine than Arginine	
TOMATO	0.62
COTTAGE CHEESE	0.56
APPLE	0.50
CHOCOLATE(MILK)	0.50
WHOLE MILK	0.50
MANGO	0.50
ICE CREAM	0.47
BUTTER	0.46
MILKSHAKE (Vanilla)	0.45
OVALTINE	0.45

For the full lists, go to Appendix 5, where the same Table numbers have been retained for ease of reference.

CHAPTER 4

The Food 'Goodies'

In a Nutshell: There is evidence that many different chemicals have a beneficial effect on artery 'furring' and therefore heart disease. Among them are the following: the amino-acids L-arginine and taurine, some vitamins (folic acid, B6 and B12, 'natural' vitamin E), some minerals (manganese, magnesium, selenium, zinc), and an assortment of others: linoleic, linolenic, and oleic fatty acids, lycopene, garlic, phytosterols, polyphenols, and soy protein. Although many people believe in them, vitamins C and A, are of no proven value to human artery and heart disease prevention, even if they are anti-oxidants.

Food, in general, is a relatively poor source of the 'goodies', but a rather good source of the 'baddies', although many foods contain some of both. We have taken a look at the 'baddies', now consider the antidotes to artery 'furring' and high blood pressure, the 'goodies'.

HOW CAN WE KNOW WHAT IS GOOD FOR OUR ARTERIES?

First we need to know which particular food chemicals are thought to be good for our arteries – many are thought to be good us, but few stand up to scrutiny. In this chapter we will take at look at the front-runners – those chemicals for which there is scientific evidence of a cardiovascular benefit. Having identified them, we will want to know where to find them in food.

To be considered good for artery 'furring' and heart disease – a 'goody', or beneficial food chemical, must either have been shown:

(1) **to prevent, or slow down, the formation of cholesterol (atherosclerosis, or 'furring') in arteries, or**

(2) **have been shown to prevent heart attacks, strokes, and death from cardiovascular diseases.**

It must also have been shown:

(3) **not to be dangerous to eat (in usual portion amounts).**

Let's take a closer look at what makes a 'goody'. Take the first qualifying statement – showing that any food chemical prevents, or slows down, the formation of cholesterol (atherosclerosis or 'furring') in our arteries.

Animal experiments on arteries, and various 'before and after' experimental trials on human arteries, using ultrasound or a coronary angiogram, have been used to examine this question. The aim is to study the individual effect of various chemicals in food on the process of artery 'furring'. Results of such research are given later in this chapter when we consider the beneficial substances individually.

Some chemicals can be shown to prevent the 'furring' process in animals, yet, paradoxically, fail to prevent heart attacks and strokes in humans. How can that be? Heart attacks are due to blocked arteries but the process is much more complicated than a simple build up of cholesterol in artery walls. Plaques of 'furring' are not all the same; some are inactive and full of chalk, others are active like an abscess. Like an abscess they can burst; an event that often leads to arterial blockage due to blood clot. To have a beneficial effect on heart attacks, some, or all, of these processes may have to be inhibited. Simply inhibiting the 'furring' process alone is not good enough.

The relevance of animal experiments to human beings is an important subject. Animals and humans are different, but not as different as all that, when it comes to the functioning of arteries.

Since the advice given to us about medicines and chemicals may be based on the results of animal experiments, several important questions need to be asked –

- Have the chemicals been shown to be effective in both animals and humans?

- When a beneficial effect has been shown in animals, what is the equivalent beneficial dose for humans?

- Over what period would the chemicals need to be taken, in order to achieve benefit?

THE CLINICAL TRIAL

To show that a particular chemical can prevent heart attacks, strokes, and death from cardiovascular diseases, better than any inert and biologically inactive substance like chalk, we have to undertake a clinical trial.

Because it is so easy to fool ourselves into thinking that medicine works, the effects and side-effects of all medicinal products have to be put to the test and compared to a placebo, that is, an inert blank substance like chalk. During a clinical trial, neither the patient nor the doctor giving the trial medicine to the patient may know which is which. When neither party knows which is which, it is called a double blind trial. The scientists conducting the research know which is which of course; they would have secretly coded the tablets beforehand. The object of such secrecy is to limit bias towards one pill or the other in the mind of the patient. It would be very easy for a doctor who knew which pill was active and which inactive, to subliminally impart that knowledge. Because belief (the placebo effect) is so important to the effectiveness of medicines, the final result could also be biased.

It is somewhat difficult to believe, but inert pills such as chalk, will help 20% of those who take them, whether it is for headache, impotence, anxiety, or joint pains! This surprising result means that the placebo effect is a very valuable one indeed, and it is for this reason that so many 'therapists' come to fool themselves into thinking that they have a magic cure. After all, if one in five of your patients claim an improvement, that is not bad going. A placebo helps, with no risk to health, but when it comes to changes in our arteries, subjective benefit is not the issue; what needs to be shown is that the chemical under test, actually prevents artery 'furring' more than the placebo.

To prevent heart attacks we would have to put a stop to artery 'furring', plaque rupture, and clotting – as early in life as possible. Many individual food substances have been tested in clinical trials, to see if these benefits can be achieved.

The results of clinical trials can be illustrated by the research on aspirin and vitamin E. Aspirin reduces both heart attacks and some strokes, by reducing the clotting tendency. The same is true of the Mediterranean diet and natural vitamin E (but not synthetic vitamin E). Both aspirin and vitamin E partially prevent clotting, so one might expect them both to have one nasty side-effect – bleeding. Trials on vitamin E do, in fact, show a slight excess of strokes due to bleeding, so the safety of both vitamin E and aspirin is of concern. Those with high blood pressure, who are more likely to have strokes due to bleeding, are one group in particular, who might be at greater risk when taking such medication.

Is there always a price to pay? Aspirin, given to 22,000 healthy doctors (The Physicians' Health Study, 1988), was seen to reduce heart attacks (by 44%), but to increase strokes due to bleeding. So there is a cost. For those who have had a heart attack already, the advantages are of great value, because their chances of a further heart attack are substantial, and their need for preventative treatment that much greater.

CAN A 'GOODY' BE TOO MUCH OF A GOOD THING?

None of the chemicals I have considered to be beneficial have been shown to be dangerous in recommended daily amounts. **Eat too** little, or too much food, and you will kill yourself – in these two cases – 'you are (or will be) what you eat'! Consume vast quantities of selenium or copper and they could prove to be toxic; Recommended Nutritional Intake's (RNI's) were therefore devised as a guide to healthy nutritional consumption. Toxicity levels are usually very much greater than the RNI level, so I have limited consideration here only to quantities of substances available in our usual diet. We could overdose on zinc (more than 150mgs of zinc / day), but we would have to eat 3 or 4 oysters every day – not the usual daily food for most of us these days, but still possible!

FINDING FOOD SUBSTANCES THAT MIGHT PREVENT HEART ATTACKS.

How can we identify the substances found in food that might prevent, stabilize, or reduce the 'furring' process in our arteries? I chose to do a computer search of a medical database which lists all of the relevant artery and heart research undertaken since 1966 (Medline). By asking the computer search engine to find all the research publications mentioning artery 'furring', it was possible to identify which substances had been used in experiments. After sifting through over 2000 references, I came up with about 200 of real interest. What follows is a brief appraisal of what I found.

Many substances have only been tried in animals, and then only on the early 'furring' processes within their arteries. Their effect on more advanced 'furring' remains largely unknown. It is feasible that some of these dietary factors, started early enough in life and, taken for long enough, could beneficially influence long-term 'furring'-related outcomes in humans, but this has to be proven. We need to find the front-runners, so let's review all of those in the race and explore where to find them in food.

There are five main groups of substances to consider – vitamins, amino-acids, minerals, fatty acids, and an assorted group of different substances, all of which are chemically very different.

The Vitamins

Vitamins have been widely studied. Only the B vitamins (folic acid, B6, and B12), and natural vitamin E, have any real claim to be cardio-protective, so in this chapter I have made little or no mention of any others.

Vitamins are substances that cannot be made by the body, but are essential to health. The double Nobel Prize winner Linus Pauling predicted in the early 1960's, that taking vast doses of vitamin C, would have many beneficial effects on some diseases not caused by vitamin deficiency. He inaugurated the Linus Pauling Institute to work on his ideas.

Vitamin C

Just a small amount of vitamin C is enough to prevent the deficiency disease scurvy, but do vast doses really prevent heart disease and cancer? There are many publications detailing the results of animal research, various types of animal cell research, and the beneficial effects of vitamin C on their biochemical processes. So far, however, little beneficial cardio-preventative effect in humans has yet been demonstrated for vitamin C. In particular, it has not been shown to stop artery 'furring'. Despite this, in the UK, £20,000,000 is spent every year by the public on vitamin C! £208,000,000 is spent on all the other vitamins, indicating that belief, and not proof, is a salesman's best friend!

Top Food Sources of vitamin C

Vitamin C: Orange juice, grapefruit juice, papaya, strawberries, kiwifruit, red pepper, cantaloupe melon, tomato juice, broccoli, mango, oranges, brussel sprouts, peapods, green pepper, cauliflower, kale, cabbage, collard greens, clams, squash and butternut.

While there is no evidence for a protective effect of vitamin C alone, in combination with the vegetable-based amino-acid l-arginine (found in nuts etc), it has been said to have a place in the treatment of coronary artery disease.

Vitamin E

There is evidence that vitamin E may slow the progress of early 'furring' in the main blood vessel of both rabbits and humans (the CLAS and ARIC studies). Despite this evidence, four major clinical trials of synthetic vitamin E supplementation, have failed to show any benefit in humans, when death and heart attack outcomes are measured.

Synthetic Vitamin E does appear to reduce the incidence of non-fatal heart attacks, but there is concern about its use, since several studies report more cardiovascular deaths, due mainly to brain haemorrhage (vitamin E given in a daily dosage range of 100 – 1000 I.U., or International Units). One possible explanation, as mentioned before, is that the vitamin may have a signi-ficant anti-coagulant (anti-clotting) effect. If this is correct, its combination with aspirin (also an anti-clotting agent), might have further adverse effects. Studying human neck arteries with ultrasound, the CLAS study showed that synthetic vitamin E, but not vitamin C, reduced the progress of artery 'furring'.

> ❤️ *Technical Point:*
> *Natural vitamin E is a mixture of four types of tocopherol and tocotrienols. Synthetic vitamin E is something quite different, namely: dl-α-tocopherol. The latter has been used in most clinical trials. Current evidence shows it to be ineffective in preventing fatal heart attacks. The CHAOS study however, showed a very highly significant reduction in heart attacks when natural vitamin E was taken by those with proven coronary artery disease (i.e. a very high risk group indeed), but unfortunately, this work has not been repeated and reproduced.*

Some animal experiments have revealed a beneficial effect of vitamin E alone, and the vitamin in combination with high-dose selenium. Other experiments in rabbits have shown little or no effect of vitamin E.

Top Food Sources of vitamin E

Vitamin E (natural): Wheat-germ oil, sunflower seed kernels, filberts (hazelnuts), sunflower oil, hazelnut oil, peanuts, almond oil, brazil nuts, grape-seed oil, almonds, pistachio nuts, peanut butter, turkey liver, cod liver oil, corn oil, canola oil, salmon oil, wheatgerm, white tuna, mango, and clams.

The 'B' Vitamins

Folic acid is given to pregnant women to prevent foetal abnormalities, but could it also prevent heart disease?

♥Technical Point: Some people with a raised blood homocysteine are smokers, some have impaired kidney function, some have high blood pressure (hypertension), and others have an inherited genetic enzyme defect. Homocysteine levels are reduced by exercise training, and by taking folic acid, B6, and B12 supplements.

The defect of a specific enzyme in a family, might explain the heart attack risk in a few of the families that I have investigated with normal blood fat levels.

Reduced blood levels of folic acid, and vitamins B12 and B6, have been found in association with artery 'furring', and a raised blood homocysteine level. The routine blood test for homocysteine is relatively new and could help provide a clue as to why those people with normal blood cholesterol, and other normal cardiac risk factors, have artery 'furring'.

We now know enough to say that routine blood testing for homocysteine, should be considered for all those who want to know if they have a significant heart attack risk, and for all those who have any evidence of artery 'furring' (a positive carotid artery scan, coronary artery disease, claudication, or cerebrovascular [brain blood vessel] disease).

The practical point here is that folic acid helps reduce homocysteine blood levels, and thus coronary artery disease risk. It is important to know that naturally-occurring folic acid has only half the effectiveness (bioavailability) of the synthetic form. One example, at least, of 'natural' not being the best!

Trials are underway to see if folic acid is of benefit to groups with a significant heart attack risk, that is, those who already have angina and heart disease. There is evidence to suggest that the beneficial dose is no greater than 800 micrograms per day. So far, I have used it in several doses but it doesn't always reduce blood homocysteine levels. The addition of B12 and B6 however seems to give better results. Keep your eye on this important front-runner, since it has been calculated that it should reduce ischaemic heart disease ('furred' heart arteries or coronary artery disease) by 16%, clots in the legs (deep vein thrombosis) by 25%, and strokes by 24%.

Top Sources of B vitamins

Folic Acid: Chicken, turkey, veal, and beef liver. Brewer's yeast, lentils, okra, black beans, black-eyed peas, kidney beans, spinach, green soybeans, white pasta, beef kidney, peanuts, flour tortilla, collard greens, asparagus spears, navy beans, sunflower kernels, romaine lettuce, orange juice, pinto beans.

Vitamin B6: Liver as above, Brewer's yeast, banana, salmon, chicken breast, herring, turkey, beef kidney, potato skin, baked beans, prune juice, hazelnuts, halibut, shrimp, beef, roast chestnuts, tomato juice, walnuts, veal, sweet potato.

Vitamin B12: Liver as above, steamed clams, beef kidney, oysters, heart, herring, crab, trout, pollock, catfish, salmon, beef, lamb, fish, tuna, shrimp, yogurt, cottage and feta cheese, milk.

Amino-acids

Arginine is an amino-acid – a building block, from which proteins are made. Proteins form the fabric of every tissue in our body. Just four amino-acids, in many and various combinations, make up all of our genes.

♥♥*Very Technical Point:* Something *rather odd goes on in the inner lining of our arteries. The inner lining of our arteries (called the endothelium), produces a gas called nitric oxide. This is not to be confused with 'laughing gas', or nitrous oxide (N_2O). Nitric oxide (or NO, in chemical shorthand), has the effect of expanding arteries. How well the arteries contract and expand, is a measure of how healthy they are. When they are 'furred', they respond less well. Nitric oxide reduces the cholesterol formation in the inner artery lining – an effect that seems linked to folic acid, B12, and B6. Perhaps more importantly, it stops the oxidization (equivalent to iron rusting), of the bad (LDL) cholesterol, which is thought to initiate the 'furring' process.*

Oxidized cholesterol forms irritant crystals within the artery wall, so it is beneficial to stop cholesterol combining with oxygen. Arginine is the substance from which NO is made (it is the so-called substrate for NO). Folic acid and the B vitamins, ensure that the process of NO production from arginine, keeps going. In their absence, free oxygen radicals are produced, instead of NO; cholesterol becomes more easily oxidized (perhaps crystallized), and the 'furring' process progresses. Arginine, folic acid, and the B vitamins are clearly very important to artery health.

Arginine is an anti-oxidant of sorts – while it is producing nitric oxide in the artery lining, no oxygen free-radicals are being produced. That is a process dependant on the presence of folic acid, B6, and B12 vitamins. Anti-oxidants should be beneficial if they remove, or mop-up, free oxygen radicals and limit the production of cholesterol crystals (oxidized LDL). Well, that is the script many have learned. So far, the theory is not holding up too well, since heart attack prevention has not been seen to result from taking antioxidants (Vitamin C, Vitamin E, etc.). One problem may be that anti-oxidants simply don't reach the parts where they could do some good. They should work in theory, and they can be shown to work in experiments using cells and artery tissue, but they don't seem to work when given as a medicine. The history of medical science is littered with similar examples of treatments that 'should' work, and don't; and those that 'shouldn't', and do. That's life!

When arginine is given to patients with known cardiovascular disease, it improves their symptoms. Angina, leg pain due to 'furred' arteries (claudication), and shortness of breath due to heart failure, are all improved, to some extent, by arginine supplementation.

Top Sources of Arginine

Red wine, shrimp, whelks, pumpkin seeds, white wine, walnuts, wild rice, lentils, crab, soy-beans, pine nuts, sunflower flour, cod, tuna, hazelnuts, black-eyed peas, octopus (calamari), haddock, sesame seeds, brown rice.

It has been suggested, that those with a high risk of artery and heart disease, and those who actually have coronary artery disease and heart failure, might benefit from long-term arginine administration. Theoretically, it should help, but the evidence, so far, is not overwhelming.

One study showed no reduction in coronary heart disease mortality in men aged 64 – 84 years; another showed that those with leg pain (claudication) increased their pain-free walking distance by 66%, and their total walking distance by 23%. In another study, the exercise tolerance of patients with angina was improved by 20%. Impressed? Well, to be able to walk 166 yards instead of 100 yards when you have leg pain, and 120 yards instead of 100 yards when you have angina would hardly impress me, and it certainly does not impress patients. Nevertheless, it is a worthwhile result and worthy of the time and trouble taken to do the research because it does demonstrate some benefit. How easy it is to be dismissive!

Others have found that people given arginine as a supplement, do show a significant reduction in both cholesterol formation (68% ± 6%) and inner artery lining thickness (intimal thickness), when compared to those fed a vitamin alone. Although the evidence is mixed, there are some good reasons to believe that arginine supplementation is beneficial for our arteries.

Taurine

The name taurine is derived from the source of its first discovery in an ox over 160 years ago (the Latin name for an ox is Taurus – the same as the bull of astrological fame). In the human body, taurine is found in high concentration in heart muscle, where it significantly affects the functioning of heart muscle cells, in the brain, and at the back of the eye (the retina). It is actually manufactured by the body and is, therefore, called a 'non-essential' amino-acid.

In food, the amino acid taurine is found mainly in seafood, fish, and the brown meat of chicken and turkey. Food supplementation with taurine significantly reduces the 'furring' (atherosclerotic) process in animals. Mice fed with a taurine-supplemented diet (2%) accumulated 31% less fat in their main heart valve. Similar benefits have been shown in rats, a result thought to be due to the enhanced elimination of cholesterol from the body.

Top Sources of Taurine

Shrimp, mussels, crab, chicken (dark meat), octopus, baked beans, roast leg of lamb, roast leg of pork, beef sirloin, heart, beef kidney, chicken breast, walnuts, pigs liver, pine nuts, peanut butter. Some 'energy' drinks.

It is interesting to note that the daily taurine intake in rural Japan, from fish and shellfish, is the highest in the world (200 to 2,500 milligrams per day), and the incidence of their heart disease is the lowest.

Some of the shellfish sources of taurine are also sources of cholesterol, less of which exists in food than you might have been led to believe. (See previous chapter).

The Minerals

Manganese, magnesium, zinc, and selenium, are all in the running for a 'good for our arteries', or 'cardio-protective' title. They are all metals, found in the body in very small amounts, and in the food we eat. Because they are all essential parts of enzymes – those active chemicals within all living organisms, that accelerate the way our vital chemical reactions work – we cannot do without them.

As with vitamins, there are some important questions we must ask. For instance, can we get enough of them from food? And, by taking more than a trace amount, can we better protect our arteries? Nobody really knows for sure, but experiments on animals, and some human studies, suggest that they may all have an important role to play in artery health. We also need to ask, 'can too much be dangerous'?

Manganese

There is not a lot to say about manganese. Manganese is the metal component of a very important enzyme within the body (manganese superoxide dismutase or MnSOD), known to reduce the 'furring' process in rabbits.

Top Sources of Manganese

Wheat-germ, pecan nuts, whole wheat pasta, soy-nuts, walnuts, pumpkin seeds, almonds, hazelnuts, oatmeal, peanuts, sweet potatoes, pineapple, oyster, molasses, tomato juice, blackberries, grape juice, spinach, brown rice, roast chestnuts.

Magnesium

Magnesium is involved in many important cellular functions. A lack of magnesium causes heart rhythm defects, but usually only in the context of the critically ill who are being sustained long-term on an intravenous drip. A lack of magnesium can lead to cramps and high blood pressure. When I was first qualified, I looked after a lady who had been drip-fed for weeks. She suffered very disturbing hallucinations that were completely cured by injections of magnesium.

Magnesium can become depleted in the body by a very high roughage diet because it gets bound to vegetable material in the bowel. In those with coronary heart disease, magnesium supplementation (15mmols/day) can cause a decrease in the so-called 'bad' cholesterol (LDL) in the blood, and an increase in the 'good' cholesterol (HDL). How it does this is not known, but that is the observation.

There is some interesting, if macabre, evidence about the amount of magnesium in our arteries. The magnesium content of the artery 'furring' in humans, dying from either a heart attack or a road traffic accident, has been compared. The researchers found that the magnesium content of the 'furring' in the arteries of those who had had a heart attack was much less than that in the arteries of those who died in a road traffic accident. Could it be that a lack of magnesium in the inner artery lining of our arteries promotes the clotting that leads to heart attacks?

Studying over 13,000 subjects, F. Liao and co-workers (1998), showed that blood magnesium levels were related to the amounts taken in the diet. That much was not surprising, however, they also concluded that a low magnesium concentration might contribute to heart attacks from clot formation in the heart arteries. In another study, R.B. Singh and colleagues (published in 2000), found that those taking a diet of less than half a milligram every day (low intake), were worse off than those on a diet of 2.3 milligrams of magnesium per day. **Overall, the low magnesium intake subjects, had a 50% greater chance of dying.**

Top Sources of Magnesium

Pumkin seeds, almonds, soynuts, hazelnuts, Brazil nuts, cashews (and most other common nuts), tofu, unsweetened chocolate, artichoke, spinach, black beans, oatmeal.

And here are some relevant research results. Cholesterol-fed, 'furring-prone' mice, receiving magnesium-fortified water, develop less artery 'furring' than those drinking plain water. Mice and men are rather different, but pigs are thought to have similar arteries to our own. The coronary arteries of pigs were examined following various intakes of magnesium. Dr M. Ito and co-workers (1986), concluded that moderate magnesium deficiency is associated with 'furring' and chalk accumulation in the artery walls. One of the more advanced features of the 'furring' process within our arteries is the formation of a substance, similar to common chalk, within its structure (calcium apatite).

It could be that this calcium compound, which is actually found in bone, strengthens and stabilizes the 'furring' in arteries. Better not to have it in the first place, of course, but if you do have any 'furring', then this compound could possibly make it stronger and safer. It is the fat-rich collections that are dangerous – the so-called vulnerable plaques (see Fig 5b), because they are more likely to rupture and cause clotting. EBCT scanning – an X-ray scan of the heart, can actually show these chalky patches (like that in Fig 5a), and can be used non-invasively to grade the amount of atherosclerosis present in our coronary arteries. You can read more about this interesting test in Chapter 2, on investigating the heart.

Selenium

Selenium is also an important metallic part of one of our enzyme systems. Because it is not found in all soils, selenium may be deficient in the food chain of some countries. Those with a notable deficiency are Russia, China, New Zealand, and Scotland (Aberdeenshire). High selenium levels are found in North American soils, but it is estimated that the available selenium in the EEC may have halved over the last 25 years.

A low blood selenium level is associated with a three-fold risk of cardiovascular death and coronary artery disease. Reviewing coronary angiograms, some have seen that low selenium blood levels relate to a greater average amount of arterial 'furring'.

Top Sources of Selenium

Brazil nuts, oysters, liver, clams, sardines, pork, crab, salt water fish, whole wheat pasta, chicken meat, white pasta, lamb, sunflower seeds, bagel, processed fish and crab, beef heart, oatmeal, flour tortilla, roasted soybeans.

Using carotid (neck artery) ultrasound, Dr. J.T. Salonen and co-workers (1992), showed that the progression of inner artery lining thickness (intimal thickness) over two years was associated with a low blood selenium, a higher blood copper level (a pro-oxidant), and a raised 'bad' (LDL) cholesterol level.

Zinc

Our bodies are made up of an unimaginably large number of individual cells. Zinc is a metal, essential to the healthy maintenance of the cell walls. It has anti-oxidant effects, and may protect against artery inflammation. Deficiency seems to promote artery 'furring'. It is thought that an imbalance between zinc and copper may result in a raised blood cholesterol and be important in the development of coronary heart disease.

Dr A. Reunanen and co-workers (1996), placed the blood of large numbers of patients in long-term cold-storage, and waited. They later analysed the blood of those who died, for both zinc and copper content. They found a significantly lower blood zinc level, and a higher blood copper level, in the stored blood samples of those patients who went on to suffer a cardiovascular death. In fact, their risk was nearly three times higher, than those with normal blood levels. The association of risk with dietary iron and copper, was mentioned before. Both of these metals carry oxygen, and so might aid the manufacture of oxidized 'bad' cholesterol (LDL), which is known to be so important to the initiation of the 'furring' process.

Top Sources of Zinc

Oysters, beef, liver, crab, turkey, veal, pumpkin seeds, blue crab, beef kidney, soy-nuts, lamb, almonds, peanuts, pecans, brazil nuts, cashews, dark chicken meat, steamed clams, pork, wheat-germ.

The optimal daily dose of zinc could be critical – another Goldilocks situation – it must not be too little, not too much, but just right! If too high, it could have 'furring' potential, since it may be associated with a raised blood cholesterol. Although I did try, I could find no direct studies of the effect of zinc on the actual 'furring' process.

Dietary Fat and Fatty Acids

Polyunsaturated fats (PUFA's) are fats that contain unoccupied, or un-saturated, chemical sites. They are usually liquid at room temperature, while saturated fats (no free sites i.e. all saturated), are solid.

Fish oils are rich in so-called PUFA's (omega-3 etc) and have long been known to provide protection after a heart attack (GISSI-Prevenzione Trial, and the DART study, both show this).

There are two important omega-3 fatty acids: **eicosapentaenoic acid (EPA), and docosahexaenoic acid (DHA)**. EPA and DHA are both components of omega-3 fish oil. They are known to reduce free blood fat (or triglyceride), to reduce blood coagulability (prevent clotting), and to reduce the progress of artery 'furring'.

PUFA's have been recognized to have anti-arrhythmic properties – that is, they can stop dangerous heart rhythms. In a study of 20,551 US male physicians, Dr C.M. Albert and co-workers (1998), found that the risk of sudden death was halved in those who consumed fish just once every week. Unfortunately, heart attacks when the patient survived, and non-sudden deaths, were not reduced, although all-cause mortality was significantly reduced. A lack of oleic acid (a fatty acid found in olive oil), but not omega-3 oils in the diet, has been found to be associated with an increase in the number of strokes that occur.

These rather long words are actually derived from Greek numbers. Take EPA – eicosapentoic acid – eicosa = 20, and penta = 5. Why chemists still use Greek for naming chemicals, I'm not quite sure. Contrary to the popular view, Greek not Latin, is the language used for most medical terms. The reason is historical. Once upon a time doctors had to be Latin scholars, and some very clever scholars were given ancient Greek to learn – as a treat! Doctors now have no time to fortify their souls with the delights of Greek poetry, they are just too busy reading the gobbledegook of governmental and managerial directives!

A coronary angiogram study of Japanese patients, with evidence of coronary artery disease, found them to have a lower 'good' cholesterol (HDL) and higher blood levels of both eicosapentaenoic acid (EPA) and docosahexaenoic acid (DHA), than normal subjects. EPA was related to the amount of brown-meat fish the subjects consumed, and DHA to the amount of soybean product consumed. This evidence suggests that eating omega-3 oils is associated with coronary artery disease! Alaskan Eskimos have less artery 'furring' than non-natives, but there is a dispute as to whether this is due to a higher intake of omega-3 fish oils, or to a greater intake of seal and whale meat than fish. Back to Goldilocks again – perhaps an excessive intake of fish oil is not the best thing. Clearly, more study is required to clear up this important inconsistency.

In the last 40 years, many group studies have suggested a reduction in risk from coronary heart disease, high blood pressure, and stroke, in those who consume omega-3 oils. The question is, how much fish would we need to eat in order to get the right dose? Even one fish meal per week, has been shown to be better than a non-fish diet. Dr S. Brewer (2002) suggested that, in order to eat enough poly-unsaturated fat derived from fish, we would need to eat at least 100 grams of fish per week. (Polyunsaturated fat is found mainly in oily fish such as herrings, pilchards, salmon, sardines, and mackerel.) This advice would necessitate each of us, on average, increasing our fish consumption ten-fold; advice that conflicts in opinion with the conclusions of Dr C.M. Albert and co-workers (1998), whose research suggested no further benefit, beyond one fish meal per week.

The latest dietary suggestion for cardiovascular risk reduction, the Polymeal, suggests eating 456 grams (13.8 ounces) of fish every week. However, the presence of highly poisonous dioxins in some fish could make large amounts dangerous – depending, of course, on the origin of the fish. (Salmon wars are likely to rage when such a thing is even suggested!) Perhaps supplements will prove safer than fish? Then, all we have to ask is –'what is the origin of the oil in the supplements?'

The Mediterranean diet (salads, seafood, fish 2 –3 times/week, nuts, wine, vegetable oils, and meat once per week) undoubtedly reduces heart attacks and death from cardiovascular causes. It can provide twice the intake of whole grains, fruits, vegetables, walnuts, and almonds, than other diets. In those who have heart disease already, it has been shown to reduce further cardiac events by 73% (so called secondary prevention), and to reduce total deaths by 56% over 4 years. (See references: De Lorgeril, 1997 and 1998.) It may achieve this for a number of reasons, some of which may include a substantial benefit from the many chemicals already mentioned. It is certainly not effective because of its low fat content – the French simply refuse to give up their cheese and creamy sauces!

The advantages of the Mediterranean diet, suggest that vegetable derived fatty acids are as good as the fish-derived ones. So what are these vegetable-derived fatty acids? Two very important ones are linolenic and linoleic fatty-acids. These fatty acids have been tried in rabbits with established artery furring. Dr D. Kritchevsky and colleagues (1985), found that conjugated linoleic acid (CLA) was capable of both reducing 'furring' and able to partly reduce 'furring' (by 30%), over a 90-day period.

In the National Heart, Lung, and Blood Institute Family Heart Study of 4584 participants, the intake of two vegetable-derived fatty acids – linolenic and linoleic acid, was associated with a reduced number of cardiovascular problems. In another study, the intake of linolenic acid in the intervention group was twice that of the control group (those not on the diet). The intervention group eventually went on to develop half the cardiac problems, half the non-fatal heart attacks, and almost one third fewer sudden deaths. At the same time as this was published, the UK Food Standards Agency concluded that vegetable-derived fatty acids were of only equivocal benefit in comparison to those derived from marine sources!

Top Sources of Fatty Acids

Linolenic Acid: Wheat-germ oil, walnut oil, pumpkin seeds, white rice, lettuce, peanuts, oatmeal, swordfish, brussel sprouts, spinach, almonds, corn oil, strawberry, mackerel, cauliflower.

Linoleic Acid: Pumpkin Seeds, wheat germ oil, oatmeal, corn oil, peanuts, almonds, sunflower oil, peanut butter, walnut oil, brown rice, sesame seeds, turkey dark meat, sunflower flour.

Oleic Acid: Pumpkin seeds, almonds, peanuts, oatmeal, peanut butter, wheat-germ oil, Brazil nuts, corn oil, herring, palm and olive oil, sesame seeds, turkey dark meat, potato flesh, brown rice.

VEGETARIAN FOOD

There are undoubted benefits and disadvantages for those who eat a vegetarian diet. The advantages are that blood cholesterol is generally lower than that of meat eaters, and there is likely to be a greater intake of atheroprotective substances. Nuts, for instance, contain arginine, selenium, and linolenic acid – all of which are protective. Soy protein intake reduces blood cholesterol when it is high and fruit containing phytosterols reduces the absorption of cholesterol from the bowel.

The absence of meat denies the vegetarian an adequate intake of vitamins B12 and B6, both of which are essential for the normal functioning of the intima (the inner lining of arteries). As a consequence, vegetarians generally have a raised blood homo-cysteine, now thought to be a significant risk factor for coronary heart disease. Despite this, M. Thorogood and colleagues (1994), found that **over a 12 year period, UK vegetarians had 40% fewer cancer deaths, and 30% fewer cardiovascular deaths, than meat eaters.** It could be, that homocysteine levels are not as important as we thought; or it could be that vegetarians eat many other atheroprotective substances of greater importance than B vitamins. We have to be careful with our conclusions, because vegetarians could be different from meat eaters in other ways. They might exercise more, smoke less, drink more water than coffee, and get less stressed! And these could all exert a beneficial influence.

The intake of nuts, rich in arginine, selenium, and fatty acids has been studied in many communities and found to reduce cardiovascular mortality for all age groups and races. Furthermore, the beneficial effects do not appear to be undone by other factors (J. Sabate 1990).

The World Health Organisation now recommends unsalted nuts as cardioprotective. If you cannot eat nuts, there are alternative supplements (containing arginine, selenium, and fatty acids).

NON-DRUG, BLOOD CHOLESTEROL LOWERING AGENTS

There are at least four to consider: dietary fibre, soya, phytosterols, and phytostanols. The last two are now added to artificial butter spreads and some milk. Naturally occurring chemicals, similar to 'statin' drugs (which lower cholesterol), do exist in food, but little information exists about them at present.

Dietary Fibre

Top Sources of Dietary Fibre
Dietary Fibre: Oatmeal, Bran Flakes, Lima beans, soybeans, Shredded Wheat, garden peas, black-eyed peas, hazelnuts, lentils.

Fibre is important, because it has been shown to reduce the uptake of cholesterol and other fats, from the bowel. Ten to twenty-five grams of soluble fibre every day are recommended. From a statistical point of view, any measure that lowers the average blood cholesterol of a population, will reduce the heart disease mortality of that group. Whether it will help you or me, is much less certain.

Phytosterols

These are plant-based chemicals (sterols and stanols) that share a similar chemical structure with cholesterol. They reduce the absorption of cholesterol from the bowel, by competing with it for absorption. Two grams every day have been recommended as a worthwhile supplement to a low fat diet.

The three most abundant, of the 40 or so known phytosterols, are called: sitosterol, campesterol, and sigmasterol. Neither the sterols, nor the stanols, are very well absorbed from the digestive tract. This is a good thing because, like cholesterol, they have the potential to 'fur' arteries. However, only 5% of sitosterol; 15% of campesterol, and less than 1% of stanols are absorbed. By contrast, 50 – 70% of the cholesterol in food is normally absorbed. When any of these other sterols is ingested, along with cholesterol, about 50% less cholesterol is absorbed through the bowel. The result is a reduction in blood cholesterol of about 20% (13% lower LDL). Two and a half grams of phytosterol per day is said to lower the blood cholesterol by 0.5 (mmols/litre). However, they can also reduce the absorption of fat-soluble vitamins, such as vitamin E and vitamin K, so these may need to be supplemented.

For those patients with high blood cholesterol, sterols could be an important dietary component, either taken as a butter substitute spread (Flora Pro-Active, or Benecol in the UK), or in the naturally occurring forms listed in the top sources given below. Phytosterols and stanols are a useful dietary supplement to those patients already

---

Top Sources of Phytosterols

Phytosterols: Sesame seeds, Flora Pro-Active (phyto-sterol), Benecol (phyto-stanol), peas, sunflower seeds, blackeyed peas, walnuts, almonds, corn oil, peanuts, taramasalata, pine nuts, brussel sprouts, thousand island dressing, peanut butter, onion, wheat-germ oil, pappadoms, almond oil.

---

taking a 'statin' drug. Very little research on the direct arterial affect of phytosterols has been done, but there is at least one report of stanols reducing the 'furring' in the aorta in some animals. Their most important effect, however, is on the reduction of cholesterol absorption from the bowel. (Ezetimibe is a drug that inhibits cholesterol uptake in the bowel. Its effect is, therefore, similar to that of stanols and phytosterols.)

For those with a further interest, refer to the article written by Malcolm Law in the British Medical Journal (2000), on: Plant Sterol and Stanol Margarines and Health.

Soya Protein and Isoflavones

Soy protein is capable of reducing high cholesterol (total and LDL cholesterol). Twenty-five grams per day of soy protein are a useful adjunct to a low fat diet.

Soya proteins have many different structures, and research is continuing to refine their most useful components – the so-called '75 component' is the most important, according to Prof. Cesare Sirtori of Milan University.

♡♡ *Very Technical Point*: soya protein up-regulates the LDL receptors (by 60%), while milk protein inhibits, or down-regulates, the LDL receptors.

If you add 500 milligrams of cholesterol (3 – 4 prawn cocktails) to a diet containing soya protein, it fails to raise the blood cholesterol. How can this be? Soya protein has a unique effect on certain cells – it makes cells mop up bad cholesterol, while milk protein has the reverse effect. Could this adverse effect be due to the amino-acid lysine in milk, and the good effect be due to the arginine in soya?

It has been calculated (science-based guesswork) that a 10% average reduction of blood cholesterol in a population, could reduce coronary events by 20 – 25%.

Soya protein can reduce blood cholesterol by 20% in those with raised cholesterol (i.e. greater than 8 mmols/l). 25 grams of soya protein per day will lower the LDL (bad cholesterol) and raise the HDL (good cholesterol), an effect that could significantly reduce the overall occurrence of coronary heart disease. For these reasons, soya products should be promoted in our diets. That raises a very important question. Should those with evidence of artery 'furring' switch from animal derived milk, to soya milk? I think that would be sensible.

Soya contains chemicals called isoflavones – sometimes referred to as phyto-oestrogens, that is, female hormone-like chemicals. The effect of oestrogen in women was said to reduce heart disease incidence, but this has now been challenged. At least one of these plant-derived oestrogens (genistein), has been shown to reduce the 'furring' in arteries.

Routine hormone replacement therapy (oestrogen + progesterone) in both healthy women, and those with a history of heart disease, can slightly increase the risk of heart disease in the first year. There are no cardioprotective effects after five years, even when oestrogen is taken alone (the HERS and WHI studies, 2004).

> ## Wine and Alcohol

> ### NEWS FLASH!
> The WHO (2003) recommends one glass of wine per day!

Wine is said to loosen the tongue and warm the heart! It has been used as a medicine for millennia, and still occupies a prominent place in the life of many nations. It has long been thought to be good for the heart, and bad for the liver. A daily glass or two of wine (150 – 300mls – a bottle contains 750mls), decreases heart attacks.

Wine forms an important part of the Mediterranean diet and probably contributes to its cardio-protective effect, although heavier drinking is known to increase mortality. **It has been said that 20 – 30 grams of pure alcohol per day, taken from whatever source (while disregarding other significant consequences), could reduce coronary heart disease by 40%.** This amounts to approximately two cans of 5% alcohol beer (880mls contains 44mls of pure alcohol), or to 1/4 – 1/3 of a bottle of 14% alcohol wine. One mechanism involved is that wine can raise our good cholesterol (HDL), and reduce our bad cholesterol (LDL)(Gaetano, G. 2001).

One of the reasons why all alcoholic drinks may be beneficial is that the alcohol itself reduces the reactivity of those sticky little clotting components in blood called platelets. Pilot studies have suggested that the average platelet activity in France (lowish heart attack rate) is lower than that in Scotland (high heart attack rate)! Beware, though, the French also consume less beer, less Iron Bru, and whisky than the Scots, so the cause of the difference might not be that straightforward!

Immediately following the ingestion of spirits and beer, but not wine, there is an increase in blood coagulability. This has been suggested as the possible cause of those strokes that occasionally follow big binges.

When I was a medical student, pathologists performing autopsies could reliably recognize the arteries of big drinkers and alcoholics. Their arteries were often seen to be completely free of 'furring'. Unfortunately, alcoholics die prematurely of many other alcohol-induced diseases – pancreatitis and cirrhosis of the liver, to name but two. For this reason the medical profession is conservative in its approach to recommending alcohol as a preventative treatment for the 'furring' of arteries.

There are several chemical ingredients in wine, other than alcohol, which could make it atheroprotective. Red wine has at least three: reservatrol, arginine, and polyphenols. White wine has mainly arginine. All of these have been shown to have anti-oxidant and anti-platelet effects. The concentration of these chemicals in wine depends, of course, on the chemistry of the soil in which the vines were grown. There are now products on the market, which contain them, without the alcohol – the so – called non-alcoholic extracts of red wine (RWPE or the Red Wine Polyphenolic Extracts). **Grape juice, because it also inhibits platelet function in a way that orange and grapefruit juice do not, is a useful alternative to wine. Red grape juice has more anti-oxidant effect than white grape juice. Fortunately for non-alcohol drinkers, the advantageous chemicals in wine also exist in fruit and vegetables.**

Brazilian scientists (Luz, P. L and colleagues, 1999) gave some rabbits a cholesterol-rich diet then gave them red wine; others they fed with non-alcoholic wine products. Both reduced the 'furring' in arteries (by 45% and 32% respectively), and reduced the inner artery lining thickness (intimal thickness or IMT), by 77% and 35% respectively. So the alcohol is beneficial, but so also are the other chemical components of wine.

So which wine is best for our arteries? Red is better than white, dry is better than sweet; but which grape, and from which country? I don't know, except to say that the Chardonnay grape has lots of arginine. The Chardonnay grape is used to make Champagne and many other wines, so if you have ever needed an excuse to drink Champagne, this is the least motivating one I can think of! If you have no taste for wine, drink red grape juice.

Garlic

Experiment: *If you take the blood of patients with proven coronary artery disease, then mix the yellow serum (left after the blood has clotted) with normal artery cells, cholesterol accumulates within the cells – the basis of the 'furring' process. If the experiment is repeated with blood taken two hours after eating 300mgs of water extract of garlic, cholesterol does not accumulate within the cells. (Orekhov, A. N., 1995).*

Garlic is available in several forms – garlic plant, and various extracts. The effects of each could be different. Garlic is known to lower blood cholesterol, increase HDL (the good cholesterol fraction), and reduce clotting. It acts as an anti-oxidant (the equivalent of an anti-rusting agent) on cholesterol.

Dr R.M. Steiner and colleagues (1996), found that aged garlic extract (7.2 grams/day), taken for six months, reduced the blood cholesterol of those with a high cholesterol by 6 – 7%. The dangerous fraction of the cholesterol (LDL) was reduced by 4%, and blood pressure by 5%. These are only small changes, but I guess they are worth having. If your blood pressure is 150/80, six months of this garlic preparation might lower it to 142/76. If this were the average for a large group, it would reduce the number of strokes in that group, but in an individual, it is hardly impressive. Blood pressure swings around all day long: one minute it can be 110/60 when you are relaxed, and then 165/90, the minute you get angry. At which point in time does the 5% apply? After lying in a darkened room for 20 minutes, or just having completed a roller-coaster ride?

When I was a lecturer at Charing Cross Hospital in London, I was involved in many academic conferences. At one conference on high blood pressure, my boss, Dr Peter Nixon, whose insight into the effects of stressors on the heart was decades ahead of his time, asked: 'How long is a penis?' 'Like blood pressure', he said, 'it depends entirely on the circumstances under which it is measured!' Much better to say: my blood pressure ranges between 110 and 160, over 80 to 90, than to say that it is exactly 135/85!

Aged garlic extract has been shown to stop the early changes of fat accumulation in the arteries of rabbits, and to stop the growth of some cells that contribute to the 'furring' process. The degree of change observed is very impressive. Garlic must therefore be taken seriously as a therapeutic agent. Unfortunately, many human studies have failed to bear out the promise of such experiments, and we are not sure why. One reason could be that there is certainly more to heart attacks and strokes than just artery 'furring'. A lot of life, and a lot of chemistry are involved.

Out of interest, ginko biloba, has similar anti-clotting effects to garlic, but I know of no definitive studies on its effects in heart disease. Ginseng has neither the anti-clotting nor the cholesterol lowering effects of garlic, so I have not considered it further. There are almost as many suggestions for other supposedly beneficial substances as there are food enthusiasts, but without experimental proof of their direct value to arteries and the heart, I have had to give them all a raincheck for now.

KNOWING WHAT IS GOOD FOR OUR ARTERIES

I have identified 16 'front-runner' food chemicals, likely to be protective against artery 'furring'. Seven of them at least are components of the latest food recommendations of the World Health Organisation (2003).

So which foods contain most of what is good for our hearts and circulation? To find an acceptable answer, we can take each food and either add together all 16 substances that I have identified, or just the 7 World Health Organisation related recommendations.

The score I have developed to represent the protective effect of food chemicals on the 'furring' process in our arteries, I have called the **Atheroprotective Index, or API** for short. The API score using all 16 substances, I have called the API_{16} (see Table 8). One based on only seven of the 16 substances, I have called the API_7.

Table 8 is a list of how good each food is likely to be as an artery 'furring' protector. **The higher the API_{16} score, the more 'furring' protection it should provide.**

This index makes no reference to the atherogenic index of food (AGI, or a measure of the food 'baddies' and their 'furring' effect). For this reason you will see that a cheeseburger, which tops the list for 'baddies', is actually 10th in the protective API list, because it also contains a lot of 'goodies'.

Table 8

The Atheroprotective Index of Foods

The portion sizes are taken to be 'usual' ones,
and are taken mostly from E.S.Hands, Nutrients in Food (2000).

Food	Portion Wt (g)	API 16
LIVER (PIG)	54	107.2
LIVER (BEEF)	85	104.5
KIDNEY (BEEF)	85	56.1
PUMPKIN SEED	57	53.1
OYSTERS	70	35.5
HERRING	143	35.4
MUSSEL	85	32.5
LIVER (CHICKEN)	85	30.7
SESAME SEEDS	28	28.1
CHEESEBURGER (TRIP MEAT	400	27.2
MACKEREL	88	27.1
WHELK	85	26.9
EEL	136	26.7
SALMON (PINK/BAKED)	150	24.2
CHICKEN BREAST (ROASTED)	196	23.7
SAUSAGE (PORK)	100	23.7
HEART (BEEF)	85	22.1

Food	Portion Wt (g)	API 16
WALNUTS	28	21.5
PANCREAS (SWEETBREAD)	85	21.0
TUNA	150	20.5
CRAB (STEAMED)	118	20.4
HAZELNUTS	28	19.9
OIL (WHEATGERM)	14	19.4
AVOCADO	100	19.2
OIL (WALNUT)	14	18.6
OIL (SUNFLOWER)	14	18.4
LOBSTER	145	18.3
ALMONDS	28	17.2
CHICKEN (LEG)	114	16.9
OIL (CORN)	14	16.9
SUNFLOWER SEEDS	28	16.8
PEANUT BUTTER	32	16.1
HALIBUT	150	16.1
SOYBEANS (DRY-ROASTED)	50	15.8
PEANUTS	28	15.3
COD	180	15.1
CUTTLEFISH	85	14.6
DUCK (ROASTED)	85	14.5
SOLE	127	14.2
HADDOCK	150	13.9
SWORDFISH	106	13.9
HAMBURGER (DOUB MEAT)	250	13.9
BEEF (rump) COOKED	100	13.8
OCTOPUS	85	13.4
OIL (PALM)	14	12.1
LENTILS	100	11.6
SCOLLOP	120	11.1
LAMB (LEG ROASTED)	85	10.8
BRAZIL NUTS	28	10.4
SARDINES	50	10.1
TURKEY (LEG)	85	10.0
PORK (LEG ROASTED)	85	9.9
TURKEY (BREAST ROASTED)	85	9.2
SUNFLOWER FLOUR	28	8.2
ANCHOVY	85	8.1
OIL (COD LIVER)	14	7.9
SHRIMP	50	7.8
BLACKEYED PEAS	80	7.7
LIMA BEANS	78	7.2
MONKFISH	85	7.1
PINE NUTS	28	7.0
RICE (WILD/DRY)	100	6.6

Food	Portion Wt (g)	API 16
OIL (OLIVE)	14	6.4
CAMEMBERT	62	6.3
BREAKFAST CEREAL:BRAN FLAKES	50	6.0
OIL (HAZELNUT)	14	5.6
OIL (ALMOND)	14	5.6
RICE (BROWN)	100	5.5
EGG (YOLK)	17	5.5
CHOCOLATE: PLAIN	44	5.4
CHOCOLATE: WHITE	44	5.2
COTTAGE CHEESE	100	5.1
HONEY	33	5.0
MILK (SEMI)	245	4.7
CHEDDAR	28	4.5
POTATO (FLESH)	100	4.0
BEANS (BAKED)	100	3.8
TOFU	100	3.6
MILKSHAKE (Vanilla)	200	3.5
OVALTINE	200	3.2
SPINACH	100	3.1
PEAS (GARDEN)	80	3.0
HORLICKS	200	2.9
RICE KRISPIES	25	2.7
BRUSSEL SPROUTS	78	2.5
COCONUT	23	2.5
PEPPER (GREEN)	74	2.2
ASPARAGUS	60	2.1
BUTTER	5	2.1
EGG (WHITE) CT33	33	2.1
CHOCOLATE: MILK	44	2.0
LETTUCE (ICE BERG)	55	2.0
BREAD (WHOLEWHEAT)	28	1.9
PARMESAN	6	1.9
CRISPS (POTATO)	30	1.9
ALCOHOL: BEER (average)	500	1.9
CAULIFLOWER	50	1.8
ICE CREAM (VANILLA)	66	1.8
BANANA	75	1.8
POTATO (SWEET)	100	1.8
BREAD (WHITE AVE)	30	1.8
WINE: RED	100	1.8
PEAS (PROCESSED)	80	1.7
BROCCOLI	44	1.7
MANGO	100	1.7
APPLE	138	1.7
STRAWBERRY	83	1.6

Food	Portion Wt (g)	API 16
TOMATO	100	1.6
WINE: WHITE	100	1.6
CABBAGE	75	1.6
ONION	50	1.5
TEA	200	1.5
FLORA PRO-ACTIVE	5	1.5
PAPAYA	100	1.4
ORANGE JUICE	124	1.4
CARROTS	50	1.3
COFFEE	200	1.3
DIET COLA	250	1.0
COLA	250	1.0
WATER	1000	1.0

If we look for food groups that contain the top 10 amounts, of each of all the 16 atheroprotective substances (the 'goodies') (Table 9), we can form a list of those food groups which contain most, down to those which contain least. If one food group contained all of the top 10 foods for each of the 16 protective substances, it would score 10 x 16, or 160. The nearest group to this is fish, with a score of 31. Fruit and confection do not make it to the top ten for any protective substance, and score zero. In Table 9 below, you will be able to see which food groups contain most of the top ten protective chemicals. The number in each box shows how many foods of each group are featured in the top ten foods for that protective substance.

Table 9

Number out of top 10 food sources for each of 16 protective chemicals

Chemical	fish	shlf	nuts	off	brk	oils	meat	prep	puls	veg	alc	dairy	fruit	conf
linoleic acid	2	1	1	1			1	1		1	1	1		
B12	2	2	6											
oleic acid	5	1		1		2	1							
arginine	5	2	1				1	1						
linolenic acid	4	2		2			1				1			
omega-3	6	1			3									
Selenium	4	5	1											
Zn	1	3	1	1			1	2	1					
folic acid				2	2			5		1				
taurine		4		2			4							
Vit E			4		1	5								
B6	1	1		1	3		2	1		1				
Mg	1		3	1				1	2	2				
fibre					5				3	2				
Mn		1	2	1				1	3	2				
phytosterols			5			5								
TOTALS	31	22	18	16	14	13	12	13	9	9	2	1	0	0

(Key: shlf = shellfish, off = offal, brk = breakfast cereals, prep = prepared meals, puls = pulses, veg = vegetables, alc = alcohol, conf = confectionary.) Zn = zinc, Mg = magnesium, Mn = manganese.

Explanation of Table 9: The figure '2', for the linoleic acid in fish means – of the top 10 food sources of linoleic acid, '2' are fish. The figure '5' for phytosterol in nuts, means that, of the top ten food sources of phytosterol, five are nuts.

Considering that we are asked to eat five portions of fruit and vegetables per day, it may come as a surprise that among the top ten food sources for all of the 16 protective chemicals, none are in fruit, and only nine are in vegetables. They are, however, a source of some fibre and some potassium, which help keep blood cholesterol and blood pressure down (in some people), but they are largely water. At least, while you are eating them, you are not eating cakes, sweets, and fatty foods! Whatever else they are good for, fruit and vegetables are simply not good sources of the substances that will protect us against artery 'furring'.

These conclusions make such an important point, that it is worth comparing the above results to the top ten sources of each of the seven substances, derived from World Health Organisation recommendations (see Table 10).

Table 10

Number out of top 10 food sources that supply each of the
7 protective chemicals derived from the WHO recommendations.

Portion Analysis

Chemical	nuts	fish	shlf	oils	off	brk	puls	meat	prep	veg	alc	fruit	dairy	conf
oleic acid	**6**	1			1	1			1					
linoleic acid	5			4	1									
omega-3	1	6		3										
folic acid					2	2	3		2	1				
linolenic acid		4	2					2	1			1		
fibre						5	3			2				
phytosterols	6			**4**										
TOTALS	18	11	2	11	4	8	6	2	3	3	1	1	0	0

(Key: shlf = shellfish, off = offal, brk = breakfast cereals, prep = prepared meals, puls = pulses, veg = vegetables, alc = alcohol, conf = confectionary.)

Explanation of Table 10: The figure '6' above, for the oleic acid in nuts, means – of the top 10 food sources of oleic acid, '6' are nuts. The figure '4' for phytosterol in oils, means that of the top ten food sources of phytosterol, four are oils.

On this basis, nuts are the most beneficial group, containing 18 of the top ten food sources for each of the 7, WHO recommendation based protective chemicals (out of a maximum possible score of 70). Fish and oils are second, with a score of 11 out of 70. Out of a maximum score of seventy, for the top ten food sources of all seven WHO derived chemicals, vegetables score only 3, and fruit only one.

Comparing the two scores (API$_{16}$ and API$_7$), there is agreement that nuts and seeds, fish and shellfish, are all good for our arteries. Where the two scores differ, is in the calculated value of offal and meat. The API_{16} score values these higher than the API_7 score. The other difference is that the WHO derived score is much more conservative than the more speculative API_{16} score. You are free to choose which score you wish to follow. Because all of the chemicals involved are virtually harmless, there is no particular downside to being speculative.

There is another rather large problem to face. How many calories must we consume to get these 'goodies', and how many portions of food would that entail eating? Obviously, food is not of much use for cardioprotection, if you have to eat many kilos of food with thousands of calories, just to get one recommended daily amount of a 'goody'.

What follows next is the consideration of just one score, derived from both the 'furring' or atherogenic score (AGI) and the protective score (API), that balances all the 'goodies' with all the 'baddies' in food.

CHAPTER 5

The Cardiac Value
of Food

In a Nutshell: Chemicals in food are 'good' for you if they prevent artery 'furring', keep down your blood pressure and help control diabetes, and 'bad' for you if they promote the 'furring' of arteries, increase your blood pressure and worsen diabetes.

I have developed a single score that balances all the 'good', against all the 'bad' chemicals in food. I have called this the Overall Cardiac Value of Food, (or CVo for short). Pure water, which is completely neutral because it contains neither good nor bad substances, scores '1'. Foods that are 'good' for our arteries score more than '1' ; those that are 'bad' for our arteries, score less than '1' – it's that simple!

If you want to know which food has a high cardiac value and is a good source of a particular constituent such as omega-3 fatty acids, you can refer to the specific cardiac value of foods for that chemical.

Healthy foods are those which allow you to eat enough of the 'goodies', in one or two portions, with not too many calories and not too much salt, fat, or carbohydrate.

No one food can supply all of the cardio-protective

chemicals that might help prevent artery 'furring'. After all, natural foods have not evolved to protect our arteries!

The best of high cardiac value foods can only supply 9 of a possible16, protective chemicals; the other seven can only be obtained by combining the contents of carefully chosen individual foods. To obtain all 16 protective substances, monotony of choice and a strong preference for shellfish, offal, nuts, seeds, and fish are essential.

Are vitamins, supplements, and food additives the easy and reliable way to achieve maximum daily protection without food monotony, too many calories, and too much fat, salt, and sugar? Could be!

Could it be that heart disease is a pandemic made worse by eating too much fat and by not eating sufficient protective chemicals?

In the last two chapters I described scores for both the artery 'furring' potential of food – the atherogenic food index, or AGI, and the cardiovascular protective value of food – the atheroprotective index, or API. But I don't want to leave you with them, because they are of limited value on their own.

- What we need is one figure, which, at a glance, will tell us whether any particular food is 'good' for our heart and arteries; 'bad' for us, or somewhere in between.

- By combining the AGI and API, we can forget them. As far as the heart and circulation is concerned, the only figure we really need is:

The cardiac value of food

My grandmother used to say that fish was good for the brain – OK, I know, I should have eaten more of it! In fact, omega-3 fatty acids from fish have been shown to improve mood, behaviour, and sleep

– so my grandmother was right! Put it down to native wisdom, handed down from generation to generation and put to the ordinary test of time to see whether it works. Or is all this just folklore, a romantic myth, and my grandmother was correct, but only by chance? I'll go for the handed down wisdom. How about you?

> Cardiovascular disease is the commonest cause of death in the western world, and food plays a major part!

The question that concerns many of my patients, and some cardiologists, is: 'could there be 'Heart Food'? If there is, it will have to be good for the arteries, the heart itself, blood pressure, and diabetes – all at the same time!

If we look at food from the point of view of how much bad stuff it has in it, and how much good stuff there is in it, there are four possibilities:

Food that has: all good and no bad chemicals.

Food that has: all good with all bad chemicals.

Food that has: no good and all bad chemicals.

Food that has: no good with no bad chemicals.

When it comes to protecting ourselves against artery 'furring', no food is exactly any of these, but what comes nearest is:

Food that has: mostly good, with a little bad – wine, nuts, and some fish.

Food that has: mostly good, with some bad – seafood.

Food that has: very little good, and mostly bad – cheeses.

Food that has: not much good, and not at all bad – salads.

How is it possible to arrive at these conclusions? We previously calculated the overall 'bad' (AGI) score, and then the 'good' (API) score for individual foods. Combining the two will account for both the 'good' and the 'bad' components at the same time and give a **Cardiac Value Score**, but for artery 'furring' alone. For cardiovascular disease in general, that is not good enough, because diabetes and high blood pressure are also major causes of heart and artery trouble and must be taken into account. This necessitates adding in sodium salt and potassium factors for high blood pressure, and a sugar ('glycaemic', or carbohydrate) factor, for diabetics. When we do, the resulting score, I have called the **Overall Cardiac Value Score (CVo)**. To keep things as simple as possible, I will only refer to this value from now on.

Food Fact: Glucose, sucrose (table sugar), and starch (bread and potatoes), are said to be **'glycaemic'** because they raise our blood glucose level. In diabetics they may raise blood glucose a lot. Fructose, or fruit sugar, does not do this, and is safer.

The *overall cardiac value score* will allow us to say – which is the overall best, and which the overall worst, food for our arteries and heart – based on chemistry, not guesswork. Using this score, we can directly compare one food with another. The overall cardiac value

♥**Some Technical Points**: There are two overall cardiac values (CVo), depending on the number of protective substances we wish to recognise. From the World Health Organisation (WHO) recommendations, we have only to include 7 of the 16 substances (the foods they recommend contain at least seven of the 16 substances). I'm going to refer from now on, mainly to the value calculated by using these 16 substances, together with lysine as a 'baddy' (the shorthand for this score is CVo16). The WHO based calculations (CVo7) take no account of lysine, and are given in the Appendices if you are interested. The lists are different in detail, so you can choose which one you want to value most, remembering that the CVo7 calculations are based on the most conservative research, and those based on the 16 chemicals are more speculative.

THE CARDIAC VALUE OF FOOD

for red wine is for instance, twice that of white wine – that tells us, that red wine has twice as many good chemicals, as white wine. Therefore, a glass of red wine is likely to be twice as good for your heart as the same size glass of white wine.

Not all red and white wines have the same chemical composition, of course; that depends on the soil in which the vines were grown, the grape variety, the age of the wine, the year in which it was produced, and many other factors. The problem with wine is that you have to drink quite a lot of it to get enough of the 'goodies'. Good news for some, but drinking too much risks liver damage and obesity. The World Health Organisation (WHO), which is not prone to taking chances in its recommendations, has been bold enough to suggest that one glass of wine every day is cardioprotective.

OVERALL CARDIAC VALUE

You may not like this idea much, but one major biological purpose of our existence (from the evolutionary point of view that is) is to procreate, in order to further our species. Biologically, we need sufficient calories, regardless of the risk, to get us to the minimum age for sexual activity. The food available (when available) is capable of doing this easily, albeit with the downside of possible heart disease later on. What is not necessary for us to do, under this biological rule of purpose, is to survive much beyond the minimal age for procreation, to old age. This may now be our mission, but it is not that of our biology.

> ### Cardiac Value – What does it mean?
>
> A high score will mean lots of 'goodies', and few 'baddies.
>
> A low score will mean few 'goodies', and lots of 'baddies'.

If we are to follow a personal mission aimed at longevity we will need all the protection we can get, with minimal risk, and from the very earliest possible age. If we start in life eating food that has no protective cardiac value (and the sort of stuff that babies and children consume, is hardly good for the heart), even though it is good for growth and health in many other ways, we start off heading for trouble. This trouble, in the form of atherosclerosis or artery 'furring', is accumulative, so, *the longer we ignore all the beneficial dietary and lifestyle factors, the worse off we may be later on in life.*

The top 10 cardiac value foods are:

For all 16 protective substances (CVo16) – liver (pig and beef), walnuts, beef kidney, whelk, oysters, mussels, sesame seeds, cuttlefish, and hazelnuts.

If you want only to follow the WHO recommendations (seven protective substances), the top ten are: walnuts, sesame seeds, hazelnuts, walnut oil, almonds, sunflower seeds, salmon, corn oil, and tuna.

There are two important caveats to this view. The first is that we are not all prone to atherosclerosis: some of us will never get it, whatever we eat or do. The second is that the 'furring' process is probably dynamic, that is, it doesn't just accumulate, but partly comes and goes.

Technical Point: In CVo16, sixteen 'furring' protective substances, together with potassium (the 'goodies'), are calculated in ratio to the total fat, lysine, glycaemic sugar, and sodium salt content (the 'baddies') of food.

In CVo7 (WHO based), seven 'furring' protective substances, together with potassium (the 'goodies'), are calculated in ratio to the total fat, glycaemic sugar, and sodium salt content (the 'baddies') of food. Lysine is not recognised as a 'baddy' by the WHO.

You cannot however compare the CVo16 score to the CVo7 (WHO based) score, since the basis on which they are calculated is very different.

In order to derive an overall cardiac value, we need to know the sum of all the 'goodies', and a sum for all the 'baddies' in food. The overall cardiac value will then reflect, not only what is good for our arteries, but what will keep our blood pressure low and diabetes in check. Appendix 1, Tables 1 & 2, list the best foods, based on the overall cardiac values. These scores take 'furring', blood pressure, and diabetes into account – all in one figure.

WHAT ARE THE BEST FOOD GROUPS TO EAT?

I have not analysed that many foods in each food group but let us see how the averages compare. In Table 11, the average cardiac values of the foods in each food sub-group are given. The cardioprotective food scores, are listed from best to worst, based on both 16 protective chemicals (CVo16), and the WHO based 7 chemicals (CVo7).

Table 11

Food Group (WHO based)	CVo16	Food Group	CVo7
Offal	17.4	Nuts & Seeds	4.9
Shellfish	8.2	Oils	2.3
Nuts & Seeds	6.2	Fish	1.8
Pulses	5.0	Pulses	1.7
Fish	3.8	Vegetables	1.4
Oils	2.6	Fruit	1.2
Breakfast Cereal	2.0	Offal	1.1
Vegetables	2.0	Breakfast Cereal	1.1
Alcohol	1.8	Alcohol	1.1
Fruit	1.5	Shellfish	0.9
Meat	1.4	Dairy	0.8
Prepared Food	0.9	Meat	0.7
Dairy	0.2	Prepared Food	0.6
Confection	0.2	Confection	0.1

Looking down the two lists, there is good agreement about which food groups are worst: confection, prepared foods, dairy, and, meat products. There is some disagreement over which food groups are best. Taking all 16 protective substances into account, offal and shellfish score highest. Nuts and seeds, fish, oils, and pulses, appear in the top 6 of each list. The scores allow you to measure one group against another. In the CVo16 list, nuts and seeds are four times better than fruit; in the CVo7 (WHO based) list, nuts and seeds are six times better for us than dairy produce.

CARDIAC VALUE SCORES AND THEIR MEANING

Here is a guide to how I interpret the overall cardiac value scores:

CVo16	CVo7	(WHO based) Meaning
3 or more	1.6 or more	Best for the heart and circulation.
1.0 to 3	1.0 to 1.6	Neutral to just OK.
1	1	The neutral value of water
Less than 1	Less than 1	Not good for the heart and circulation.

If we eat food of low cardiac value (scores less than '1') for 35 years, perhaps it is not surprising that those prone to the problem will get artery 'furring', high blood pressure, or diabetes. The effects of diet on 'furring' are likely to be accumulative, and not reversible, but having said that, a lot more research is required to be sure.

What protective substances have I left out of my calculations? Every nutrition expert will have their own favourite list. One problem is, that not every substance has been tested for its effect on the 'furring' process. All we can do, then, is to dismiss them or to reserve judgement on many of them for the moment. Among the many possible protective substances are: lycopene, flavinoids, vitamin K, carnitine, and Q10, but at present these substances either need to be further researched or data on their concentration in various foods is not available. Garlic has a unique chemical composition of its own and is a valuable cardioprotective foodstuff in its own right. Because its active ingredient (allicin) is not a component of other foods (as far as I know), it would be inappropriate to include it, at this stage, in the calculation of cardiac value.

As I mentioned before, one of the most fundamental limiting factors in calculating cardiac value, is not knowing the actual strength of influence of each food chemical on the 'furring' process. *The big assumption I have had to make is that all the chemicals included in my calculations have an equal influence on our heart and arteries – even though this is very unlikely to be the case.* It might turn out, for instance, that selenium is twice as protective as magnesium in the prevention of the 'furring' process. That would mean that the formula I have used to calculate cardiac value would have to have a double value for selenium. Similarly, if saturated fat turns out to be four times worse for our arteries than cholesterol, then the saturated fat factor will have to be multiplied by four. Too little is known about these relative strengths of influence to make such adjustments just now – future research must aim to find out.

Then there is the problem of individual biological variation. Put another way – we are all different, so saturated fat might be very bad for you, but not that bad for me. However, it could be that saturated fat 'furs' the arteries of everyone equally, with other factors like exercise and smoking influencing us differently. If I have no tendency to clot, and you do have – you might get the heart attack and I might not, even though we have an equal amount of 'furring'. Because there are many and various factors contributing to heart disease, its cause is said to be 'multi-factorial'. For all of us, our genetic traits and some of our lifestyle habits (smoking and exercise), will play major, but different, roles for each of us.

RECOMMENDED AMOUNTS OF THE GOOD STUFF

The unit used to measure our daily need for zinc or selenium, is called an **RNI, or Recommended Nutritional Intake**. By trying to balance 'good' with 'bad' units, I have made a very big assumption: that one unit of 'good' chemical will balance the adverse effects of one unit of a 'bad' chemical in food. I will return to this point later.

An Ideal Food for Arteries and the Heart

If we eat ten portions of ideal foods per day, each on average would have to contain one tenth of all the daily 'goodies' needed, and 150 Kcals (or less) per portion, with a minimal amount of the 'baddies' (lysine, fats, glycaemic sugars, and sodium salt). No food actually exists that contains all the necessary daily 'goodies' in one portion, but benefit can be had by combining foods into a daily diet. Different daily diets are examined in the next chapter.

HOW BIG IS A PORTION?

Nutrition experts like the idea of measuring the chemistry of 100 grams (3 ounces) of each food. We don't usually eat as much as 100grams of mustard in one go, although most of us could easily eat 100grams of fish at one sitting. To be more practical for consumers, I have chosen to use portion amounts. So what amount should we accept as one portion? This will be subject to enormous variation between people; nevertheless, it is obvious that there is an average, or reasonable, portion of say olive oil, honey, caviar, or walnuts that would weigh less than an average portion of tuna, porridge, or beefsteak. We could argue about what an ideal, reasonable, or average portion is, so I have been guided by the edible portion sizes suggested by Elizabeth S. Hands in her comprehensive compilation of food chemistry called 'The Nutrients in Food' (see references).

The weight of food we consume is of vital importance. There is a strong argument for saying that we all eat too much, and too much of the wrong things. *Weighing our food is not a routine we are used to, but it could be a strategy for those who want to lose weight and have found it difficult.* Since an excessive body-weight is itself an important risk factor for heart disease, portion size is a vital issue. Portion size is also vital when it comes to calorie intake. 'Going Large' could mean just that, as far as your weight is concerned.

If we accept the notion of acceptable portion sizes, we can then ask several questions: How many calories are there in each portion? How many portions do we need to eat, in order to get enough zinc, magnesium, or vitamin E etc? A food may have a wonderful cardiac value score, but if we have to eat twenty portions and hundreds of calories, just to get just one RNI of any protective substance, it would fail the test of good value for the heart. It wouldn't matter so much if we all did enough exercise to burn off the excess calories, but these days we don't.

Historical Point: *The nutrition of pregnant mothers and heart disease: During the Second World War, there was a time when the pregnant mothers of Holland were subjected to enforced starvation. The babies born to these women were underweight, but after birth they rapidly put on excessive weight, and then went on to adulthood with more coronary heart disease than those born to mothers who had eaten normally during their pregnancy. The very latest information confirms this.*

HAVE WE PROGRESSED BEYOND OUR BEST?

In Paleolithic or Stone Age times, after the last Ice Age (about 40,000 years ago), families led a nomadic existence, hunting and gathering in order to acquire food as best they could. Could that lifestyle have provided them with an optimal diet and exercise regime? Are we, in fact, biologically adapted only for such an existence? We do see ourselves now as 'never having had it so good', but that may not be true for our health. Could the food we now eat be doing us more harm than good, especially if we desire a long life free from heart disease?

Ray Mears is an expert in bushcraft – the ability to survive using only the natural resources of the land, forest, and shoreline. In a fascinating collaborative TV programme (BBC 2), he combined his knowledge with that of paleontologists in order to reconstruct the likely Stone-Age existence. He showed that arrows could be fashioned with flint tools from hazelwood and finished with

The Metabolic Syndrome: *Some overweight people easily raise their blood glucose level when they eat sugars and starchy food and more easily elevate their blood fat levels when they eat fatty meals. The main reason for this is that their insulin is less effective than normal – they have, in fact, become resistant to it. One consequence of this is that they may more readily 'fur' their arteries and more commonly suffer from coronary heart disease. The best foods for them are those with a high Overall Cardiac Value.*

sharpened flint tips, stuck and bound to the arrows with pine resin. He demonstrated how meat and shellfish could be cooked to perfection in a pit lined with previously-heated stones, and how fish could be caught using multiple hawthorns hanging from one fishing line. He had little time to talk about possible vegetable gathering, but did mention plants that would have been available for use – fungus for fire-lighters, moss for absorbent bandages and nappies, roots and tubers to eat. The picture he painted was one of plenty for those with the hunting and gathering skills to acquire it.

One conclusion from my analysis is that many of us would need to return to a shellfish, nuts, seeds, fish, and offal based diet, in order to have any chance of keeping our arteries healthy in the long-term. Even though it is possible to construct such a diet, it is quite difficult to get all of the required substances for artery and heart protection, without too many portions, and too many calories. Stone-Age man must have done a lot of exercise, and used a lot of calories – perhaps as many as 4 to 5000 calories per day. If he also ate an equivalent amount of food, he might have gained lots of protective micronutrients. By contrast, the cardiac value of our modern diet barely reaches the lower limit of cardioprotective value. At the same time, our modern motorised existence means that we eat many more calories than we can easily burn off with exercise.

Stone-age peoples may not have lived long enough to get heart disease, but that doesn't mean to say that their diet was not perfect for heart disease protection. There are still a few tribes leading a similar existence, and much has been learned from studying them.

In Papua New Guinea the hunter-gatherer Kitavan people have a lifestyle comparable to that of Stone-Age man. Strokes, heart disease, and diabetes, are virtually unknown. Could it be that it was not until humans started to domesticate animals and drink their milk, as well as grow and eat cereals, that cardiovascular diseases first made their appearance?

Dietary Revolutions: The first big change in human nutrition occurred after agriculture and the domestication of animals began; the second occurred quite recently with the advent of processed food, containing lots of fat, salt and sugar. With it, came a health impact more damaging than the first. What we need now, is a third big change – back to a diet of more substantial cardiac value, which will contrast little with that of our Stone-Age ancestors.

There is another fundamental aspect to the change from hunter gathering to agriculture. If hunting is thought of as exciting, agriculture by contrast, could be thought of as arduous, lengthy, and dull. A hunter needed few possessions, but once he pursued the growth of crops, he would have come to appreciate the advantage of having his own land. With possession would come the need to defend it against others, something the free-ranging hunters might not have thought important. With acquisitiveness might come selfishness and the striving for more land, more possessions, workers to help with the heavy work, and a need for security. Develop that a little bit further, with like-minded people grouping together into societies in order to protect mutual rights; leaders to rule, bankers to fund the purchase of more land, lawyers to legalise the claims, private doctors to care for the owners, and NHS doctors to care for the workers, and you have the structure of a modern western capitalist society, along with its major killer – cardiovascular disease!

Those societies that are more relaxed about personal possession and where, traditionally, a contribution to the common good is highly valued, have less heart disease. Many years ago Professor Geoffrey Marmot studied Japanese people as they moved from a traditional lifestyle to an American lifestyle. What he found was that as the Japanese became more American, they developed more heart disease.

To get the best diet for our circulation, the important points to observe are: –

- First, minimize the 'baddies'– that means eating less fat, less sodium salt, and fewer carbohydrates (sugars and starch).

- Maximise the 'goodies'.

- My calculations show that a diet full of fat, salt, and carbohydrate, with few protective substances, cannot be reversed at all by adding cardioprotective supplements to food – it's that bad!

- The first priority must be to eat the best cardioprotective diet available (like the Mediterranean diet).

- Because such a diet is expensive, unacceptable to some, and not universally available, should we consider routinely adding positively protective substances to our diet, or encourage the taking of specifically formulated daily supplement tablets?

One obvious conclusion from my research is that the best protection cannot be easily had from food alone. For some substances, there are either too few foods available (phytosterols, taurine, fibre, and vitamin E), or an insufficient choice of healthy foods (those without fat, salt, carbohydrate, and calories), that contain them.

The Mediterranean diet has yielded impressive results for heart patients. This suggests that the presence of cardio-protective substances (in which it is rich), outweigh the 'furring', or atherogenic effects of fat and lysine, in which it is *not* deficient. From my own analysis, I would guess that we should be able to do even better. To do so, we would have to include all of the known cardio-protective substances in our diet, on a regular daily basis. All theories need proof and this important one is no exception. Heart disease is such a big problem in the western world that we need to do something. The drug companies would prefer us all to take 'statin' drugs of course – especially now that they have succeeded in making them available 'over – the – counter'.

The prevention of early artery 'furring' should be our highest priority. Because it is virtually impossible to get a fully cardio-

protective diet, suitable to all tastes, while restricting calories to 1500 per day, we need to seriously consider food, or tablet supplementation.

The results of my research conclude, that only the best diet, combined with either food or tablet supplementation, will provide the best regular daily intake of all cardio-protective substances. This is contrary to the current advice of nutrition authorities, all of whom support a low fat, so called, 'balanced' diet, rather than supplementation. The alternative is for us all to become serious athletes and to each burn off many more than 3000 calories every day. Let's all run or cycle to work and play a sport every day then we could all eat enough food to fill our heart protection needs. I don't see that happening, do you?

So what else can we do? What might work is to build car parks a long way away from the shops. Fewer and slower elevators in buildings might induce us, through frustration, to use the stairs more. These measures, complemented by fewer adverts for unhealthy food, might make any plans for a healthier existence work faster. (A very heavy emphasis on the word 'might', is required here!)

INDIVIDUAL CHEMICAL CARDIAC VALUE SCORES

This subject will be of importance to nutritionists, most of whom will want more detail. If you are a general reader, you may want to skip what follows, unless you have a specific interest in individual protective chemicals and where to find them in food.

If you have a raised blood homocysteine and want to lower it with foods of cardiac value, rich in vitamins B12, B6, and folic acid, or you believe that selenium is good for you and want to know where to find it in food – read on.

Suppose you need one RNI of each protective chemical substance every day. And suppose you are allowed ten portions of food per day, the choice of which is entirely yours. One RNI of each substance needs either to be concentrated in one portion, or spread over ten portions of different foods. If there are only ten portions and 16 protective substances of importance, most portions must contain more than one substance. **It is obvious from food analysis that only a few foods are good sources of all sixteen cardioprotective nutrients, although, arginine, vitamin B12, magnesium, and some fatty acids, are not difficult to source in a complete daily diet.** Finding such food would therefore require very careful food selection from a very limited list of healthy food groups. In reality, few single food portions contain more than one RNI of any protective substance. One food portion that does contain more than one RNI of zinc is oyster. By contrast, many foods are a very good source of calories and adverse substances like fats, sodium salt, carbohydrate, and lysine.

Why only one RNI for cardioprotection? There is no reason to assume that the recommended amounts for healthy eating have anything to do with artery protection. It could be that we need much more than one RNI of each protective substance per day. However, if the Mediterranean diet can reduce second heart attacks by 70%, then one RNI of each protective substance might just be sufficient.

♥ *Technical Point: Individual Cardiac Values for each protective chemical:*

The cardiac value of each of 16 protective substances can be calculated. Let us take a practical example. If a portion of oysters is 70grams, there are 127.7 milligrams of zinc in one portion. That's a lot of zinc, and a cardiac value for zinc in oysters of 5.8 . Any score between 1 and 2 is good for individual substances, and more than that is excellent, therefore oysters have a very good cardiac value for zinc. The same consideration for the zinc in white chocolate, leads to a cardiac value (CVzinc) of 0.11 (anything less than '1' is bad). So as far as zinc is concerned, white chocolate has a very poor cardiac value.

In Appendix 3, you will find a list of foods and the protective substances they can supply. Only those foods that can supply a substance with better than a minimum individual cardiac value of 1.2, with less than 150Kcals per portion, are included. If there are only 50 calories per portion, two to three portions could be eaten in the place of one, while keeping the total daily calorie content of ten portions under 1500 calories (Kcals). What we don't want to do is eat too many calories every day. Most of us do of course, but with the obesity problem growing the way it is, that should be avoided.

Only 52 of the 130 foods I studied are useful sources of one or more protective substances – that is, they have a minimum individual cardiac value, and no more than 150 calories per portion. Tuna contains more atheroprotective substances than any other food, but even so, tuna is a source of only four: arginine, oleic acid, B12, and selenium. There are 14 foods that can supply 3 protective substances, 14 that can supply 2, and 23 that can supply only one. It can be seen from this list that there are lots of good sources of arginine, vitamin B12, oleic, and linoleic acids. For zinc, linolenic acid, and taurine, there are very few food choices. For vitamins B6 and E, phytosterol, fibre, and manganese, there are no sufficient single food sources in my list having less than 150Kcals per portion.

The cardiac values for individual substances allow us to compare one food with another. As far as zinc is concerned, one portion of oyster (70 grams – just over 2 ounces), has 81 times more cardiac value for zinc, than one portion of Camembert cheese (62grams). However, one cannot be too critical when considering one chemical – all of the 'good' and 'bad' factors have been taken into account. And before deciding never to eat Camembert again, consider that one small enjoyable portion may not be that bad, if eaten just once a week! The overall cardiac value for red wine is 6 times better than Camembert, so at least have them together!

I suspect Marie Harel, the recognised originator of Camembert cheese, might have had something to say about this . . . 'Il y a beaucoup de . . . there is much more to life than knowing what to avoid!'

Here is the fallback situation:

**If you cannot keep away from the bad things,
eat them sparingly.**

**If you must eat the 'baddies' – eat them
with lots of 'goodies'.**

From the list of cardiac values for taurine, only shrimp scores more than 1.2 (1.56 actually), with only 28 Kcals per portion. No other food has a taurine cardiac value greater than 1.2. The conclusion is therefore, that no food, apart from shrimp, can give you enough taurine, while avoiding too much lysine, too much fat, or too much sodium salt. To get enough taurine without eating shrimp, you must either take a supplement, or have it added to your food.

Key Point: *It is not good enough to know the cardiac value score of food alone, the number of portions needed to get the 'good' substances, and the number of calories involved, are both crucial to health.*

When it comes to arginine, 47 foods are able to deliver the goods, without too many calories. Whelks have the best cardiac value (CV arginine = 9.24), whereas pine nuts just qualify (1.21).

The Table that follows (Food with the best of the 'Goodies'), addresses the question: which are the best sources of individual substances? I have omitted the foods with too many calories per portion (more than 150 calories). A high individual cardiac value means that the food contains lots of that particular 'goody', with only a little fat, lysine, sodium salt, and sugar.

Food with the best of the 'Goodies'

Cardiac Value scores for individual 'goodies' are listed if their score is greater than '1.2' – ie good for the heart (individual scores shown in brackets), and if they are low calorie (less than 150 Kcals per portion). Where no individual food choice is available, the daily diet may provide enough by combining small amounts from each of several choices.

The Amino-acids:

Arginine: Whelk (9.2), cuttlefish (6), lentils (5.8), soybeans (roasted)(5), walnuts (5), black-eyed peas (4.2), crab (3.6), haddock (3.5), shrimp (3.2), cod (3.2), halibut (3), octopus (3), scollop (2.9), tuna (2.7), sole (2.6), salmon (2.5), mussels (2.5), sunflower flour (2.2), tofu (2), lima beans (2), garden peas (2).
For full list see Appendix 1B.
Taurine: Shrimp (1.57).

The Vitamins:

Vitamin B6: NO INDIVIDUAL FOOD CHOICES
Vitamin B12: liver (pig 29), (beef 26), beef kidney (13), mussels (7.7), oysters (7.2), chicken liver (4.8), whelk (4.5), crab (3.7), cuttlefish (3), mackerel (2.3), heart (2.2), herring (2), sardines (1.9), salmon (1.7), tea (1.4), sole (1.3), shrimp (1.2).
Folic acid: Asparagus (1.5), spinach (1.3).
Vitamin E: NO INDIVIDUAL FOOD CHOICES.

The Minerals:

Magnesium: Spinach (1.3). Red wine (1.3), although it has too many calories.
Manganese: NO INDIVIDUAL FOOD CHOICES
Selenium: Cuttlefish only (1.4).
Zinc: Oysters (4).

Fatty Acids:

Linolenic Acid: Walnuts (3), lettuce (1.4), walnut oil (1.2).
Linoleic Acid: Walnuts (10.5), sesame seeds (3.5), sunflower oil (4.1), walnut oil (3.8), sunflower seeds (3.5), corn oil (2.9), wheatgerm oil (2.44), almonds (2), hazelnuts (1.5).
Oleic Acid: Hazelnuts (6), almonds (7.17), peanuts (4.4), sesame seeds (4.3), walnuts (4), avocado (2.9), potato flesh (2.5), peanut butter (2), sunflower seeds (1.9), sunflower oil (1.6), peanuts (1.6), walnut oil (1.6), corn oil (1.5), corn (1.3), pink salmon (1.3), brazil nuts (1.23), tuna (1.2).
Omega 3 oil: Walnuts (2), but just fail on calories (222KCals per portion).

Cholesterol Uptake Reducers:

Phytosterol: NO INDIVIDUAL FOOD CHOICES (Flora Pro-Active is best) (1.13).
Fibre: NO INDIVIDUAL FOOD CHOICES.

CHAPTER 6

The Cardiac Value of Different Diets

In a Nutshell: Which daily diet is best for the heart? It is possible to add up all of the 'goodies', and all the 'baddies' of a daily diet, and calculate a cardiac value score for the day. Only two diets are of sufficient cardiac value to be considered highly beneficial: the Polymeal Diet and the Mediterranean Diet.

How good are your daily food choices? Are you protecting your arteries, or damaging them every day? By identifying typical diet types, it is possible to identify the best and the worst. What are the results?

Junk food, really is junk! Eaten over decades, those prone to heart disease, could die as a result – it's that bad! If you are to eat the best diet, it helps if you like shellfish, nuts and seeds, fish, and offal, or at least some of them. Without including some of these, a positively healthy diet for the heart and circulation, is just not possible.

We all know what 'Junk Food' is, don't we? Is it what teenagers eat? Are gourmet meals with creamy sauces any better? Is vegetarian food the best? So many questions in search of an answer.

If you want to measure something you have to have a ruler, and preferably one that everyone else agrees to use. No point in asking an American how many litres of gas he would like in his Chevy; no point in asking a Frenchmen how many gallons of fuel he would like in his Renault. Gallons and litres are both good measures of petrol, but only if they are understood. I have invented a measure of how good food is for the heart and circulation – *the overall cardiac value*, but this will only be of use, if everyone recognises what it means. You are one of the first to hear about it, so you know as much about it as anyone else. To my knowledge it is the only all-in-one measure available of cardiac food value, so unlike the arguments that might arise over the use of gallons and litres, there is no competition, except from the complicated but very incomplete measures of the salt, fat, and sugar content shown on processed food packets.

We now have the overall cardiac value of each individual food, but what about our complete daily diet? How good or bad are all those personal daily food choices in protecting our heart and circulation when eaten together?

To find out how much fat there is in a processed food, all we have to do is look on the packet. That will tell us how much fat there is in every 100 grams. Then all we have to do is work out what that is per portion, add up all of the fats in all of the foods we eat in a day, and voilà – a measure of how bad is our daily diet. Can't be bothered? I guessed not! For a start, do you have any idea what one 100 grams of porridge looks like? What you need to know is how much fat there is per portion, and not any old portion, but the portion *you* want to eat. That is admittedly difficult to provide, because there is no agreement on what measure represents a portion. That depends on individual appetite, of course. That is why 100 grams of each food has become the measure used on food labels.

So what about sodium salt in food? Too much could raise your blood pressure (not in everyone though). And what about potassium, carbohydrate, omega-3 fatty acids, and magnesium? We are going to need a whole bunch of figures to represent them all! I prefer the overall cardiac value – but then, I suppose I would. At least you only need one figure to look at. There is, however, a problem with acceptance. Some ideas never break through into public consciousness and in the big business of food there are those who would keep us ignorant of the dangers, while exaggerating the benefits. What would happen to profits if we did know the truth? Profits from certain items might suffer initially, but the truth might then stimulate a new generation of healthier and even more profitable products.

With one score to look at, we could go around a big supermarket, easily and quickly making the correct 'healthy heart' food choices. I think I had better pay Tesco's a visit. My guess is that they might have more influence on food manufacturers than a whole bunch of doctors and politicians!

The relative inaction of politicians to minimize the further availability of smoking and some food products, given their contribution to premature death, is reason enough to be disenchanted with them. Freedom of choice, is at stake, of course. People must be free to choose their poison! The problem is – how many of us know what the poisons are and where to find them? Forget politicians – better that we, the public, come to know what is best for our health and start making demands! If that sounds all too reactionary, you must know that the medical profession has for decades, tried to influence processed food manufacturers to remove excessive salt and sugar from their products, but worry about profitability and an apparent lack of political will have been reasons for failure, although there is movement afoot – it is now possible to buy some low salt and sugar versions of standard products like baked beans – if you look long and hard enough for them.

THE CARDIAC VALUE OF DIFFERENT DIETS

Let's take a look at several different daily diets. Let's add up all of their bad points, and all of their good points, to see which diet has the best overall cardiac value score.

You will remember that individual foods that are good for the heart and arteries have an overall cardiac value score (CVo16) greater than 3.0. Water scores '1' and is neutral. Foods with a score between '1' and 3.0 are of neutral value. Daily diets that score between 3.0

and 7.6 are 'acceptable as beneficial' and those with a score greater than 7.6 are very beneficial. I have not used any foods with a score less than one (bad for the heart and arteries) in the diets that follow.

The Ideal Cardiac Protection Diet

It is really quite difficult to construct an ideal cardiac diet. You will see why when I tell you that this daily diet must have:

- Fewer than 1500 daily calories (Kcals).

- No excess fat, carbohydrate, or lysine.

- A low sodium, high potassium, salt content.

- As many chemical artery 'furring' protectors (atheroprotective micronutrients) as possible.

There are only two diets that come close to providing what is necessary:

- the Polymeal diet and

- the Mediterranean diet.

THE MEDITERRANEAN DIET

To provide the necessary ingredients for a beneficial daily diet of high cardiac value, food choices will be few and unlikely to keep us satisfied for long – food fatigue is a real problem for any diet plan. In Table 12, I have constructed a Mediterranean style cardiac diet. The ingredients include foods of high individual cardiac value, balanced by others that are complimentary, but barely of acceptable beneficial cardiac value.

Table 12

A Mediterranean Diet

Cardiac Diet Analysis Food	Portion Wt (grams)	Portion Wt (ozs)	Calories/ Portion	CVo16 Cardiac Value
TUNA	150	4.5	150	6.81
MUSSEL	85	2.6	88	11.74
WALNUTS	14	0.4	96	11.72
SUNFLOWER SEEDS	28	0.8	160	6.75
BLACKEYED PEAS	80	2.4	93	5.20
BRAN FLAKES	50	1.5	135	3.10
SESAME SEEDS	14	0.4	84	3.70
ASPARAGUS	60	1.8	15	2.08
LETTUCE	55	1.7	7	1.98
RED WINE	100	3.0	68	1.81
BANANA	75	2.3	87	1.54
TOMATO	100	3.0	17	1.70
BREAD (WHOLEWHEAT)	28	0.8	61	1.17
ORANGE JUICE	124	3.8	56	1.33
BEVERAGES: COFFEE	200	6.1	0	1.29
MILK (1% FAT)	200	6.1	92	1.33
YOGURT	100	3.0	56	1.08
FLORA PRO-ACTIVE	5	0.2	68	1.46
WHOLE DIET	1468	45	1333	2.35
DIET (Without Milk and Yogurt)	1168	35	1185	3.70

By adding all of the individual fats and protective substances together, we arrive at a score for the day. This is the equivalent to taking all of the daily ingredients, mixing them together in a large bowl and analysing the result, as if it were one portion of food. As a whole, that bowl of food would have a cardiac value of only 2.35 with milk products (of borderline cardiac value), and a cardiac value of 3.7 (just acceptable cardiac value), without them. Unlike individual foods, your daily food bowl would have to have in it all of the protective substances, a minimal amount of fat, lysine, and salt, and should contain less than 1500 calories for the day.

What is the minimum daily score we need for artery and heart protection? To be good for your heart and circulation, the minimum daily cardiac score should at least equal 7.6 (CVo16). This Mediterranean diet scores only 2.35, despite the fact that it contains only 57 grams of carbohydrate (just OK for diet controlled diabetics), 89% of the minimum daily fat requirement, 96% of the daily sodium salt requirement, 112% of the daily potassium requirement, and nearly every micronutrient of value apart from phytosterol (which blocks the uptake of cholesterol from the bowel).

Why then, is the cardiac value of this diet so low? Quite simply, it's a matter of the ratio between the 'goodies' and the 'baddies'. As we add foods together, the total 'goodies' divided by the total 'baddies' (the cardiac value), changes from a high individual score of 11.7 for mussels, all the way down to 2.35, for the diet as a whole. So perhaps we should only eat mussels? That would be good for the heart, but not exactly a balanced diet for total health.

Let's try withdrawing a few items. Table 13 has one result.

Table 13

Alternative Mediterranean Diet Analysis

Portion Analysis Food	Portion Wt (grams)	Portion Wt (ozs)	Calories/ Portion	CVo16 Cardiac Value
MUSSEL	85	2.6	88	11.74
WALNUTS	14	0.4	96	11.72
SUNFLOWER SEEDS	28	0.8	160	6.75
BRAN FLAKES	50	1.5	135	3.10
LETTUCE	55	1.7	7	1.98
RED WINE	100	3.0	68	1.81
BANANA	75	2.3	87	1.54
TOMATO	100	3.0	17	1.70
ORANGE JUICE	124	3.8	56	1.33
BEVERAGES: COFFEE	200	6.1	0	1.29
FOR WHOLE DIET:	831	25.2	715	9.9

In Table 13, as an experiment, I have taken away all dairy produce and tuna, the black-eyed peas and sesame seeds, the asparagus and bread. This successfully brings the daily cardiac value score for the diet up to 9.9 – a very beneficial overall cardiac value score. However, this diet would be very uninteresting if eaten more than once a week, it is too low in calories and short of phytosterols, calcium, and zinc.

THE WHAT IF'S?

Suppose you don't like fish and prefer to replace the tuna with something else? In Table 14, I have recalculated the figures with tuna replaced by turkey breast, beef liver, and leg of lamb. Not much change is caused by replacing tuna with turkey, but the other two cause some quite large changes. Replacing tuna with liver improves the overall cardiac score from 2.35 (just acceptable) to 8.3 (very beneficial) – a healthy heart and circulation daily diet score. Leg of lamb though, because of its saturated fat content, takes the score for the diet to a much lower level. **This leads to an important conclusion: the whole daily diet can be greatly improved, or ruined, by one main course choice.**

The problem is that good food choices are quite limited. By referring to the list of cardiac values for individual foods in Appendix 1, you can guess that if the cardiac score for that food is above 3.0, using it to replace a food with a low score will make it a healthier food choice.

Table 14

Food Replacements for the Mediterranean Diet:
their effect on the overall cardiac value score

| | | | WHOLE DIET FEATURES | |
	Portion grams	Portion ozs	Calories	CVo16 Cardiac Value
CARDIAC DIET WITH TUNA	1468	45	1333	2.4
TUNA REPLACED WITH				
Turkey Breast	85	2.6	1313	2.6
Liver (beef)	**85**	**2.6**	**1327**	**8.3**
Lamb (leg)	85	2.6	1370	1.6
MUSSELS REPLACED WITH				
Cheddar Cheese	28	0.8	1361	1.1
Cuttlefish	85	2.6	1245	2.7
Shrimp	50	1.5	1295	2.6
ALL 3 NUTS & SEEDS REPLACED WITH				
Broccoli	44	1.3	1176	1.12

Suppose you don't like mussels. How about replacing them with cheddar cheese, cuttlefish, or shrimp? You can see in Table 14, that the scores are not much altered by alternative seafoods, while the cheese option reduces the whole daily diet score to an unacceptably low level. **The conclusion: unless you like nuts and seeds, seafood, offal, or fish, a healthy cardiac diet will be difficult to construct.**

What about those of us who dislike nuts and seeds, or have allergies to them? You can see in Table 14, that replacing the nuts and seeds with broccoli in the cardiac diet, leads to a deterioration in the overall cardiac score, because both linolenic fatty acid and zinc, will be lost to some extent.

DIETARY SUBSTITUTIONS

Experimenting with substitutions would be a very laborious business without a computer program to help you do it. If you want to experiment and put your own diet ideas together, you can. I have written a special computer program for the purpose. These programs will run on your home or office PC, and are available for home and professional use. To obtain them, log on to: www.cardiaccentres.co.uk and follow the links to **HeartShield Products.**

THE POLYMEAL DIET

A recently published cardioprotective diet is based only on those foods with evidence of their cardiovascular benefit. Franco and colleagues (see references), recently published details of their Polymeal cardiac diet in the British Medical Journal (2004). Let's put it to the test by calculating its cardiac value (CVo16), using chemical

💜 *Technical Point: Using data from two different sources leads to different final results for CVo16 and gives an insight into the magnitude of variation that can come from failing to standardise the data.*

data sets from two independent sources. These are shown with and without the chocolate in Tables 15a and 15b respectively. Compare the calculations based on the two separate data sets by observing column CVo16 A versus column CVo16 B.

Table 15a

Cardiac Value of the Polymeal with chocolate

Portion Analysis Food	Portion Wt (grams)	Portion Wt (ozs)	Cals/ Portion	CVo16 A	CVo16 B
ASPARAGUS	88	2.7	22	2.48	2.12
PEPPER (GREEN)	74	2.2	39	2.03	2.06
ALMONDS (unsalted, blanched)	68	2.1	416	24.96	18.84
RED WINE (Burgundy)	150	4.5	102	2.04	1.56
PAPAYA	100	3.0	39	1.34	1.36
PLAIN CHOCOLATE (unsweetened)	100	3.0	510	0.16	0.39
LETTUCE	55	1.7	7	1.98	1.90
STRAWBERRY	83	2.5	22	1.67	1.72
TUNA (smoked/fresh)	65	2.0	150	3.96	2.14
FOR WHOLE DIET:	783	23.7	1308	4.91	8.32

Table 15b

Cardiac Value of the Polymeal without chocolate

Portion Analysis Food	Portion Wt (grams)	Portion Wt (ozs)	Cals/ Portion	CVo16 A	CVo16 B
ASPARAGUS	88	2.7	22	2.48	2.12
PEPPER (GREEN)	74	2.2	39	2.03	2.06
ALMONDS (unsalted, blanched)	68	2.1	416	24.96	18.84
RED WINE (Burgundy)	150	4.5	102	2.04	1.56
PAPAYA	100	3.0	39	1.34	1.36
LETTUCE	55	1.7	7	1.98	1.90
STRAWBERRY	83	2.5	22	1.67	1.72
TUNA (smoked)	65	2.0	150	3.96	2.14
FOR WHOLE DIET:	683	20.7	798	36.17	21.38

The Polymeal diet as published, advises 114 grams of fish four times a week (equivalent to 65 grams, or 2ozs per day); 400 grams of fruit and vegetables per day (3/4 of one pound), and the above amounts of almonds, chocolate, and wine. They also suggest 2.7 grams of garlic every day, the beneficial effect of which is unique, and therefore additional to that represented by the cardiac value score. Garlic would make this diet even more valuable than suggested by the above calculation since it has been shown to reduce cardiovascular risk by 25%.

If we take the CVo16 column A as correct, the diet needs only 3.5 RNI's (recommended daily nutritional intakes) of protective substances to raise its cardiac value to the minimum of 7.6. For column B, no supplements are needed, since the CVo16 is greater than 7.6. Both diets are somewhat deficient in the minerals manganese (by 34%), selenium (by 14%) and zinc (by 68%), and could do with some more B6 (43% extra), B12 (23% extra), omega 3 fatty acid (39% extra), fibre (28% extra), phytosterol (96% extra), and taurine (it has none). It also has far too much saturated fat (2.6 times the advisable amount) unless especially low fat chocolate is consumed. It is, however, very low in sodium (only 15% of minimum requirement) and potassium, with a 5:1 potassium to sodium salt ratio.

Without the plain chocolate, which itself contains a large amount of saturated fat (16.8 grams) and cholesterol (6 milligrams) (it is possible to obtain chocolate without much of these) – the cardiac value of the Polymeal becomes highly beneficial indeed with an overall cardiac value score of 36.17 (column A) or 21.38 (column B). By taking out the 'baddies', the ratio of 'goodies' to 'baddies' changes dramatically for the better. This qualifies it, even without garlic, as a very valuable cardiac diet indeed, although it could benefit from some supplements. Without doubt, it would be impossibly boring to eat every day.

OTHER DIETS EXAMINED

Instead of attempting to find the ideal diet, let us take a look at some examples of different everyday eating styles, to see how they score. I have used my imagination here because I am no chef and, with a limited choice of foods, it is difficult to represent all the different eating styles. Nevertheless, I have tried to imagine what a teenager, a person dieting to lose weight (on a low calorie or Atkin's diet), a vegetarian, and a gourmet, might eat in a day. There are lots of possible variations, but these examples will serve to illustrate how easy it is to construct a diet that is bad for the heart and circulation, and how difficult it is to improve its cardiac value.

The Teen Diet

Table 16

Teen Diet Analysis Food	Portion Wt (grams)	Portion Wt (ozs)	Calories/ Portion	CVo16 Cardiac Value
CHEESEBURGER (triple meat)	400	12.1	1036	0.11
BEANS (BAKED)	100	3.0	84	2.22
EGG (YOLK)	17	0.5	58	1.88
APPLE	138	4.2	65	1.48
HONEY	33	1.0	109	1.05
CORN	100	3.0	111	2.13
CRISPS (POTATO)	30	0.9	137	0.39
RICE KRISPIES	25	0.8	70	1.79
BEER (average)	500	15.2	145	1.88
PASTA	57	1.7	164	1.93
LETTUCE	55	1.7	7	1.98
BEER (average)	500	15.2	145	1.88
DIET COLA	250	7.6	0	1.01
TOMATO	100	3.0	17	1.70
BREAD (WHOLEWHEAT)	28	0.8	61	1.17
DIET COLA	250	7.6	0	1.01
TEA	200	6.1	0	1.50
MILK (1% FAT)	200	6.1	92	1.33
ICE CREAM	66	2.0	117	0.26
MAGARINE	5	0.2	37	1.62
FOR WHOLE DIET:	3054	93	2455	0.05

For a start, no foodstuff in my teenage diet has a cardiac value over 2.2 (over 3.0 is definitely good for the heart and circulation). This 'teen' diet has too much fat (4.5 times too much), too much salt (more than twice the recommended level), too much carbohydrate (twice that recommended) and lots of calories (although an active teenager might easily make use of them if very active). It also lacks fibre, phytosterol, and linolenic acid. As a consequence, it has a low anti-furring cardiac value, and an overall cardiac value (CVo16) of only 0.05. If 3.0 is the minimum value for a cardioprotective daily diet and over 7.6 is necessary for good protection, this diet is very unhealthy indeed.

If (and it is an unproven 'if') supplements are capable of neutralising the bad effects of fat, salt, and carbohydrate, you would need 495 RNI's (daily requirements) of each protective substance, to bring its cardiac value score up to the minimum of 7.6!

In cardiac terms, this diet is a 'no hoper'. *Add to this, other risk factors such as – a lack of exercise (perhaps associated with computer use), and smoking, and this will provide an efficient killer combination.*

The effects of such a diet, eaten over decades, are accumulative – and since 'furring' starts early in life, and mostly gets worse with age, an adverse outcome is highly probable. Diets like this will contribute to the cardiac problems of any nation.

Gourmet Diets

The chief characteristic of a gourmet diet is its diversity of choice. In Tables 17a and 17b, I admit to having done no justice to such diversity because of my self-imposed limitation of food choice. Here are two different daily assortments.

Table 17a

Gourmet 1 Analysis Food	Portion Wt (grams)	Portion Wt (ozs)	Calories Portion	CVo16 Cardiac Value
ASPARAGUS	60	1.8	15	2.08
PEPPER (GREEN)	74	2.2	39	2.03
TURKEY (BREAST ROASTED)	85	2.6	130	2.01
PARMESAN	6	0.2	27	0.75
BRAZIL NUTS	28	0.8	191	1.97
EGG (YOLK)	17	0.5	58	1.88
RED WINE	100	3.0	68	1.81
PAPAYA	100	3.0	39	1.34
RED WINE	100	3.0	68	1.81
PASTA	57	1.7	164	1.93
LETTUCE	55	1.7	7	1.98
STRAWBERRY	83	2.5	22	1.67
ANCHOVY (in oil)	85	2.6	162	0.80
TOMATO	100	3.0	17	1.70
BREAD (WHOLEWHEAT)	28	0.8	61	1.17
LAMB (LEG ROASTED)	85	2.6	187	0.79
TEA	200	6.1	0	1.50
MILK (1% FAT)	200	6.1	92	1.33
LOBSTER	90	2.7	260	2.75
BUTTER	5	0.2	37	0.56
FOR WHOLE DIET:	1558	47	1645	0.14

The first daily combination (Table 17a), is truly terrible, with a cardiac value for the day of only 0.14.

You would need 240 RNI's (daily requirements) of each protective substance, to bring its cardiac value score up to 7.6!

Table 17b

Gourmet 2 Analysis Food	Portion Wt (grams)	Portion Wt (oz)	Calories/ Portion	Cardiac Value CVo16
SWORDFISH	106	3.2	147	2.91
TURKEY (BREAST ROASTED)	85	2.6	130	2.01
ASPARAGUS	60	1.8	15	2.08
BROCCOLI	44	1.3	24	1.56
PINE NUTS	28	0.8	193	1.40
ONION	50	1.5	18	1.53

Gourmet 2 Analysis Food	Portion Wt (grams)	Portion Wt (oz)	Calories/ Portion	Cardiac Value CVo16
APPLE	138	4.2	65	1.48
EGG (YOLK)	17	0.5	58	1.88
BRAZIL NUTS	28	0.8	191	1.97
STRAWBERRY	83	2.5	22	1.67
LETTUCE	55	1.7	7	1.98
RED WINE	100	3.0	68	1.81
TOMATO	100	3.0	17	1.70
BREAD (WHOLEWHEAT)	28	0.8	61	1.17
ORANGE JUICE	124	3.8	56	1.33
BEVERAGES: COFFEE	200	6.1	0	1.29
MILK (1% FAT)	200	6.1	92	1.33
FOR WHOLE DIET:	1546	46.8	1232	1.93

The second combination (Table 17b), is almost 14 times better (Cardiac Value or CVo16 = 1.93), because it does contain a lot of 'goodies'. It is not too far removed from the Mediterranean diet which research has proven to be so cardioprotective (see references: Michel de Lorgeril). It has three times more fat, and 2.7 times more sodium salt, than recommended, and could do with more fibre, phytosterol, linolenic acid, taurine, and vitamin E.

You would need an additional 10 RNI's of all the protective substances, to bring this diet up to the beneficial overall cardiac value score of 7.6. Doubling the quantity of food doubles the cardiac value of the gourmet diet from 0.14 to 0.28, but it also doubles the number of calories.

A Very Low Calorie Diet for Dieting

Table 18

Dieting Diet Analysis Food	Portion Wt (grams)	Portion Wt (ozs)	Calories/ Portion	CVo16 Cardiac Value
SWORDFISH	106	3.2	147	5.82
BLACKEYED PEAS	80	2.4	93	5.20
BRAN FLAKES	50	1.5	135	3.10
ASPARAGUS	60	1.8	15	2.08
LETTUCE	55	1.7	7	1.98
RED WINE	100	3.0	68	1.81

Dieting Diet Analysis Food	Portion Wt (grams)	Portion Wt (ozs)	Calories/ Portion	CVo16 Cardiac Value
TOMATO	100	3.0	17	1.70
BREAD (WHOLEWHEAT)	28	0.8	61	1.17
ORANGE JUICE	124	3.8	56	1.33
BEVERAGES: COFFEE	200	6.1	0	1.29
MILK (1% FAT)	200	6.1	92	1.33
FOR WHOLE DIET:	1103	33	691	1.40

This diet is rather low in calories (only 691 Kcals), but does quite well for anti-furring potential. It, too, completely fails to reach the minimum level for acceptable overall cardiac value. However, it is low in salt and calories, and has enough of all of the necessary micronutrients. You would need an additional 10.8 RNI's of all the protective substances, to raise its overall cardiac value score up to 7.6 .

The Atkin's Diet

Dr Robert Atkins was a New York cardiologist who well knew that weight reduction would be of benefit to his obese cardiac patients. If you have angina or heart failure, the last thing you want to do is carry extra weight around. He was, therefore, motivated to find an effective weight reducing diet his patients could follow and enjoy. Because he couldn't find one, he created one himself. His great achievement was to create a diet that works without being boring. For more details I would recommend reading his original text ('Dr Atkins' New Diet Revolution', first published in 1992 in the UK by Vermillion).

Table 19

An Atkin's Type Diet

Atkin's Diet Analysis Food	Portion Wt (grams)	Portion Wt (ozs)	Calories/ Portion	CVo16 Cardiac Value
ASPARAGUS	60	1.8	15	2.08
TURKEY (BREAST ROASTED)	85	2.6	130	2.01
PARMESAN	6	0.2	27	0.75
BRAZIL NUTS	28	0.8	191	1.97
EGG (YOLK)	17	0.5	58	1.88
RED WINE	100	3.0	68	1.81
LETTUCE	55	1.7	7	1.98
STRAWBERRY	83	2.5	22	1.67
ANCHOVY (in oil)	85	2.6	162	0.80
TOMATO	100	3.0	17	1.70
LAMB (LEG ROASTED)	85	2.6	187	0.79
TEA	200	6.1	0	1.50
MILK (1% FAT)	200	6.1	92	1.33
BUTTER	5	0.2	37	0.56
FOR WHOLE DIET:	1109	33.6	1274	0.19

The principle of the diet is very simple – zero, or at least, a very low carbohydrate content. If we virtually strip the gourmet diet of its carbohydrate, we get what approximates to an Atkin's Diet (Table 19).

Many patients have asked me, not how to lose weight, but 'what is best to eat for my heart?' Because I could not find an evidence-based answer, apart from low fat, low salt options, I too have had to find my own solution.

Despite the fact that my Atkin's style diet has 1274 Kcals, one will still lose weight, because eating carbohydrates actually switches off weight loss. When we eat carbohydrate, we don't burn fat – we burn carbohydrate. Because liberal fat is allowed, it is not constructed for cardiac prevention, indeed it scores very badly on both anti-furring potential, and on overall cardiac value (CVo16 = 0.19). It is almost three times better for us than the 'teen' diet, but ten times worse than the gourmet diet.

The diet in Table 19 needs an additional 120 RNI's of all the protective substances, just to bring it up to the beneficial overall cardiac value of 7.6.

Health Warning! This diet has only 3 grams (1/10 ounce) of carbohydrate, three times more fat than is healthy, 2.6 times more sodium salt than recommended, not enough potassium or fibre, and is deficient in phytosterol, linolenic acid, vitamin E, taurine, and manganese. *If you want to follow this diet, and you have any 'furring' in your arteries, do it for short periods only. If you have no evidence of 'furring', and no other adverse risk factors, follow it as you wish.*

I admit that I have not done full justice to the Atkin's regime which is much more complex than the daily diet given here, so do read his books if you wish to know more.

The Vegetarian Diet

Table 20

Portion Analysis Food	Portion Wt (grams)	Portion Wt (oz)	Calories/ Portion	CVo16 Cardiac Value
PASTA	57	1.7	164	1.98
BROCCOLI	44	1.3	24	1.56
BANANA	75	2.3	87	1.54
HONEY	33	1.0	109	1.05
ONION	50	1.5	18	1.53
BLACKEYED PEAS	80	2.4	93	5.20
BRAN FLAKES	50	1.5	135	3.10
CAULIFLOWER	50	1.5	14	1.54
ASPARAGUS	60	1.8	15	2.08
LETTUCE	55	1.7	7	1.98
RED WINE	100	3.0	68	1.81
COTTAGE CHEESE	100	3.0	101	2.01
TOMATO	100	3.0	17	1.70
BREAD (WHOLEWHEAT)	28	0.8	61	1.17
ORANGE JUICE	124	3.8	56	1.33
BEVERAGES: COFFEE	200	6.1	0	1.29
MILK (1% FAT)	200	6.1	92	1.33
FOR WHOLE DIET:	1406	42.6	1061	1.44

This variation of a vegetarian diet has too much carbohydrate and not enough potassium. It could do with more fibre, and has no phytosterol; it is deficient in manganese, selenium, zinc, taurine, and vitamin E.

The diet has some anti-furring value, but fails to meet overall cardiac protection requirements (Cardiac Value or CVo16 = 1.44). You would need an additional 8.7 RNI's, of all the protective substances, to bring this diet up to the beneficial overall cardiac value of 7.6 .

SOME CONCLUSIONS

Once your arteries are 'furred', the process is unlikely to be reversed, even with the latest medication. Unfortunately, the damaging effects of a poor diet are mostly 'one-way' – accumulative.

'Furring', started in early life, may lead to trouble in middle life; therefore, teaching children what food is good for them must become a top priority.

The unfortunate conclusion for those who cannot eat them, or do not enjoy them, is that shellfish, fish, nuts and seeds, and offal, make for a diet that is healthy for the heart and circulation. Grazing on snacks full of sugar, salt, and spice, and all things nice, is just not good for us!

As mentioned in the last chapter, the best diet could be the sort of thing eaten by palaeolithic people (around 40,000 years ago), before agriculture and the domestication of animals took place. They did eat fish and hunt for meat, but had no sugar, milk or wheat. I doubt that our metabolism has changed much since then, and has not yet evolved far enough for us to cope with the hamburger, ice cream, or the toasted cheese sandwich!

For the heart and circulation, the Mediterranean diet and the Polymeal diet without chocolate, are clear leaders; something, in retrospect, my analysis could have predicted!

If you want to keep to foods that are good for the heart and circulation, try to eat several portions every day of food with a high overall cardiac value (CVo16 greater than 3.0).

Refer to the two lists given in Appendix 1. Table 1 lists the foods in order of cardiac value; Table 2 lists them alphabetically. These lists are admittedly very limited, given the fact that there are many thousands of separate foodstuffs available to us from all over the world. From these lists you can easily get a clear sense of which foods have a high cardiac value, and which do not. If the food you favour is not listed, the next best thing is to choose something similar or, at the least, from the same food group. That will give you a reasonable idea of its cardiac value.

CHAPTER 7

Food Choice for Patients – A Simple 100 Unit System

In a Nutshell: This chapter is mainly for those with a problem. It is aimed at those with artery 'furring' and at diabetics controlled by diet alone, as well as a diet with tablets. (Insulin dependant diabetics must follow their doctor's advice and ignore what is written here). Those with high blood pressure, and those who wish to lose weight, may also find this chapter useful.

To make things as simple as possible, I have given the daily requirement for each food chemical a number of units – 100 Units per day is the magic number. Diabetics are allowed up to 100 units of carbohydrate (starch and sugar) per day; high blood pressure subjects are allowed up to 100 sodium salt units per day, and should aim for more than 100 potassium units per day. Those who want to lose weight, should aim for 100 calorie units (= 1000 calories), or less. Those with 'furred' arteries can check that they are getting at least 100 units of each protective substance, and not more than 100 units of fat per day.

When a food has a high overall cardiac value, it is good for 'furring' prevention, for high blood pressure, and for diabetes, so if you do nothing else – eat foods with a high overall cardiac value, and leave it at that. If you want more detail to fine-tune your choice, refer to the Tables in Appendix 2.

The fact that food has a high cardiac value does not mean that it contains all of the micronutrients you need daily. The 100 unit system allows you to see at a glance whether or not your food choices contain the advisable quantity of all the 'goodies' and the 'baddies'.

For health maintenance, you should try keeping to a certain amount of salt (sodium), potassium, fat, and carbohydrate in your diet. If you eat pre-prepared food with nutritional information on the packets, all you have to do is add up all of the sugars, the fats, and the salt . . . but then that is simply not very practicable is it? Instead of referring to the number of milligrams of this, or that substance, I have simplified all your requirements into 100 units per day. With this system you are allowed up to 100 units of salt and carbohydrate (diabetic), although more than 100 units of potassium is not only beneficial for those with high blood pressure, but for most of us. Potassium is not safe for some patients with kidney disease. If you are known to have kidney disease consult your doctor on this point.

Those with high blood pressure may find that sodium salt restriction helps to control their blood pressure, although it doesn't always. They should aim for less than 100 units of sodium salt per day, but should also be advised to have more than 100 units of potassium every day. The advice to eat five portions of fruit or vegetable per day, comes partly from the need to eat potassium. The cardiac diet, given in Table 21, is low in salt (84 units ie less than 100 units) and has just sufficient potassium (101 units).

For those who want to lose weight, 100 calorie units = 1000 Calories. If you choose a tough calorie weight reduction regime, you might aim for 80 units. If you do a lot of exercise, 100 – 120 calorie units will be sufficient for weight loss, but without much exercise, you will not lose weight unless you drop your calorie units to less than 100 per day. The cardiac diet (Table 21) has 119 calorie units.

In the case of other substances such as folic acid, vitamin B6, and vitamin B12 etc, we all need at least 100 units of each, every day – (100 units = one RNI or recommended nutritional intake per day). The cardiac diet provides much more than that i.e. 275 units, in the case of folic acid. It has been suggested that 350 units per day (800 micrograms) of folic acid, is the beneficial daily requirement for heart and circulation protection.

If these considerations interest you, go to Appendix 2, Table E, where you can look up how many units of vitamin B6 or folic acid, omega 3 or linoleic acid are contained in each food. Aim to get at least 100 units of every cardioprotective substance every day.

My conclusion from the analysis of many different diets given in the last chapter, is that you will need a lot more than 100 units of each of these substances daily, to raise the cardiac value of the food you eat to a protective level. As many as 400 units, of each protective substance, might be required daily for optimal cardiovascular protection. This remains to be proven however.

DIABETES AND CARBOHYDRATE UNITS

Diabetics not on insulin rarely get to grips with what they should and shouldn't eat. As well as disturbing diabetic control, a high intake of carbohydrate may contribute to artery 'furring', in diabetics and non-diabetics alike.

WARNING: *Those on insulin have to match their carbohydrate and insulin to their physical requirements, and cannot use the carbohydrate units described here.*

It is now known that the more sugary drinks we consume, the more we are likely to develop diabetes; therefore, even non-diabetics need to watch out for their carbohydrate intake. Women who drink two or more cans of sugar – sweetened drinks per day, over several years, have twice the risk (1.8 times the risk actually) of developing diabetes. In the USA the consumption of soft drinks – the leading source of sugar in the

American diet – doubled in children and increased by 61% in adults between 1977 and 1997 (the reference if you want it is: *JAMA* 2004; 297:927).

Depending on physical activity, the minimum amount of carbohydrate in the form of starch and sugars, allowed for non-insulin diabetics, is about 50 grams (1.7 ounces) per day. In order to see what is good for diabetics and what is not, all you have to do is to look at the carbohydrate or diabetic units given in Appendix 2, Tables A and B. If you are a sedentary person and are a diet controlled (or tablet and diet controlled) diabetic, your usual daily quota should not add up to more than 100 units in all. **Advice from your doctor or dietician is always advisable to check the suitability of any regime to your individual requirements.**

Table 21

Calorie and diabetic units with units of saturated fat (Sat fat), sodium and potassium salts.

Cardiac Diet Food	Portion grams	Portion Wt (oz)	CVo16	Calorie Units	Diabetic Units	Sat. Fat Units	Salt Units	Potassium Units
TUNA	70	2.1	6.81	15	0	5	27	6
MUSSEL	85	2.6	11.74	9	0	9	19	4
WALNUTS	14	0.4	11.72	10	0	0	0	2
SUNFLOWER SEEDS	28	0.8	6.75	16	0	19	0	7
BLACKEYED PEAS	80	2.4	5.20	9	27	2	1	31
BRAN FLAKES	50	1.5	3.10	14	35	3	25	10
SESAME SEEDS	14	0.4	3.70	9	0	13	0	3
ASPARAGUS	60	1.8	2.08	2	1	1	0	5
LETTUCE	55	1.7	1.98	1	1	0	0	3
RED WINE	100	3.0	1.81	7	0	0	0	4
BANANA	75	2.3	1.54	9	17	1	0	10
TOMATO	100	3.0	1.70	2	2	0	1	8
BREAD (Wholewheat)	28	0.8	1.17	6	16	4	10	3
ORANGE JUICE	124	3.8	1.33	6	12	0	1	6
BEVERAGES: COFFEE	200	6.1	1.29	0	0	0	0	0
FLORA PRO-ACTIVE	5	0.2	1.46	7	0	0	0	0
TOTALS	**1088**	**33**	**3.70**	**119**	**110**	**57**	**84**	**101**

Let's take a practical example. In Table 21, the column for diabetic units allows you to see at a glance which foods contain the carbohydrate. Bran flakes and black-eyed peas contain a lot of carbohydrate – between them, 62 units, or 62% of the suggested daily amount. This diet contains a bit more than the recommended 100 units of carbohydrate, and would suit someone doing no particular physical work. In the same table, fat and sodium salt (Na) units, are also given. These 'baddies' must be kept to fewer than 100 units per day, whereas for potassium (a 'goody'), more than 100 units per day is best. This diet is healthy from a high blood pressure point of view, because it contains more units of potassium (135 units) than it does sodium salt (85 units).

We can follow the same method for all the important elements in the diet. Those that are 'baddies' (fat, sodium salt, and carbohydrate), we must try to keep under one hundred units per day. Those that are 'goodies', we should try to exceed 100 units per day. It's that simple.

All the tables of units are given in Appendix 2. I have divided the tables into those for diabetics (Tables A and B); those for high blood pressure patients (Tables C and D), and in Tables E – G, the other factors important to those who need be concerned about artery 'furring' (those who have been shown to have artery 'furring', those who have angina, a history of heart attack, or narrowed arteries in the legs – claudication). Some Tables have a low to high listing of values, others an alphabetic listing, to help you find the food you would normally choose.

PART 3

Are we . . .
Just What We Eat?

Other Killer Causes.
Other Killer Cures.

CHAPTER 8

Other 'Baddies'

In a Nutshell: If your aim is to be a survivor from artery disease (the cause of heart attacks and other forms of cardiovascular problem), to be in with a chance, you will need to know all about the 'furring' of your arteries. Don't worry about other people's arteries, worry about your own. What is bad for their arteries, may not be bad for yours. Other than certain foods, do you know what else is bad for your arteries, and your heart?

Here is a list of the non-food 'baddies':

- Smoking (*inhaling the smoke from burning leaves etc*), as well as giving-up smoking (*no, not a joke!*).
- Poverty (*having less resources than you feel you need*).
- Stress that causes energy depletion (*any factor, psychological or physical, that makes you spend more energy than you have to spend: especially the feeling of not being in control, but also anger, resentment, and an obsessive anxious nature.*
- Weight problems (*too much, or too little – enough to affect your health*).
- Diabetes (*absent or ineffective insulin, that affects your fat and sugar metabolism*).
- Excessive alcohol and alcoholic binges.
- Insufficient exercise.
- Your attitude: *controversially – a disinterest in looking before you leap; an arrogant approach to ignorance in matters of prevention and trouble avoidance, and a tendency to make subjective rather than objective judgements – all are characteristics of the potential non-survivor.*

Weapons of mass destruction are just about everywhere these days. We the public and those in power, have not yet taken sufficient notice, otherwise they might have been removed years ago. The secret services of both the US and UK missed them in Iraq. Even the Iraqi's didn't realize how many they had stored away. The idea that they could be deployed to kill in 45 minutes was of course nonsense – they actually take a good 45 years to kill. They are called cigarettes!

You have seen the adverts. You have been told the bad news a thousand times. You may have even turned a blind eye to it and ignored every warning about it, even though every packet is now covered with death threats. It is the only really successful weapon of mass destruction: it's SMOKING!

There are many other factors, though, some of which you might not have guessed. Your attitudes and behaviour, your socio-economic and educational status and, bizarrely, whether or not you have gum disease or dental root infection – the infection, and therefore the inflammation, could also affect your arteries. The latter possibility may seem a little far-fetched but it has been seriously suggested because the 'furring' itself is an inflammatory process.

STOP SMOKING

Get fit.

Limit stress, if you feel tired or exhausted, by

limiting your energy spending, and increasing your energy saving.

Lose weight, if advised.

The Atkin's Diet does work – keep to it for short periods, otherwise weigh all of your food to make sure you are not eating too much.

Limit alcohol to two units per day

(two small wine glasses or one pint of beer).

Control diabetes by all means possible.

Cardiovascular disease has many possible origins, and perhaps a combination of different ones, for each of us. It turns out that there can be a lot more to preventing heart attacks than just eating the right things and simply avoiding the wrong things.

Every factor has its advocates. You don't really need to know about them all, just those relevant to you. Medical screening examinations should, but do not always, tell you which are yours. Unfortunately, this is a subject, like so many others to do with prevention, which gains recognition the moment *after* catastrophe strikes! Learning about 'medical catastrophe', and what causes it well before it occurs, has the potential to maximize your chances of avoiding and surviving it – if you are prepared to take heed.

Survival is a serious business. Survival is also a frivolous business – it depends on your attitude. To survive like the late Bob Hope and our Queen Mother to 100 years of age, without heart attacks, strokes, cancer, lung disease, or fractured bones, takes some doing. It is beyond our technology to guarantee it but with inside knowledge, you can maximise your chances.

You will need to know enough about the pitfalls to avoid them. As Bob Hope said on his 100th birthday: "If I'd have known I was going live this long, I would have looked after myself better!" **How do you look after yourself better? That is the question.**

Quality and quantity of life are different, but not mutually exclusive issues. You can do all the wrong things and live to 100; you can do all the right things and die at 40! Perhaps we should all decide what it is we want to go for. Deciding on your objective is the first step; acquiring the knowledge to achieve healthy survival can then follow.

SO YOU WANT TO TRUST TO LUCK?

Cardiovascular disease can seriously damage your health and can affect both your quality and quantity of life. For these reasons it is definitely worth preventing. In general, doctors enjoy a good

Ken Says: 'I'd sooner die young and happy, than give up cigarettes and the food I want to eat. I don't want a long miserable life – no way!'

emergency; not surprisingly, most patients don't! Why then would those who have no taste for emergencies, wish only to trust to luck? 'To hell with it', they say, 'I'll take my chances'. Good luck to them! It's their choice, and rightly so – my guess though, is that their fear is inhibiting them, or, that they are locked into the – 'it won't happen to me', conviction.

Survival behaviour is a skill. James Bond, and Rambo, although fictional characters, were both cast with a fantastic knowledge-base of survival skills, few of which are needed in everyday life. But for everyday survival, you do need some knowledge-based survival skills, few of which are taught in school.

To survive as well as James Bond, you would need to know what works, and how. James had 'Q'; you have a number of writers (including myself), trying to sell you what they believe to be the secrets of success. Believing that something works, although a powerful force to be reckoned with, is not usually good enough for survival; you need to *know* what works and what doesn't. The irony is that your life, like that of James Bond, may depend just as much on proven survival skills – **there is no place for myth, unsubstantiated belief, and fantasy in this game.**

You will need commitment, to find out what works for you, and what does not. You are likely to have some mistaken ideas, so be prepared to learn, and steel yourself to unlearn. Anyway, what is so bad about being wrong? Nobody can be right all of the time, and to expect perfection is becoming politically incorrect. As our disillusionment with politicians grows, even they are retreating to a mid-field position – where good enough, is good enough!

Be careful with the "everyone knows that . . . ." type of conviction. You might have to find the courage to actually disbelieve some of the dogma. Examples: 'you are what you eat!' 'Vitamin C is good for you!' 'Wrap up warm, you'll catch a cold!' 'The rich and famous must be happy!' If you unquestionably accept any of these statements – you may have a survival problem. Only objective observation, judgement, and a readiness to change your mind count

---

Four little f's: Fantasy, Fashion, Fame, and Fanity (OK, **V**anity).

Because these are all built on myth and ego, dependency on them will lead to unhappiness when they fail to work for you. And since unhappiness can hasten demise, they are not intrinsically healthy, except that is, for the bank balances of those who market them as necessities.

---

when it comes to maximising your chances of survival. And all of them count whatever the type of survival, be it economic, social, or biological. A lack of objectivity, and an undue fascination with fantasy and vanity, cause both businesses and lives to fail. Could this be why the well informed, and the rich, pay to seek the advice of the well informed?

I have found over the years, that the stimulus required for most people to seek a heart check is not the warning on cigarette packets but the premature death of a close friend or relative. That is not to say that warning words don't have their place, they do – but the wise get checked anyway. A medical check can induce anxiety, that is undoubted, but to the potential survivor, it is clearly better than death! Those who are survivors by nature have the courage to face fear and anxiety, and to deal with whatever is needed to overcome them. Non-survivors tend to run away whenever the possibility of fear or anxiety looms. They don't want to die, but their inability to face up to reality can expose them to danger. It's for you to choose how you wish to play this game of life but, in choosing, you define your survival potential.

When the general population has been surveyed, few seem to know what is actually good or bad for their heart, although most of those interviewed think they know! In general, women thought they were five times more likely to die of breast cancer than heart disease. This is not true, of course, but the perception does do wonders for promoting self-examination and screening for breast lumps.

It is common to want to maximize your chances of survival in some ways (changing eating habits), but not in others (giving up smoking). The choice is yours, but at least try to base all your decisions on evidence, not on hearsay.

THE SMOKING GUN

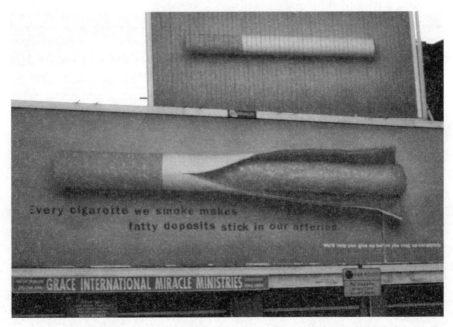

Fig 12 British Heart Foundation anti-smoking advert: UK, January 2004.

Here is that advert again, just to remind you of the sort of thing that smoking can do to your arteries. Although not anatomically correct, it gets the message across – something very nasty is going on in the arteries of many smokers.

When it comes to considering other 'baddies' there is no better place to start than at the deep end. Are you a smoker? Are you looking for anti-smoking ammunition to help you give up the habit? What follows is a veritable arsenal of ammunition, and it is an arsenal you need, because smoking has been more deadly to the human race than all wars of the last 100 years put together!

STOP SMOKING

If you want to prevent heart and artery disease and you are a smoker, forget everything else – **stop smoking**.

See: www.givingupsmoking.co.uk

Here is a rule of thumb calculation. Assume that there are one billion adults alive. If 20% smoke, half of them (10%), will die as a result of smoking. Ten percent of one billion is 100 million – an equivalent number to all those killed by all the weapons used in the last 100 years. In the Second World War alone, it is estimated that a total 61 million soldiers and civilians lost their lives. On the field of battle there can be honour in death, but there is no honour and no dignity in death from smoking, only an ignoble profit for tobacco companies!

Allow me to be even more uncompromising: **You have to be completely crazy (medically) to smoke, *and* to think that you can maximize your chances of survival.** Chances are, unless you are very, very . . .very lucky, you can't do both! Some lucky people do, of course, survive machine-gun attacks, mid-air aircraft collisions and land mines, so there is always hope!

There will, of course, always be exceptions, but where is there a mention in the newspapers of all those poor souls who did not survive, and have died as a result of cigarettes?

In September 2004 the British Medical Journal (BMJ) reported that smoking six to ten cigarettes per day doubles the risk of heart attack, twenty cigarettes per day quadruples the risk and, for those who smoke forty per day, there is a nine-fold risk. Also recently reported was the finding that for men, passive smoking, can almost double the risk of coronary artery disease but not of strokes (BMJ July 2004).

> **What Ken says**: *Ken knows lots of people who smoke 100 cigarettes every day, and have lived a long and happy life. Sure he knows one or two, but where are the others? Already gone up in smoke!?*
>
> *In fact, Ken took a cutting from a newspaper for me, just to prove his point. This is what it said:*
>
> **Half a million fags ... and she lived to 105.** *Ciggie-loving Marie ... was laid to rest yesterday – after living to 105, despite smoking nearly half a million fags. (The Sun, December 15, 2004)*

Surviving smokers *are* simply the lucky ones. There is, of course, more to life than death. So what of the survivors? What state are they in?

> In a study of 1400 office workers (aged 40 – 65 years) who engaged in vigorous exercise, but did not smoke, there were 12 fatal coronaries in 12,000 man – years of observation. *This number was five times more, in unfit smokers.*

Smoking is the single most serious amenable risk factor for artery and heart disease. Smokers have half the chance of reaching the age of 65 years! That's not to say that smoking WILL kill you, it's just that an early death is twice as likely if you smoke. Because hope springs eternal, many smokers get to think that they won't be among them. This attitude is fortified in the young by a feeling of invincibility, by the idea that their youth will protect them against all ills, and by the conviction that dying is too far off to be contemplated seriously.

We are talking about odds here, not facts. Nobody, and I mean nobody, has a crystal ball to see what the future holds for any of us. The future is simply not predictable, whatever anyone says. We can, however, express what might happen in terms of likelihood. If you are a self-confessed gambler, you won't mind chancing your luck. The problem is, that in the game of life we are all unwitting gamblers, whether we like it or not. Every decision we make is playing the odds, and this is never more so than when making the decision to smoke another cigarette.

> **Ken says:**'smoking doesn't affect me – I don't inhale!'

The difference in smoking prevalence between different socio-economic groups runs in parallel to other lifestyle differences, which together help explain the great inequalities in both health and disease status that exist in our society.

> If doctors did nothing else but stop people smoking, they would have more impact on the incidence of disease and life expectancy, than anything else they do.

Professionals smoke least of all (15% of males, 4% females); employers, and managers are next with 24% and 32%, male and female smokers, and then come the manual workers who smoke more than all other groups (29% and 42%, male and female smokers). In the UK, one third of girls, and one quarter of teenage boys smoke. In all other groups, women are said to smoke less, but I have to say that is not my impression. Impressions, like all anecdotal evidence, are limited to individual experience, and do not necessarily reflect the complete picture.

Cigars and pipes are said to be less risky than cigarettes, but then cigar and pipe smokers are far fewer in number and consume less tobacco. In any case, people who smoke cigars and pipes are different; they tend to be richer and generally have a lower risk profile than cigarette smokers. Like cigars, low-tar cigarettes are said to be less risky than the high tar; so if you can't give up your cigarettes, at least switch to cigarillo's, or to low tar cigarettes as a first move.

Forget heart bypasses, heart transplants, and road traffic accident emergency doctoring, all of these are a relative waste of time, while so many people continue to smoke! I don't know how many jumbo-jet loads of smokers die from smoking-related diseases in the UK every day, but it is a good few!

A word of caution though – one-sided stories will always be unbalanced. The pursuit of truth requires that both sides of every story be told. So is there anything good to say about smoking?

Smoking helps relaxation, aids concentration, and keeps body-weight down. Smoking used to be advised by Victorian doctors to treat asthma, and because cigarette smoke 'poisons' the tubes of the lung into a form of chemical submission, a cigarette can help the asthmatic temporarily. Surprised? Well, this is something every ex-smoking asthmatic knows well. For asthmatic smokers, there would seem to be a short-term gain, to be traded against a long-term disaster. You will also be surprised to know that when smoking asthmatics give up smoking, their condition often deteriorates badly. One of my patients spent months in hospital, requiring oxygen most of the time, in her first year of giving up.

Yet another surprise is, that **soon after stopping smoking there is a temporary increase in the risk of a heart attack.** When first found, this conclusion was deliberately suppressed by the researchers who discovered it because they disbelieved it themselves. They were so convinced that it was a mistake they decided not to publish it! When later data supported the finding, the Framingham Study researchers had to admit their omission. Mistakes can easily be made in scientific analysis, so their caution was entirely understandable. Better to omit than to mislead.

A Case History: Ralph's Dad was one of those smokers who had survived into his 70's, dragging every last bit of nicotine from each of his hand-rolled cigarettes. He came to me because he was breathless at rest and wanted help. First, I asked him for his expectations. He replied, stopping to gasp between phrases, "all I wanna do . . . ...is to get to that #### betting shop". The betting shop was only five doors away from his home but it was a bit too far for him to walk. I would have given him a pull-along oxygen cylinder, but that would have been too heavy. In the end, some special expectorant tablets helped him. There was no point in telling him to stop smoking; after all, smoking was probably keeping his airways open! To stop, might have meant a closedown reaction and a sudden deterioration in his breathing. Unfortunately, he did not last too long, but long enough to make a few more bets . . .with his money this time, not his life!

A few years later I was examining his son, Ralph, one of the funniest men I have ever known, when, without my knowing it at the time, I influenced him to give up smoking. I said, having examined his chest, "Ralph, I think your lungs are going the same way as your Dad's!" When I saw him six weeks later, I asked him how many cigarettes he was then smoking. "Smoking", he exclaimed in loud astonishment, "smoking . . .. after what you said to me!" I was baffled, and had to ask: "But, what did I say?" He replied, "You said to me, that my lungs were going the same way as my father's. After that, I'd have been mad to smoke another one, wouldn't I?"

Half a century ago, smoking used to be a fashion accessory. To smoke elegantly, you had only to copy your favourite film stars and become one of the 'in crowd'. Nowadays, camaraderie and product loyalty are a big part of the social acceptability game that many play. While many are prone to say: 'you're not still smoking those cheap old cigarettes are you?', peer pressure will remain an unstubbed economic driving force.

In some parts of the world, it is now considered seriously anti-social, and in bad taste to smoke. Well done, Ireland! They first had the guts to ban smoking in pubs and restaurants, with no loss in sales! Scotland will soon follow, an even more apt decision, given their top position in the international coronary league. Bhutan in the Himalayas has decided to go one further and ban the sale of cigarettes altogether, so there is well-informed intelligent life on earth after all!

The outcast, addicted followers of fashion, now found smoking on the office steps, summer and winter, rain or shine, need our sympathy, even if it is tinged with a touch of self-righteousness. Don't feel too sorry for them though; the steps are the new meeting place, where many newly gained friends are to be found –

reinforcing one another's habits. These smokers are either addicted (need treating), ill informed (need educating), or think themselves clever enough to buck the odds (need listening to – they only rarely listen to the facts)!

The fact that smoking and lung cancer are related was established in Nazi Germany in 1939. A case-controlled study of smoking had shown that heavy smoking, in particular, was strongly related to lung cancer (see George D. Smith 2004). Before Doll and Hill's report in 1950, also relating smoking to lung cancer, one of the other prevailing theories had been that car exhaust was a cause. To investigate this possibility, Doll chose to study two separate populations: those living a few metres from the traffic on a dual carriageway in London, and others living in farming communities. The theory predicted that it would be those living next to the traffic who would more often suffer the terrors of lung cancer. As it turned out, the important factor was not where they lived, but whether or not they smoked.

The relationship between lung cancer and smoking is still argued about but, as a consequence, very few doctors now smoke. At every large conference at the Royal College of Physicians in London, however, there are always a few knowledgeable physicians to be seen (on the front steps, well out of sight), yielding to their addiction.

Quite recently we have seen tobacco-advertising reduced, tobacco linked in adverts to artery disease, tobacco sponsorship restricted, low-tar cigarettes, and various aids to smoking-cessation, but no U.K. law completely outlawing it. Are we slowly getting the message, or could it be that world governments are worried by the economic realities of smoking reduction? If large numbers of smokers do give up smoking and increase their life expectancy, there will be more pensioners; the more pensioners, the higher the pension bill! With less tobacco tax revenue, who will pay?

Let's look on the bright side! If you do smoke, you are performing a great service for your country – reducing the burden of the elderly upon the young. Fewer old people, less burden! Now there's something to justify the smoking habit! This cruel outlook is so strongly supported by the facts about smoking that we have to be cruel to be kind. What we seem unable to do is be objective about it. If we do take it seriously, we face the opposition of industrial giants, allied to bench-loads of faint-hearted politicians heard around the world muttering that liberty, and the right to choose, is what democracy is all about. Now how cruel is that?

> **Ken Says**: *"I'm not a child, you know!" "You can't tell me what to do! In any case, I'll take my chances!" In more mellow moments he has been known to say "I'd like to give up smoking, but it's impossible. I just feel so bad". After a heart by-pass, and two leg by-passes, he still refuses to give up smoking! Mad, or what? Because his arteries are so bad now, giving up smoking (one of the few pleasures he says he has left'), will definitely make him miserable, and will hardly help his life expectancy. So perhaps he is right to continue smoking after all!*

Some smokers (and other addicts) say that giving up is easy – keeping off it is difficult. Many smokers want to give up (so they say), but cannot. OK, it's an addiction, and we ought to be helpful, not cynical. As with all addicts, though, help only works when they have first committed themselves to giving up. Without the will to give up, excuses will be constantly invented. Those not proficient at excuses, get angry and argumentative.

Liberty means the unhindered right to pursue one's chosen way of life – without hurting others, or their way of life. Smoking does harm others, so should it be banned in public places?

Passive smoking has become a big issue, so I have taken a look at the evidence. It is now largely accepted medically that passive smoking is a cause of serious disease in adults

Jamrozik (2005) reports that 2 employed persons per day, die as a result of passive smoking in the UK (617 deaths per year, 54 of whom had worked in the hospitality business). Smoking at home accounts for another 2,700 deaths, in persons aged 20 – 64 years, and another 8000 deaths among those older than 64 years of age.

(Jamrozik, K. BMJ: April 2005). The evidence supports the view that if you live with a 70 per day smoker, your attendant risk is the same as if you smoked 10 per day – you carry one seventh of the risk. This is likely to be of crucial importance to innocent children who unknowingly have to suffer the disregard of smoking parents and their friends. To trap their children in the confines of a car while they smoke is unforgivably selfish. The disregard these smokers have may be based on ignorance that might almost be forgivable; more likely, it is based on arrogance, and that is not.

GIVING UP THE HABIT

For good advice about giving up smoking log onto:
www.givingupsmoking.co.uk.

There you will find many methods listed: 'cold-turkey', hypno-therapy, nicotine replacement, and a drug called buproprion (Zyban). I have seen all of these help different individuals. The key point here is that the method must suit the individual.

INFLUENCING DESTINY?

Those who wish to avoid accidents and catastrophes have to have a certain attitude towards prevention if they are to have any chance of success. Such an attitude may be rooted in anxiety or obsessionality, because it attempts the impossible – to prevent all disasters, and to put off the inevitable. Having been a member of the medical profession for over 40 years, I have seen all sorts of health and disease-related behaviour that is unlikely to aid self-preservation. In the field of prevention, fear and disinterest are the main antagonists of intelligent avoidance behaviour, although there are other human characteristics worth considering.

We have all heard of the proverbial horse led to water: it will only drink if it feels like it, right? But can it, or should it, be made to drink?

After all, it might be about to travel and need water? Horses are not capable of much forethought, but you and I should be. Mostly, we trust to luck or put faith in what our friends tell us, but that is not much better than herd behaviour. In this life game there is no safety in numbers and too much at stake to chance in luck. There are those who are happy to think for themselves, do their own research, verify the information, make a decision, act on it, and move forward. This is good survival strategy, and it is what the smart guys do.

If you are depressed, angry, resentful, arrogant, happily ignorant of the facts, bloody minded, or just a little silly, survival behaviour may not be within your grasp! Take heart though – you will still have luck to rely on!

If you were to recognise your lack of survival potential, and wanted help, how could we help? The first and biggest step would be to get you some insight. Speaking to a good friend (one you can really rely on to tell you the unpalatable truth), and with whom you share many values, could give you a valuable start. After that, you might need someone more experienced: a doctor, priest, counsellor, parent, grandparent, accountant, bank manager, even your hairdresser and manicurist, can all have valuable experiences and insights to share with you. Anyone who has the time for you, and who knows you well, may hold a valuable view. Experience is always of value, although it may not always be pertinent. Views you don't like can be especially valuable – by coming to know what you disagree with, your own views may gain strength.

IGNORANCE AS A CULTURE

We live in a society where the acquisition of goods and status is more desirable than the acquisition of knowledge.

Patients have a right to expect their doctors to be knowledgeable and informative – their lives could depend on it. Doctors have no right to expect their patients to be knowledgeable even if their lives may depend on it.

> I hold that there is no sin
> but ignorance.
>
> Christopher Marlowe. c1592.
> *The Oxford Dictionary
> of Quotations.*

A lack of knowledge puts us all at risk. Without knowing about the dangers that exist, we won't be on the lookout for them and can only avoid them by chance. A lack of knowledge can also disadvantage us. Without knowing about the benefits available, we won't be on the lookout for them either and won't be able to take advantage of them, except by chance. Knowledge on the other hand only has power if its significance is recognised.

When Watson and Crick published their findings on the structure of DNA, from which all our genes are made, they concluded that the significance of what they had discovered had not escaped them. Prophetic words indeed!

> 'The vain presumption of understanding everything can have no other basis than never understanding anything. For anyone who had experienced just once the perfect understanding of one single thing, and had truly tasted how knowledge is accomplished, would recognise that infinity of other truths of which he understands nothing.'
>
> Galileo, *The Two Chief World Systems.* Quoted by Edmund B.Bolles in *Galileo's Commandment.*

A common characteristic of truly knowledgeable people is humility – they are humbled by what they don't know and are modest about what they do know. That is not to say that some very knowledgeable people cannot be arrogant; it's just that their arrogance suggests insecurity. For the less knowledgeable arrogance is sometimes a defence against those who might find out just how little they do know.

There is so much information being generated every day that nobody can keep abreast of it – there aren't enough hours in the day. What we have to do, in order to select the vital information we need for healthy survival, is be able to separate the helpful from the irrelevant. This requires judgement, focus, an ability to avoid distraction, and an ability to ask the appropriate inquiring questions.

Einstein was humbled by not understanding how time and gravity work – his search for that understanding led to his works of genius.

Ignorance may be bliss, but a lack of wisdom can be dangerous when important decisions have to be made. Not everyone, however, would want to pursue wisdom and become learned or academic – you can certainly lead a very happy life without learning, and learning cannot guarantee a happy life.

> **Lady Bracknell:** "I have always been of the opinion that a man who desires to get married should know either everything or nothing. Which do you know?"
> **Jack:** "I know nothing Lady Bracknell."
> **Lady Bracknell:** "I am glad to hear it. I do not approve of anything that tampers with natural ignorance. Ignorance is like a delicate exotic flower – touch it and the bloom is gone.
>
> **Oscar Wilde 1895.**
> *The Importance of Being Ernest. Act 1.*

> 'From ignorance our comfort flows. The only wretched are the wise'.
>
> **Matthew Prior. 1692.**
> *The Oxford Dictionary of Quotations.*

One generation ago, many were denied the right to knowledge. Coming from a poor background meant having to leave school at an early age in order to earn a wage. Some parents had a serious objective in having a lot of children (and some still do) – they needed enough of them to ensure their welfare into old age. Some parents may still insist that their children leave school early, get a 'proper' job and start to make a living to help support the family.

My mother is 93 years old this year and was the twelfth of thirteen children. She was unable to go to school – it became her vocation to care for her younger disabled sister. She became Polly's surrogate mother and gloried in the experience. When

> There are two extreme forms of ignorance: **simple ignorance**, where you know all there is to know, have verified your knowledge as much as possible, but still don't understand everything (which you are humble enough to admit), and **profound ignorance**, where you know little or nothing, have made no attempt to verify that you know nothing, but still think you know everything about it. When profound ignorance and arrogance combine, bullshit results – strong valueless opinions in search of someone to persuade!

Polly died in her early twenties, my mother was the one who grieved the most. She can still be brought to tears by the memories of that special love that passed between them. My mother was happy not to attend school at the time; now, she somewhat regrets the fact that she did not get that education which would have fed her intelligent mind.

A good education teaches objectivity. When it comes to healthy survival, a lack of objectivity and ignorance of the facts (no need seen for reconnaissance) will put you at risk of failure. Why do so many people give up smoking, only after, but not before, their first heart attack? Either they were completely unaware of the connection, or had ignored the issue altogether and made no attempt to find out the truth about heart attacks and smoking. We all should learn from our mistakes, but how can we, if we don't recognise them? Since quite a few heart attack victims do not give up smoking, and go on to have a further heart attack, sensitive questions have to be asked: – are there some people incapable of learning from their mistakes, and, are some people ineducable? Schooling with army-styled discipline might teach some of them the merits of learning, reconnaissance, and objectivity, but I doubt it. I am sad to say that I doubt we human beings have changed much across the eons of time – it still takes a catastrophic event to galvanise our minds into 'looking before we leap', or thinking that 'prevention is better than cure'!

I sense that there is now something new and perverse about a lack of knowledge. Whereas once it was a source of unnecessary shame, it can now be a source of shameless pride. There are now very many newly-rich and famous people who are proud of the fact that they needed no knowledge whatsoever to achieve their success. Having seen no particular need for their own education they may, however, want their children to be 'top of the class' at the best schools money can buy! They have always been around of course; it's just that their number and their endless exposure in the media make them a noticeable force to be reckoned with. They have already influenced general standards of behaviour and attitude, and that is serious. Whether we like it or not, a culture of ignorance is growing, is alive and well and using its purchasing power to gain ascendancy.

From the medical point of view, some followers of this growing culture want someone, other than themselves, to 'do something', about their illnesses, many of which they may have worked hard to create for themselves. Something quick and easy fits the bill – a pill for every ill, rather than a more difficult lifestyle change, based on objective personal appraisal and enough knowledge to understand the necessary reasons for change. Whether it is obesity due to their overeating and lack of exercise, or their chronic bronchitis, lung cancer, or heart disease due to smoking, their idea is simple – 'someone should do something about my condition!'

Doctors are not unaware that they have been set up for failure. By giving them the responsibility to change the lifestyles of those who see no need for it; to cure the incurable and to magic away ill-health and disease, governments are, of course, asking doctors to achieve the impossible. By setting impossible targets for doctors, governments can measure their degree of failure and blame them for the inequalities in health that will always exist naturally in a diverse society. This does not, however, stop doctors working for governments and resigning themselves to accept targets they know to be impossible. Those who long ago committed their working lives to the system, at a time when experience and common sense prevailed, now have to comply in order to get paid.

The medical profession will never be able to help everyone. Benefiting from help does require certain attributes. To benefit from help, some insight, enough intelligence, a willingness to get educated (enough to know what we don't know) and, a motivation to comply with common sense survival strategies are required. From a political point of view, though, we the democratic electorate, must never be allowed to sense inequality – we must at all times be made to feel that we are honoured as equals, even though society is obviously made up of really bright guys, really dim guys, and the majority of us who are somewhere in between. It would not be a vote winner to admit the obvious – that the inequalities between us, in education and our outlook towards healthy survival, engendered mostly by deprivation and ignorance, underpin all of the scandalous inequalities in health and disease that exist in western societies. The unpalatable fact that we have lived with for a few decades is that there are five times more cases of heart disease and cancer where financial, social, and educational deprivation exist.

It is somewhat depressing to think that this is 'the way it is', or that it's just part of life's rich tapestry, with nobody at fault! Because a good part of the strength of a society depends on its diversity, there can be little point in asking the question – what, if anything, can be done to actually make us all equal. There will be worthy self-esteem derived from trying to answer the question of course, but in my view it would take as much energy to convert a cart horse into a race horse, as it would to change our society into one with absolute equality and perfect health!

Medicine does not exist, and cannot progress, in a vacuum. For the moment, if we are to change lives by preventing disease, our patients have to be able to understand what we are talking about and, something of what they need to do for themselves – we cannot do it for them. If, as I suspect, ignorance is to become even more acceptable in the future, more and more complicated treatments will have to be 'done' to patients without their really achieving fully-informed consent. The problem will be getting them to achieve, anything like a fully-informed status. If only the very few truly understand anything about anything, 'medical' practice will become 'veterinary' practice.

In private, most of my colleagues will predictably say: " so what's new?" After all, they work in the real world, not in government offices, where those with no direct knowledge or experience of medicine, spend much of their time dreaming up pointless targets and management objectives for busy doctors who have learned from decades of experience, what works and what does not.

There is a new light in the sky, however – the Internet. This wonderful resource provides many of my patients with a great deal of valuable medical information, although, few have enough medical discernment and insight to judge the value of all that knowledge. Many of my consultations now start with a discussion of the facts they have gleaned from medical web-sites. This can only be a good thing, although it is more likely to fuel them with irrelevant information than to empower them with understanding. Nevertheless, they are getting involved and making a worthy attempt to understand their problems. This may annoy some doctors, who still regard medical knowledge as their exclusive reserve. Others must now be prepared to discuss illness from a new standpoint: acting more like a tutor correcting misconceptions rather than having to teach students the basics from scratch.

INEQUALITY – IS THAT THE WAY IT IS?

In their book, The Bell Curve, Herrnstein and Murray (Free Press, NY USA, 1994) showed, that in the US, money for education was more productively spent on the clever than on those less well endowed. A bit like saying, it is better to give money to the rich than to the poor: the rich know what to do with it! This very unpopular, and socially indigestible conclusion parallels the daily experience of every doctor – patients who don't seem to be able to learn. Patient's may moan about their medical condition, but make no attempt to change those patterns of behaviour that may contribute to the cause. This is uncharitable I know, because not everyone has the capacity to change their circumstances. Nevertheless, **insight into our own problems, and a willingness to address those problems objectively, both remain crucial to a healthy survival strategy.** Without patients seeking insight, doctors have little chance of educating them and improving their chances of survival. Doctors are, otherwise, limited to the use of drugs.

The political pressure to create equality between socio-economic classes may have serious medical consequences. Those who once had privilege could now have lost it; those born without privilege, may now feel a new sense of value. Such **changes in life status have been shown to contribute to the occurrence of heart attacks.** Life changes associated with anger, resentment, and the feelings of loss or entrapment, can also be potent killers, especially for those with narrowed arteries, heart failure, and a tendency to clot. Self-esteem, gained from being newly honoured as important and privileged, may sustain good health.

Books like this, while prescribing what to eat and what to do, are unlikely to result in much social change for the majority. Books simply don't have that power. For instance, this book will most likely be bought, and read, by those already well on their way to maximising their survival potential. It is unlikely to be bought, and read, by those who really need it: those who let destiny, and not knowledge, direct their lives.

Behaviour-modifying techniques, which allow no options, can work well. Ban smoking in all public places; make the cost of one pack of cigarettes a real disincentive, make movies that show the rich and famous reeling away from outcast smokers – these strategies are much more likely to work. They might work because they are primitive enough to bypass thought, and strike at a softer, more vulnerable psychological target. They might not work because addicts are always strongly driven to continue their habit.

To succeed in survival, you need knowledge (especially, knowledge of what you don't know), together with some effective strategies. The most important strategy is the use of reconnaissance. To use a military analogy, you need to find and assess your enemy, and if possible get a map of his minefields, before you attack. The wise get an accurate map of the minefields before they take their first step; the foolish see no point in asking questions, and tend to proceed with unrealistic confidence. In my experience, it helps to have the right character: best suited, are those with motivation, intelligence, and resourcefulness. It also helps to have good equipment, by which I mean, a fit and healthy mind and body. Although these are largely given as genetic traits, they can be worked on.

Personal survival is not always the object of human behaviour. Modesty, respect for others, and unbounded courage in the face of overwhelming adversity, are the mark of those remarkable men, who have been awarded the Victoria Cross. Their success meant the survival of their colleagues. The first was awarded in the Crimean War and the last was announced yesterday (March 2005) to Private Johnson Beharry from Grenada for his selfless action, twice under ambush in the Iraqi War – that makes only 1355 V.C.'s awarded since 1854, only 12 of which have been awarded since the Second World War.

Those who need knowledge of survival will not always know who they are, until their first symptom strikes. A policy of regular checking is therefore essential. We somehow have to raise public awareness to the point where unidentified, but potential, victims regard reconnaissance as important. They will need courage, because fear is what stops most of us getting ourselves checked. It also takes an interest and a motivation, which has to spring from somewhere. Fear will suffice as a stimulus, but common sense and the need to know the facts are more dignified.

ENERGY BALANCE AND STRESS

> We journey outward,
> Seeking paradise.
> We journey inward,
> Seeking peace.
>
> We depart in hope,
> Journey in stress;
> Spending life's energy.
> The blessed,
> Arrive after just one step.

Stress has become a big subject. It is a major concept without doubt, but one that is impotent medically. Because it fails to differentiate those at risk from those who are not, the concept lacks practical application for doctors. Every action has a reaction, but one that varies enormously between people. What we need, in order to use stress as a meaningful medical concept, is an explanation of why responses to the same stressful situations differ between individuals.

Imagine suddenly shouting and screaming at 100 strangers (I don't recommend it by the way). Reactions to such a verbal attack would vary enormously. Some would get angry, some would shout back; others would be shocked into submission and cry. Accompanying these responses, some would get a high blood pressure, and others would raise their blood cholesterol or suffer a racing pulse. The *reaction,* not the stress, is the relevant medical feature.

DISASTER AND STRESS

When heat waves brought Athens to a halt, many people died of heart attacks. The same has happened after earthquakes and all major disasters. Even the fear of potential disasters can reap the same havoc. While Israelis awaited Saddam Hussein's SCUD missiles, the heart attack rate in Tel Aviv soared.

One major risk factor, in any stressful catastrophic situation, is the removal of our feeling that we can control the situation. Living under curfew, with no water or electricity, nobody can do what he or she wants. Some can live with this deprivation; others loot shops, get angry, or try to find someone to blame. Once the idea sinks in, though, most people settle down, and adapt. Disasters shape humanity.

A common story abounds in medical circles, that during the Second World War, a healthier diet (fewer calories and less fat), was the responsible factor for fewer heart attacks in bomb-blitzed Britain. But is it true? How could doctors have known when somebody had had a heart attack I wonder? ECG machines were few in number, based in hospitals, and far too heavy to move around – certainly not the sort of thing you could have taken into a patient's home. Death certificates written during the Second World War were likely to be unreliable, because any death certificates not based on autopsy evidence, will always be unreliable. Even now, most autopsies performed by non-cardiac specialists rarely aim to detect minor coronary artery disease, so what chance had they 60 years ago? I was quite surprised when my search through some old cardiac textbooks dating back to the 1930's failed to find much mention of heart attacks. At the time, rheumatic heart disease was a far more important issue. For these circumstantial reasons, and from what we now know to be the human effects of war, the idea that heart attack rates fell in war-time Britain, is very unlikely to be correct.

During the Second World War, it is true to say that fatty meat was rationed, and that only 2 ounces (60 grams) of butter were allowed each week. Fruit was also difficult to obtain. Dietary change affected almost everyone . . . but fewer heart attacks? This assumption remains a mainstay argument for the many experts who are convinced that the current excessive intake of fat and calories is the principal cause of heart attacks.

THE STRESS OF POVERTY

The poor and those without power have fewer choices: to buy what they want, to live where they want, and to do what they want, when they want.

In Professor Geoffrey Marmot's study of Whitehall workers, those with the most security and power had fewer heart attacks; those with no security and no power had the most. In everyday life, the feeling that we are 'in control' is important for both health and disease.

Poverty of all sorts contributes to the incidence of disease. One can be impoverished in the basic requirements of life: food and water, clean air, and sunlight. One can be impoverished in spirit, depressed, and with no will to go on. One can be impoverished through a lack of self-esteem, faith, courage, and intelligence. All affect health. How they might affect disease processes is a much more controversial matter.

Tired people react to stress differently from those brimming with energy. Over 95% of those going to have a heart attack, will have experienced progressive tiredness, in the year before their attack. What then causes tiredness? The most important cause is poor sleep, which fails to 'recharge our batteries'. Poor sleep can result from business and family worries, depression, love, hate, anxiety, perfectionism, 'Type A' personality, poverty, bereavement, hostility, aggression, and resentment . . . to name but a few causes.

A PERSONALITY ISSUE?

Not everyone believes in the relevance of the so-called Type A and B personalities, but I do. Friedman and Rosenman, back in the 1970's, introduced the idea of a complex behaviour pattern that can double heart attack risk. They described the Type 'A' person as one who is 'time urgent'; a person who might look at their watch and say: 'just enough time to see my mother, buy a present for my girlfriend, get some petrol, make something to eat, and then get off to the airport!' So far, so good – but with only 90 minutes to spare before the plane leaves! They are usually aggressive, perfectionist, and believe that there is no other way to be if they are to become a success.

In fact, Type 'B's, who have the opposite traits, are just as often successful in life. They plan relaxation, and schedule time in their diary for both lunch and the gymnasium. They have time to spare because they are very realistic about what they can achieve within any given time frame. Type A's spend energy like mad, easily run down their energy reserves, and have heart attacks twice as often. They can change, but major life shocks, or prolonged therapy is required. Long holidays and retirement often bring about a change in their personality, but not always. In any case, the effect rarely lasts.

The Energy Secret

If you save more energy than you spend, you will have reserves of energy to draw upon. If you spend more energy than you save, you will get tired. It's that simple, but not always easy to deal with.

If you are unhealthily stressed, you will be spending more energy than you are saving. Many have the cherished belief that there is some secret to personal energy, there isn't: it's just a simple equation.

In my own survey of 1000 patients investigated for tiredness, only 15 had a discernable physical cause.

A lack of energy comes in several degrees of severity: tiredness, fatigue, and even exhaustion. Let me define what I mean by these. For a start, a stress is any demand on the body, physical (exercise) or mental (anxiety or solving problems); external (environmental), or internal (pain for instance). If you take a whip to *a tired man,* he can be made to do more. The *fatigued man* can do no more – he is at his limit. *The exhausted man* is past his limit, his energy has failed, and the whip causes his performance to collapse.

It takes more to make an athletic person tired or fatigued than it does a couch potato. Tiredness and fatigue also occur less readily in those trained to deal with stress. If you get exhausted, you cannot cope with even minor demands (stresses) – mentally or physically – and that may include opening your eyes in the morning! The aim of stress management must always be to reduce both the load and the reactions to it. Coping strategies can be learned, but tired people suffer from poor concentration, unreliable memory, muddled decision-making, and an inability to learn. It is, therefore, essential to treat their tiredness first. Rest, sleep, and relaxation come first, and then, once a solution to their energy draining problems has been found, they should get fit to fight off, or avoid, future stress.

If you want to know a little more about sleep and stress, look up an old article of mine written when I was researching such things at Charing Cross Hospital, London. The article is entitled: 'Sleep Therapy: sleep that knits up the ravell'd sleeve of care.' You will find this in the General Practitioner magazine dated 25.1.1980.

CHAPTER 9

Other 'Goodies'

In a Nutshell: Sleep restores our energy and is essential to all our physiological systems. This is especially important when you are stressed. Defective sleep, resulting from fear, worry, depression, and resentment, is an important risk factor since it may be associated with the onset or worsening of many medical conditions.

A commitment to exercise, can double our chances of living to 65 years. High-intensity, short-lasting, aerobic activity is best, but even walking the dog contributes. Being athletically adapted is best.

Alcohol and the many chemicals that make wine what it is, are cardioprotective. One drink daily could reduce heart disease risk by up to 50%. Alcohol can act as a double-edged sword – heavy binge drinking can cause heart rhythm problems, and even death; drinking red wine in moderation can be beneficial. I advise my patients to consider a maximum of two glasses of wine daily (approx. 200mls). Red wine is better than white. Wine is better than beer and spirits.

'Statin' drugs and aspirin can reduce the number of heart attacks and lower the death rates from cardiovascular diseases. They may be essential, if scanning shows your arteries to be 'furred' – regardless of your blood cholesterol. 'Furring' of arteries and a high blood pressure are the main causes of cardiovascular disease, with or without a raised blood cholesterol.

A good sense of humour, adaptability, a love of life, and being loved, should be good survival characteristics, but there is little or no research to confirm it. The theory is a weak one because too many humorous people have died young. Bob Hope was a notable exception. He lived to one hundred and was said to be the only comic older than his jokes!

Exercise

> *Did you know?* Exercise is the single most powerful intervention in the prevention of artery 'furring' and coronary artery disease. It prevents strokes and delays the onset of both high blood pressure and diabetes. It might also prevent some cancers. It can be more powerful than any dietary consideration, and more effective than the much-acclaimed 'statin' cholesterol lowering drugs. Rhythmic, vigorous exercise, that gets you breathless, done at least twice every week, is just sufficient to induce a beneficial effect.

Heavy gardening isn't good enough – it may be arduous, but it's too intermittent and not hard enough. What you need is sustained rhythmic exercise like rowing, cycling, running, and swimming. And never say 'I'm too old' – not unless you want to give into the tyranny of youth!

The highest levels of consistent aerobic exercise (you have to get breathless) can reduce your chances of a heart attack by up to 80%, although 50% is a more representative figure. In some cases, the advantages are even greater for older, fatter people. The advantages even extend to smokers, diabetics, and those with high blood pressure. Exercise improves your

It doesn't matter if you are overweight.

It doesn't matter if you are old . . . exercise.

Exercise can double your chances of living to 65!

immunity, your composure, your self-confidence, your shape (not necessarily your weight), your blood pressure (but not always), and your blood cholesterol (it can decrease 'bad' cholesterol, or LDL, and sometimes increases 'good' cholesterol, or HDL). It also limits artery 'furring' in the carotid (neck) arteries, as well as reducing the clotting tendency – both of which are relevant to the occurrence of heart attacks and strokes.

There are lots of good books and videos on exercise to refer to, but let me give you a potted version of what I think to be worthwhile.

Those rich enough can join a private gymnasium and employ a personal trainer. The less well off can join a public gym and exercise with a friend who knows how to train. Alternatively, go for a brisk walk regularly and aim to get breathless.

> The vitality and health gained from exercise could be worth more than any extra years of life. Both are worthy objectives, however.

In the past, doctors have worried too much about the dangers of exercise. There is now no doubt that it reduces sudden death from heart disease, heart attacks, and strokes. Remarkably, it has even been shown to improve conditions where the heart muscle is weak (heart failure).

In the 1930's and before, many school children with a 'heart murmur' (noise arising from heart valves) were not allowed out to play during school breaks. Twenty-five years ago doctors were worried about the exercise done by patients with coronary heart disease. Even now, many patients are told to 'take it easy'. This advice is, of course, too non-specific to be of any use. 'Train . . . don't strain', I was taught by Mike Welton, who once ran a gymnasium called 'Gym and Tonic', and actually started his own gym at the Loughton Clinic in the 1970's. Unfortunately, Mike was before his time and too few patients believed that he could lengthen, or at least improve, the quality of their lives. But wait a minute! Surely one can have a very happy, healthy, and long life, without much exercise at all? True, but your chances are better if you are fit.

(A newer meaning of 'fit' is to be attractive and 'sexy'. To be good at sex, it can help to be athletically fit, so both definitions suffice!)

Everyone who wants to train should exercise to the point of breathlessness. The point at which an Olympic athlete will get breathless, and the point at which a person with heart failure will get breathless, are at opposite ends of a wide spectrum. They have one thing in common though: both will get breathless when their hearts and lungs have had enough!

Health Warning!
Make sure that you are fit to get fit. If in doubt, consult you doctor

Gymnasium instructors love pulse rates as a guide to what we should do at any given age. Written instructions about pulse rates are even written on exercise equipment. This is physiological non-sense, and completely unnecessary when **all you have to do is stop when you get too breathless**. It's that simple. **Get your heart checked properly (ECG, exercise ECG, and artery scan) to make sure that you are safe to exercise, then forget pulse rates as a guide to how much exercise you should do.** Pulse rates are just too complex to interpret – even for cardiologists. If you do have heart disease, high blood pressure, asthma or some other lung disease, your ability to exercise will be restricted and might just be dangerous. **If in doubt, consult your doctor.** Exercise is possible for all, including those with heart and lung disease, with some advantage for everyone.

A Case History – John's Tale. How being fit can't save everyone: Only rarely do doctors encounter sport-related deaths. John's story illustrates some important lessons. He was a competitive squash player, playing in the top UK club leagues. His paraplegic teenage son needed to be carried upstairs to bed every night, and John was always easily capable of doing this, without a problem, because he was very fit.

On one occasion, during a squash match, he felt dizzy, and had to excuse himself in order to run to the toilet. He had diarrhoea, felt a bit off-colour, and retired early from the match

– *something he had never done before. After several weeks, when he failed to improve, he decided to seek his GP's advice.*

His doctor took his history, examined him, did a few blood tests and proclaimed that there was 'nothing wrong with him', that he could detect. John was not happy. 'Why do I feel so lousy then?' he asked. His GP was not sure, and referred him to a hospital physician for further testing.

The hospital physician examined him, did X-rays, and further blood tests, and pronounced him 'fit'. He asked the same question: 'why then, do I feel so lousy? I'm an athlete, and I have never felt like this. So what IS wrong?' The physician became short-tempered, and implied that he might seek psychological appraisal. John became very unhappy and retorted: 'I am an athlete, I'm not well, and you are seriously trying to tell me that there is nothing wrong!

When I saw him, he kept quiet about this story. Quiet, that is, until I had found something rather surprising wrong with him: he had had a very major heart attack, sometime in the past. Because he was clearly an athlete, no ECG (heart tracing) had previously been thought necessary.

He came back with some specific questions. 'Good', he said, 'now we can begin to get to the bottom of this. I want to know what has caused my problem?' I explained that he must have had a blocked coronary artery. The artery would have 'furred' first (like central heating pipes), and then clotted. No blood getting through to the heart muscle would cause heart tissue to die, and that is what we call a heart attack. There are several areas of the heart that can be affected, the most dangerous of which, is the front wall (a so called anterior infarction – the most dangerous sort).

That same week, I found that he had coronary artery disease, so widespread and so serious, that his condition was inoperable (beyond surgery) – a very rare situation.

I had to tell John that competitive squash might be dangerous. It's a bit like armed-combat, and he did admit to playing aggressively. 'Squash is a big part of my life', he confided, 'I'm not giving it up, but I'll try to play it in a friendly way!' John died on the squash court 3 months later.

When an ex-Olympic trainer, Al Murray, decided in the early 1970's, that he wanted to exercise post-heart attack patients, he could find nobody in the medical profession to back him, except my boss Dr Peter Nixon. It was thought to be 'too dangerous'. Two hundred years before, William Heberden had reported someone with angina who 'felt all the better for sawing wood twenty minutes every day' – a clue to possible future practice that had been over-looked. Peter, it seems, was only one of a few cardiologists who knew about safe exercise. He had been a paratrooper, and had watched men exercise until they dropped! He told me: 'even the best of the best, must come to know their limitations if they are to make successful SAS men'. After many years, Al saw nobody collapse or die in his exercise class – at least with him as an instructor. So many heart attack victims benefited from the exercise experience that the idea quickly spread. Now, you would never know that there had ever been any controversy about the idea.

SOME GUIDELINES FOR EXERCISE

When some people think of exercise, they feel tired! Don't lie down until the feeling wears off – your body was designed for exercise!

Nobody, it seems, really knows whether aerobic exercise or weight training is best for our arteries, so for the moment do both. I, personally, prefer non-impact exercises of all sorts. I have seen too many footballers with knee problems, and runners with hip and back problems, to feel happy recommending these sports. Cycling, rowing, and hard swimming are the best aerobically, with no impact involved whatsoever.

Cycle or row for twenty minutes continuously, or develop a circuit that suits you – that is, a series of exercises that uses every muscle. No more than 40 minutes in all, twice a week, is all you need to start with. You need to start sensibly, within your limits of available energy and breath. In the beginning your muscles will hurt afterwards. If they don't hurt, you may not be doing enough! Do 'interval training', that is, speed up in order to get breathless, then slow down until you feel comfortable again, then push the limits again, and repeat as often as you wish.

In general, **don't worry about your pulse rate, just concentrate on your breathing. If you can't get your breath,** you are doing too much – that applies, whether you are a couch potato or an Olympic athlete! You need to get breathless, and you need to push the limits.*(Those with heart disease and high blood pressure, should be tested to assess the advisability of this advice)*. You need to get breathless if you are to travel the path from couch potato to athlete. You don't need to become an athlete of course, merely to tread the path that leads to improved fitness and well-being.

You need some exercise every day, so between work-outs walk the dog and put a spring in your step – and don't be ashamed to get breathless.

IMPORTANT NOTE

The evidence suggests that it is not necessary but, if you have doubts about your health status, get a formal heart tracing, blood pressure, treadmill exercise test, and artery scan done before you get into exercise. This is especially true if you have a family history of heart disease or are over 35years of age. These tests can spot angina, unacceptably high blood pressure, and other medical problems, before you would know you had them yourself. Your doctor may be able to advise you, but remember, not every doctor has had training in health and exercise issues, and few have a personal interest, sufficient at least, to take them to the gymnasium themselves.

WHAT IS THE TECHNICAL EVIDENCE FOR THE BENEFITS OF EXERCISE?

It would be inappropriate here to give an exhaustive account of the evidence. Some headlines from the research work of a leader in the field, Professor J. N. Morris and his group, will give you the flavour of it. His pioneering epidemiological work has been with various groups of people, comparing those who exercise, with those who do not.

An all-UK autopsy study, started in 1954, asked the question: are the hearts of those middle-aged men who have exercised a lot, different from those who have not? Men who had undertaken physically demanding jobs had fewer severe narrowings in their coronary arteries and many

Carry-home message: sedentary executives, get 2 to 3 times more heart disease than their colleagues who exercise vigorously.

fewer heart muscle scars (called myocardial fibrosis from heart attacks). Exercise also appears to delay the onset of high blood pressure by ten years in the active groups.

An analysis of 18,000 men aged 40 – 64 years of age, of executive middle-management grade in government service, with no known heart disease followed. **Only vigorous exercise, (that is, enough to induce a training effect) was found to be protective.** Gymnasium and sport related exercise proved better than intermittent heavy gardening and work around the house. Social dancing and golf proved no advantage. **Comparing the vigorous exercise group with the sedentary group, the occur-**

Older men (55 years and older) who exercise, can reduce their cardiovascular mortality by one third.

rence of heart disease overall was reduced by half (6.9% down to 3.1%), in those who exercised vigorously. In detail, fatal heart attacks were reduced by exercise (2.9% down to 1.1%), as were non-fatal events (4% down to 2%) in the two groups. The overall mortality was 0.81% for those who exercised, and 1.7% for those who did not (40 – 49 yrs old), and 1.5% for an older exercise group, compared to 5% of sedentary people of the same age (55 – 64yrs old).

The advantages of exercise extend to smokers, the obese, diabetics, those with high blood pressure, those with poor health records, and those with a family history of heart disease. A surprising result is that **obese people who exercise, gain more of an advantage than those who are slim.** Even more surprising was the finding that, in those overweight people who exercised, the heart attack rate was

> Obese men are 12 times better off – if they exercise.

only 0.7%, compared to a rate of 8.8% for the sedentary obese (a twelve-fold advantage).

Over 15 years, the survival of exercising non-smokers was 91.5%, while that of non-exercising smokers was 78.9%. **Exercise and smoking are both major, but independent risk factors, for heart disease.**

The intensity and frequency of exercise are more important to health than the amount of time spent exercising. Body-building does not appear, in one study at least (McKillop 1987), to lower cholesterol and other blood-based risk factors. For what it's worth, the only two people I have ever known to double their HDL cholesterol (good cholesterol), did so over a period of two years, by weight training alone. Both had been weight trainers in their youth. (Tablets of nicotinic acid are also said to help raise the HDL level.)

In a study of 4000 sets of twins in Helsinki (Kaprio et al 2000), only half of the twins who exercised developed coronary heart disease, in comparison to those who did not. The twins who smoked, had a 3.3 fold increase in risk, and if diabetic, they had a ten-fold increase in their risk of coronary heart disease.

Animal and human research on arteries also shows the benefit of exercise. When elderly non-smoking sportsmen (older than 63 yrs), were compared to non-sportsmen, they had less than half the amount of 'furring' in their neck arteries. In another study, a slower progression of cholesterol build-up was seen in those who exercised (Lakka et al 2001). Similar benefits have also been seen in leg arteries, which are very commonly affected in smokers (Leng et al 2000). A strange fact is that over 99.99% of patients with leg artery 'furring' are, or have been, smokers. Why this is the case, nobody really knows, since such a close association is not apparent with smoking and the coronary arteries.

In a study of patients with angina, an exercise and low fat diet regime was shown to increase the flow of blood down the coronary arteries at both one and five years. A slowed pace of cholesterol narrowing in arteries, was also shown to occur in those who exercised (Niebauer and Hambrecht 1995). This was a very valuable study because the arteries were visualized directly (coronary angiography).

Does exercise benefit high blood pressure? In older people, low-intensity endurance exercise seems most effective in lowering high blood pressure. While exercise may delay the need for treatment, it is not a reliable treatment in itself.

Alcohol

Because alcohol can be good or bad for us, depending on dose and type, I have had to write about it in both the 'goody' and the 'baddy' sections.

I have previously mentioned the benefits of drinking red wine. Wine contains lots of 'goodies' (including the alcohol itself), and no 'baddies' (as far as the arteries are concerned). Drink enough alcohol though, and you will pickle both your heart and your liver! So here we have another typical Goldilocks scenario – the amount of alcohol you choose to take must not be too little or too much, but just the right amount for maximum benefit.

The beneficial effects of alcohol depend greatly on whether it is taken as beer, spirits or wine, because the effects of the many chemicals in these drinks may be quite different. From the point of view of heart disease protection, the benefits of wine, taken regularly with food, exceed those of beer and spirits. One beneficial effect of alcohol is that it can raise the level of HDL (good) cholesterol, and that may reduce cardiovascular risk more than just lowering total cholesterol itself.

Heavy drinking is associated with increased cancer (throat, liver, and breast), liver disease, brain haemorrhage, and strokes, and, more rarely, heart muscle weakness (cardiomyopathy). The top 10% to 15% of heavy drinkers, drink half of all the alcohol drunk in the USA! These big drinkers are the ones who get the most problems.

Spirit manufacturers may claim that their particular product is somehow 'pure' and 'clean', because many dangerous contaminants of illicit drink manufacture, have been removed. Methylated spirit, or methyl alcohol, as opposed to the usual ethyl alcohol found in alcoholic drinks, is one such dangerous impurity. Unfortunately there are small amounts in some very old red wines, and quite a lot in some home-made spirits.

I believe that some Californian chemists once undertook an analysis of old wine. Their aim was to mix together the actual chemical ingredients, discovered by the laboratory analysis of wine, in order to reproduce the exact taste of rare wines. Being able to preserve the taste of the exceptional Château Haut Brion 1928 for posterity was a fantastic idea. The mixture produced in the laboratory, however, could never have been sold as wine, simply because the mixture would have to be labelled a 'poison' or 'unsuitable for human consumption', so dangerous were some of its chemical ingredients.

Over many years of storage, fine red wines can generate chemicals such as amyl acetate (nail vanish remover) and methyl alcohol (methylated spirit) – both of which may contribute to its special taste, and to the fight your brain will have with reality the morning after! Wine bottles do not have to disclose their chemical constituents and there is no way of knowing what is in any wine without opening and testing it. In the case of red wine, at least, the chemical analysis at the time of bottling might be quite different several years later when it has matured. Spirits and white wines are less likely to change with time because they contain little remnant plant material, such as the stalks and grape skins, found as dregs in some red wines.

Any analysis of the benefits of wine is made difficult by the fact that the chemistry of wine not only varies with the composition of the soil in which the vines are grown but also with age and storage technique. The analysis of wine, used in my research, is based on what has been called 'average wine data'. This is very unsatisfactory because it does not represent any specific wines. Unfortunately, it is all I have had access to. Just how representative are the chemical concentration values I have used I am not sure.

According to my analysis, one small glass of red wine (100mls) scores 1.8, and white wine 1.6, for overall cardiac value (CVo16). The minimum beneficial overall cardiac value score is 3.0 and to achieve this you would need to drink 2–3 glasses of average red wine (250mls), and 3 glasses of average white wine (300mls). **A bottle of red wine (750mls) scores 6.8, and a bottle of white scores 5.6 – very good overall cardiac value, but too much daily alcohol for safety.** Two to three small glasses of wine per day are, therefore, good for the heart. The World Health Organisation recommends one glass every day.

Both red and white wines have a protective score above that of beer. The cardiac value of 100mls of beer is 1.2 (CVo16), and you would need to drink nearly one litre (2 pints or 900mls) to get the cardiac value of beer up to the minimum beneficial value of 3.0.

Wine is complex stuff, of course. Chemically, it contains lots of arginine and many other beneficial chemicals, but no fat or lysine at all. The deep colour of red grapes, raspberries, strawberries and blueberries, comes mostly from their polyphenol content. Polyphenols, flavanoids and reservatrol are important ingredients of wine, thought to be of benefit for several reasons: all have an anti-oxidant effect, a direct affect on the arteries themselves and an ability to reduce clotting. I have been unable to introduce these chemicals into my calculations because the quantities present in food are not generally known. Including them would make red wine even more valuable than my current calculations suggest. Out of interest, polyphenols and flavanoids are not only found in wine; they are also found in other plant-based products such as tea, liquorice, olive oil, cola drinks and grape juice.

THE FRENCH PARADOX

The French eat quite a lot of fat, smoke a lot, regularly drink wine with meals, and have less heart disease than we British. This has been called the French Paradox. The fact that saturated fat can cause 'furring' is undoubted but, given the results of almost a century of animal experimentation, it would seem that **the beneficial chemicals (as analysed in this book), are more abundant in the French diet than they are in the diets of many other countries. If these chemicals are more active in preventing 'furring', than saturated fats are in producing it, then the paradox is explained.** At least, this is my explanation. Wine is only one part of it, since in the UK we now drink more wine than any other EU country but still have a high rate of heart disease.

Drink more than three alcoholic drinks per day and death from all causes rises sharply; coronary deaths, though, do not increase until more than six or seven drinks are taken daily.

Alcoholic drinks contain a certain amount of pure ethyl alcohol, and the amount of pure alcohol we drink can determine death from all causes. As a yardstick, one bottle of 12% alcohol wine contains 90 millilitres (or 60 grams) of pure alcohol. For those who consume less than 20 grams of alcohol per day (one third of a bottle of wine), death from all causes is 20% for 100 people followed up for 10 years. For those who drink between one and two thirds of a bottle of wine per day, mortality drops to 8% for 100 persons followed for 10 years. With a further increase of alcohol intake to one bottle of wine per day, mortality from all causes rises again to 20% of 100 people followed for 10 years.

> Alcohol has been shown to reduce sudden death and heart attacks, but heavy drinking kills.

For *coronary heart disease* occurrence (fatal and non-fatal), the three corresponding figures are 14%, 7%, and 5% of 100 persons followed for 10 years. It would seem that the higher the level of alcohol intake, from one third to one whole bottle of wine per day, the lower the coronary mortality (Ref: U.Keil et al 1997).

Heavy drinking is thought responsible for the excessive mortality of young adults who tend to binge rather than drink continuously. In Russia, an average of 6 years of life expectancy was lost in the five years following 1993. A similar pattern of binge drinking is now emerging among the young of Great Britain and Finland where, unlike central Europe, large quantities of alcohol are drunk only at the weekend. It is a matter of debate as to whether the hearts of the young, as opposed to the old, are made electrically unstable by alcohol. It could be that sudden heart rhythm changes induced by alcohol are the cause of some premature deaths. Illicit alcohol production might contribute because such alcohol can contain poisonous impurities such as cobalt and arsenic. Once upon a time in the USA, someone had the idea of adding cobalt to beer in order to improve its 'head'. Cobalt does improve the head on beer but it also causes heart muscle damage and heart failure. As a consequence, large numbers of beer drinkers lost their lives.

Alcohol has another side effect – it can raise blood pressure. More than half a bottle of wine per day (greater than 30 grams or one ounce of alcohol) can cause a problem. High blood pressure can cause bleeding into the brain and a haemorrhagic stroke. The occurrence of these strokes is directly related to alcohol intake – the more you drink, the more likely you are to have a stroke. Strokes due to artery narrowing are more commonly associated with light and heavy drinking, so moderate drinking would seem to confer some benefit. It has been suggested, that heavy bingeing can cause clots to form in the heart or neck arteries. If these clots detach (an embolus), they can end up in the brain, causing a third type of stroke.

Alcohol can poison the heart muscle when large amounts are consumed on a regular basis. This is one potentially curable cause of heart failure. Withdraw the alcohol, and the heart can regain its strength. The prognosis, however, depends on the damage done to other organs. Alcohol may prevent heart disease, but it has the potential to give you liver and pancreas disease!

HOW MUCH BOOZE?

In 1870, Sir Francis Ainstie, a renowned neurologist, wrote in his book, 'On the uses of wine in health and disease', that 'three standard drinks daily' was an apt limit for mature men. Current advice seems to have departed very little from his rule. According to my calculations, the daily dose for the minimum benefit is 2 – 3,

100ml glasses of wine per day (14 – 21 Units/week). This should be just about safe for your liver, but then you have to consider your weight and mental functioning! Some would have it that one unit of alcohol per day is all that is necessary to reduce all cause mortality by 50%. The amount required for benefit will remain controversial because estimating exactly how much people do actually drink, and in what pattern, is difficult to measure. A independent chemical method\for cross-checking individuals would be handy, but an accurate one is not available.

FATTY LIVER AND CIRRHOSIS

While we are discussing alcohol, let me add a word of caution about alcohol and the liver. Alcohol can damage the liver and it does so initially by making it fatty. The fat fills the liver cells and displaces an enzyme called gamma-GT out into the blood, where it can be measured. If you have a raised gamma-GT, you may be drinking too much, although, some pharmaceutical drugs can also do the same thing. Alcohol can also affect the bone marrow, resulting in the production of larger than normal red cells. If patients with a fatty liver continue to drink, they may develop cirrhosis – an incurable and serious disease with a high mortality rate. There is a big problem here of individual sensitivity – some people can drink ten pints of beer per day, and not get cirrhosis; others can drink one glass of sherry every day, and end up needing a liver transplant! This is because genetic predisposition counts for a lot. In general, though, the more alcohol you drink, the more likely you are to end up dying of cirrhosis. The actual amount of alcohol is what counts, not whether it is consumed as wine, beer, or spirits. Because you can drink more alcohol more quickly by drinking spirits, they are thought to be the more dangerous. **If you must drink alcohol and want to avoid cirrhosis, limit your number of weekly units; do not drink every day, and only drink while eating food.**

SLEEP AND RELAXATION

Is stress bad, and sleep good for the heart? Can love and contentment calm a troubled heart? My guess is that these claims are true. Although these factors can affect the way the heart works, it is much more contentious to suggest that they have anything to do with the origin and progression of heart disease.

> **Historical Point:** *The question of how the mind affects the heart has a notable history. William Harvey, the man who we think of as the first man to demonstrate that the blood circulates around the body, wrote in his book, published in 1628 (The Motion of the Heart, or, De Motu Cordis), that:* **'motus autem cordis . . . the heart's movement varies according to the different emotions and sensations of the soul. For the sensations of the soul are not caused by changes in the heart but just the opposite is the case'.**
>
> *Although he left us with a physiological demonstration of the circulation, William Harvey was disappointed to have failed in his mission – to understand just how the mind affects the heart.*

What William Harvey could not have known, was that the heart is connected to the brain (and therefore to the emotions) by two special sets of nerves, which influence its rate, rhythm and strength of contraction. One set acts like an accelerator (the sympathetic nervous system), the other acts as a brake (the parasympathetic nervous system). Unlike the set-up in a car, both work simultaneously, and are varied by emotion, and exercise. Something else he could not have known is that blood adrenaline, nor-adrenaline and cortisone, produced in response to stress, can also affect the heart. Both adrenaline and nor-adrenaline are capable of raising blood pressure, increasing the output of the heart, causing palpitations, inducing angina, and promoting clotting. Too much adrenaline can kill, even without 'furred' arteries. Like a rabbit faced with a fox, we too can die of shock. More gradual, but similar changes in the blood and tissue chemistry, may be responsible for the deaths that occur in association with a 'broken' heart. When one member of a typical 'Darby and Joan couple' dies, the other will often die within three years.

These ideas can make some doctors uncomfortable. Many still prefer to limit their work to physical disease alone and leave this aspect of medicine to psychotherapists. I once asked a colleague of mine at Charing Cross, one of the best intensive care cardiologists I have known, why he wasn't, like William Harvey, interested in how the mind affects the heart. His answer was simple and direct: 'I'm not that sort of doctor!' The moral of the tale is: be careful whom you choose to understand your emotional problems. Be even more careful when it comes to the person who holds your life in his hands in the intensive care unit!

WHAT IS STRESS?

Like alcohol, stress can be both a 'goody' and a 'baddy', so I have to repeat some of what I wrote before in order to complete the picture.

We all talk about it, but what do we mean by stress? Many and various forms of trouble and aggravation, I suspect. How do I define stress? That's easy: I think of it as *any applied force*. OK, so nobody is forcing you to do anything, but force can be a very subtle thing. When you open your eyes in the morning and have to deal with the light, the heat, the cold, the hunger and the noise – biologically, your body is having to respond to stressors. All stressors will excite a response, and your reaction will be greater if you are irritable: if you have not slept well, if you have worries, and especially if you are in fear of what is going to happen to you. These are at one end of the stress spectrum. Having a burglar break into your house at three o'clock in the morning, tie you naked and blind-fold to a chair – that is at the other end of the stress spectrum!

What matters, medically, is how you react. The possible reactions vary from sudden death, to one bead of sweat forming on the brow. Some people increase their blood cholesterol; some their blood pressure and others their blood coagulability. Each of these can make a heart attack or stroke more likely. Making these reactions more extreme is tiredness induced by poor sleep. Poor sleep can be caused by anxiety, fear, depression, disturbing life circumstances and the many medical problems that can disturb sleep. Among them are painful conditions such as arthritis and conditions that affect breathing, such as the common cold, hay fever, bronchitis and asthma. In very overweight people, sleep apnoea (obstructed breathing), disturbs sleep and can cause blood oxygen levels to drop dramatically. This is dangerous because it can lead to cardiac arrest and death during sleep. Leave the lights on and your car engine off, and chances are that your car battery will go flat: fail to sleep on a regular basis, and you will get tired, irritable and respond that much more to any given stress. At worst, *your* lights will go out!

The benefits of deep, relaxed, restorative sleep are that it induces composure and defuses the responses that might otherwise help induce migraine, stroke, heart attacks and other major medical events. We all need to preserve our sleep, but how is good sleep possible with a troubled mind?

Not everyone gets a troubled mind, of course. There are many people, loved by their family, adored by their partner, and with enough self-esteem to feel contented with their life. They have the chance of sleeping peacefully. But can this happy state beneficially influence the progress of heart disease? That is much less certain. I have seen it many times though, so I believe it can.

Joe and Bill . . . both cured by love?

Here are the stories of two older men with heart disease, both of whom found new love later in life, when they least expected it.

Joe's Story *Joe was a long-standing patient of mine. He was 65 years old when he developed angina. Soon after, he had a coronary bypass which relieved his pain. His wife then became* seriously ill with leukaemia and died soon after. They had been a 'Darby and Joan' couple and associated with his bereavement, which lasted at least two years, his angina returned, even though his coronary blood flow seemed adequate. Within eighteen months he had developed 'furring' in one of his bypasses. Angioplasty was tried, but was not successful – that was in the early days of the technique. His angina became disabling, even with full medication, so he decided to 'take it easy' from the demands of running his successful company.

Because he was unable to do much physical work, he engaged a contract gardener. One day his usual man became ill and was replaced by a 35 year-old woman. Like him, she was a no-nonsense, hard-working, achiever. They both felt something stir. 'No', he thought, 'I'm too old for this'. He discussed it with me. "I don't know why she's interested in me", he said, "I could be her father!" My advice was, 'to go with the flow'. Joe fell in love, and so did she.

Without any further intervention, and having given up all of his medication (pills under his tongue and a beta-blocker), Joe no longer seemed to have angina. Since then, I hear that he remains happy and well, and without any heart symptoms.

Was this a miracle, or is there a scientific explanation? I would like to think that it was a miracle, but it is more likely that finding love reduced his production of adrenaline-like chemicals. Adrenaline drives the heart to burn lots of oxygen – oxygen that cannot easily be delivered to the heart muscle down narrowed or 'furred' coronary arteries. With contentment lessening the need for oxygen, Joe's narrowed arteries might have been able to deliver all that his heart required, relieving him of pain.

Bill's Story Bill, died on Christmas Eve, 2004. He had heart failure as a result of 'furred' coronary arteries, although at no time did he ever have angina. The first we knew of his heart disease was when he awoke one night, short of breath. That was his first episode of heart failure (pulmonary oedema – his lungs had filled with fluid). An echocardiogram showed that his heart was dilated and not contracting well. When the heart fails, blood dams back into the lungs, causing breathlessness *while, at the same time, pumping too little blood forward into the circulation. The results, in addition to breathlessness, are: cold hands and feet, tiredness, and even exhaustion.*

By this time, Bill had come through a difficult and protracted period of separation and divorce. He was obviously stressed. Like Joe, love arrived on the scene, as if 'out of the blue'. With Joanne, he found a form of happiness, peace and contentment that was obvious to all. They were married and, in due course, Joanne gave birth to their son, Alistair, bringing them both much joy.

Bill was taking all the best medication but was worried about his outlook. A failing heart limits lifespan. To my surprise, his heart on echocardiogram looked stronger, and less dilated when I saw him last. His medication could now be lessened, I thought. Still he remained well. Could this unusual improvement, over and above the effect of medication, be due to his new-found joy? I believed it to be so. 'Bill', I said, 'your heart is improving, and that is something I can't easily explain and have only rarely seen'. 'Don't knock it', he said, 'I'm just thankful that that's the case. I'm sorry if you don't understand it, but I'm very happy about it!'

On his return from a business trip to Australia he had a virus, which took some time to shake off. At the end of an Indian meal in a local restaurant, he fell ill with gastroenteritis. Joanne telephoned me for advice. We agreed he wasn't bad enough to be admitted to hospital since his diarrhoea and vomiting had stopped. Re-hydration was appropriate, and Joanne went out for half an hour to buy him some bananas and re-hydration drinks (potassium is lost in diarrhoea, and bananas and some re-hydration drinks contain a fair amount of it). Sadly, Bill was not alive when she returned.

Bill's weak heart had improved. Could finding love and happiness in his life have contributed? I'm sure they did. Pathological processes, like 'furring' and heart muscle weakness, however, cannot be reversed by any known state of mind. Like Joe, he may have deteriorated his heart condition by producing too much adrenaline. Adrenaline can accelerate 'furring', raise blood pressure, cause clotting and induce deadly heart rhythm changes. Love and contentment, by reducing the adrenaline produced, could limit these processes and act to calm a troubled heart.

DRUGS AND THEIR USES

Prevention Strategies: For those who know nothing much about medical research in general and drug research in particular, **primary prevention** applies to 'normal' people (the disease or condition to be prevented, has yet to arise). **Secondary prevention** applies to those who already have a problem and would like to stop complications developing, or a repeat of the condition arising.

Medicated or natural sleep?

It could be said that our brains are badly designed because the more tired we get, the less well we sleep. Tiredness will lead to fatigue, fatigue to exhaustion, and exhaustion to collapse. This will happen if you over-run your energy-spending budget, and pay too little attention to your energy-saving budget.

Sleeping tablets are not a long-term solution for poor sleeping patterns but they can help short-term, through very troubled times. They can be a crutch while you get on and solve your problems. Since your judgment will deteriorate if you don't sleep, your problems could get worse if you make some bad decisions. Best to consult your doctor if you feel that this is happening; (s)he will be able to help. If your sleep problem is severe, you may be offered a sedative anti-depressant, since these drugs are non-addictive. Valium (diazepam) works well for short periods, but it is very addictive. This may be OK if you are not an addictive personality, but that can be difficult to assess.

Simple sleep-promoting measures, such as going to bed early, winding down before sleep, a comfortable bed, avoiding alcohol, a good blackout curtain and noise limiting strategies, will all help. An afternoon sleep or siesta can be invaluable. This may involve delegating the care of your child or delegating the gardening, shopping, or DIY to others, while you sleep. If you are excessively tired, grab sleep whenever you can. Forget conventional time. If you can sleep during the day – sleep. If you need to work in the middle of the night – do so, if you are awake enough. These are survival tactics. Since they are good enough for the SAS, they are good enough for you!

Relief of pain and symptoms that might stop you sleeping are essential moves. Again, your doctor needs to be involved.

One thing is for sure, if you don't sleep and you carry on spending energy on fear and worry, you will become energy deficient. As a consequence, your concentration, decision-making ability and sense of humour will suffer. What is more, you might well become a thorough nuisance to others, if only because of your irritability.

For many, slight degrees of tiredness are overcome by having a good time, relaxing and switching off with friends (now called 'chilling-out'). Holidays can be relaxing, as long as you are allowed to recharge yourself, rather than be forced to spend energy you cannot afford – trudging over mountain paths, being dragged unwillingly around shops, pottery factories, cathedrals and art galleries. The artists and architects whose work you might be encouraged to admire could not have known about your life and its priorities, so there is a time and place for your interest in theirs. Your priority is to sleep; the Uffizi and the Tuscan countryside will wait! Get your priorities in order. Without fuel in its tank, even the most powerful, expensive and prestigious car, is going nowhere. If you are tired out or exhausted – without any further supply of energy, you won't be going very far either!

Lowering Blood Cholesterol

Statistically, a nation will better off, the lower its average blood cholesterol.

Statistically, it impossible to say if an individual will be better off, the lower his or her blood cholesterol.

The only way to make sense of biological data (that is, facts about you and me) is to lump it all together in an average, and go from there. Statistics anchor us down to a general view of reality, but cast us adrift when it comes to viewing personal situations. They give us an excellent measure of the general risk we face, but no measure at all of our individual destiny.

An average, and its difference to other averages, is good solid stuff. We can even state how reliable such differences are likely to be. Such figures provide the best overview of biological data we can get. What they cannot do is give us individual detail – probabilities about what you and I should do for the best.

The variations between you, me, and the girl next door, are so great that whatever applies to me, is quite unlikely to apply to you. *You may have a low blood cholesterol and 'furred' arteries, I may have a higher blood cholesterol and clean arteries. You may benefit long-term from lowering your cholesterol, and I may not.* Those of us, who are aware of it, face this mathematical dilemma every day – to treat or not to treat a patient, on the basis of statistical results. As it happens, we doctors have too little time to worry about such a dilemma; in general we are encouraged to be guided by the statistics we are fed. Our approach is individual, but our treatment is of the group.

If you are a doctor responsible for the health of a whole nation, your job is staightforward. Based on what is known statistically, you must order that every doctor lower the blood cholesterol of all his patients. That way the national figures for heart attacks will drop – the lower the average blood cholesterol, the greater the benefit. If you are an individual doctor treating an individual patient, you have to ask whether you want to treat each patient as part of a group, or whether you want to treat each patient as a unique individual. You can make it easy on yourself and treat everyone as part of a group; all you have to do is follow the guidelines generated from statistics. You will be on safe ground, but you will not be on safe ground if your patient demands to be treated as an individual.

The ultimate way to overcome the problem will be to provide individual genetic information about each of our risks. If we had this information on our desks to-day, we would get reports like this – *you __will__ have a low blood cholesterol and __will__ get 'furred' arteries, I __will__ have a higher blood cholesterol and __will__ keep clean arteries. You __will__ benefit long-term from lowering your cholesterol, and I __will__ not.* The words used to express uncertainty have all been replaced by 'will'.

Having tested the blood cholesterol of 2000 patients, some with a lot of artery 'furring' and others with completely clean arteries, I know that you cannot relate one to the other. **In other words, in individuals, the blood cholesterol is a hopeless guide to the state of our arteries.** Whether it is a good predictor of what will happen to the arteries of individuals in the future, I cannot yet say – I haven't lived long enough! If we accept that blood cholesterol will predict future artery disease, we must lower it, regardless of any artery scanning information. My money, however, is on the fact that it will not be a good future predictor in individuals, but that needs proof.

Although we are not there yet, the genetic revolution is upon us. Until the promised benefits are with us, some of us are trying to get the further information we need to help us treat individuals, as individuals. This is why we are making use of various blood tests other than blood cholesterol (homocysteine, CRP, lipoprotein a, fibrinogen), and order tests such as carotid artery scanning, and EBCT scanning. Later on we might add PET scanning (Positron Emission Tomography), which promises to show whether or not an individual has actively inflamed and dangerous 'furring', or burned out harmless plaques in their arteries.

GREAT MISTAKES?

How many patients with normal cholesterol will die unnecessarily of heart disease, because they were thought *not* to have a problem?

Many people with a normal blood cholesterol have 'furred' arteries, and need treatment. Without artery scanning, this group is passed over because they are thought to be normal. Could this be one of the biggest mistakes of omission made by modern medicine?

How could this be? The answer is – you only need one serious artery narrowing in your coronary arteries to kill you. 'Furring' is usually generalized, but it can be very localized. No test is good enough to detect all those at risk, although progress is being made. The widespread screening of arteries is a possible solution, but it will have to meet the economic restrictions put in place by governments, medical insurance companies and individuals themselves. Here is a comic lesson for those who would apply such restrictions:

Jack Benny, one of the late, great, American comedians, was thought to be so mean, that Bob Hope said of him: 'he gave up golf when he lost his ball!' Jack told the story about being held up in his car by a highway robber. 'Your money or your life?' demanded the robber. When no reply was forthcoming, the robber repeated the question with added decibels: *'Your money or your life?'* Jack took his time (he was a grandmaster of timing), and finally said – 'Can't you wait . . . I'm thinking about it!'

Because your cholesterol blood level is only a very indirect measure of what is going on in your arteries (it's more to do with liver function), it is bound to be inaccurate. How do you find out what is in a jewellery box, without opening it? You can weigh it, shake it, listen to it, X-ray it, or ask a spiritualist! But wouldn't it be a lot easier just to open the box and have a look inside? That is *just what we are doing when we scan arteries: having a look, rather than second-guessing with a blood test.*

> ## Ken & Dr 'D':
>
> **Ken**: 'D', I've stopped taking my blood cholesterol pills.
> My doctor says I don't need them now because my
> blood cholesterol is OK!
>
> **Dr 'D'**: 'Are you crazy! You've had a coronary bypass
> and two leg bypasses. It's because you have a big
> problem with the cholesterol 'furring' your arteries, and
> not with your blood cholesterol, that you have had all of
> your problems. Forget your blood cholesterol and start
> worrying about the cholesterol building up in your
> arteries. If anyone needs treatment for their arteries, you
> do! And that need will never stop, at least not for you!

Fortunately for Ken, and those of us with the same problem, 'statin' drugs can lower blood cholesterol (by their action on the liver – like alcohol; they can also raise the gamma-GT), and stop artery 'furring'.

You have recently spent quite a bit of money on your car, your clothes, on a holiday, and on your home, and you don't have much left . . . right? Without knowing the state of your arteries though, you simply don't know how much longer you might be around to enjoy these material possessions. So have you got your financial priorities right? Well, OK, you didn't know about artery 'furring' before – but you do now!

It is important to make clear that my personal view about blood cholesterol and its relevance has been shaped by my own research and is not necessarily consistent with the official view at the moment. What follows is my personal advice – that too may not be consistent with the general advice currently available.

If you have 'furred' arteries and high blood cholesterol (raised LDL and low HDL), you are at high risk and should go for every beneficial intervention possible. Those with a lesser degree of 'furring', might decide to adopt all the non-drug measures known to benefit groups of patients in general, namely: smoking cessation, exercise, and the Mediterranean diet etc. In addition, I would advise taking all of the micronutrients known to stop 'furring' as a daily supplement. Those with severe 'furring', need all the help they can get – all the above measures, plus a 'statin' drug in a dose that can be proven to stop the progress of 'furring' in their arteries. There is only one way to know whether any of these measures are putting a stop to the 'furring', and that is to test the arteries regularly.

As we now think that the progression of 'furring' is a separate measure of risk, regular checks are essential. This requires a suitably repeatable test that is completely harmless. At the moment, only artery ultrasound really fits the bill. Magnetic resonance scanning (MRI) of the heart, may prove useful in the long run, but it is still under development and is not widely available. EBCT heart scanning is very useful, but because it involves quite a lot of X-rays, it should not be repeated too often.

'STATIN' DRUGS

So what are these 'statin' drugs that so many of us now take? They represent an enormous advance, without any question. In my opinion, you must not hesitate to take one if you have significant artery 'furring', or evidence of its progression over 1-2 years. The only problem is, knowing what dose to take. I am not convinced that normalizing the blood cholesterol is the best guide. What is my practice? My patients have their artery scans done regularly in order to see if their 'furring' process has been halted. If not, I double their dose, within the limits of safety, until it does.

'Statins' are blood cholesterol reducing drugs. There are four different varieties on the market that are difficult to choose between. In order to choose the most effective one, three important questions must be answered:

- 'do they stop, stabilize, or reverse the 'furring' of arteries?'

- 'do they reduce clotting', and,
- 'what side effects do they have?'

As with all tried and tested drugs, they do have side effects. In my experience, and from the results of published research trials, the side-effects of 'statin' drugs are very few and mainly relate to bowel problems. Others have found 20 – 30% with unacceptable side-effects. Among the problems are liver test abnormalities, alopecia (very rare), kidney problems, pins and needles, impotence, muscle inflammation (one 'statin' was withdrawn because of it), and sleep problems, all of which are quite rare. Interestingly, a recent large study of simvastatin, the Heart Protection Study, showed more side effects from the innocuous placebo (chalk), than it did for the simvastatin! Is that possible?

Over a 5 – 7 year period, the primary reduction in coronary heart disease is about 30% with 'statins'; this being achieved with no increase in overall mortality (Pignone, M., 2000). Doctors are, however more likely to prescribe for secondary prevention (Fairhurst, K., 1998) but both forms of protection are currently in use.

The Heart Protection Study was aimed at secondary prevention in those patients who had evidence of heart disease. The effect of simvastatin 40mgs daily, was to decrease overall mortality by 12%, to reduce cardiovascular mortality by 17%, and to reduce coronary events by 24%. Strokes were reduced by 27%. The secondary prevention figures for the Mediterranean diet are better, but the racial and other differences between the studies detract from making direct comparisons.

Because of cost, governments are restricting the usage of 'statin' drugs, but in the UK they have recently been made available 'over the counter'. My patients quite often buy their own, and mostly believe that the drugs are 'good value for money'. Following their first heart attack or stroke, patients who had previously decided against them, come to regard them as very cheap! The problem is, 20 – 50% of those who do decide to take 'statins', do not take them for long. Many questions remain about 'statins', the biggest one of which is the likelihood of side-effects in the long term. Time alone will tell.

Aspirin

Aspirin reduces the clotting tendency and, therefore, reduces the occurrence of clot formation in arteries. In 'normal' subjects (no known heart disease) it has been shown to reduce the number of heart attacks by one third (caused by clotting), to sometimes decrease strokes by 20%, but to increase the number of haemorrhagic strokes (caused by bleeding). The results vary a lot from one study to another. Where obvious risk factors exist – smoking, diabetes, a positive family history or a raised blood cholesterol, the advantages are likely to outweigh the risk of bleeding.

In people without coronary artery disease or any other high-risk condition like 'furring' in the arteries, taking 75mgs of aspirin daily has obvious merit, although it can more than double the risk of bleeding (2.5 – fold). For those with defined artery 'furring', those who have already had a heart attack, and those with a proven clotting tendency, 75 – 150mgs of aspirin, taken every day, has many advantages. For such patients, the advantages far outweigh the risks.

High blood pressure is a cause of haemorrhagic stroke (due to bleeding in the brain), and so is aspirin (and vitamin E). For this reason, I never suggest that my high blood pressure patients take aspirin, unless I am sure that they have very well controlled blood pressure (a satisfactory 24 hour recording). Those with certain stomach problems which may cause bleeding (ulcers, hiatus hernia etc) should also consider aspirin, even in small doses, to be dangerous until proven otherwise.

There are possible alternatives to aspirin such as clopidrogel (Plavix in the UK), for which there is good evidence of effectiveness, and perhaps vitamin E (synthetic and 'natural'), for which there is little evidence. These might be considered when aspirin is considered inappropriate, but you must seek your doctor's advice if this relevant to you.

PART 4

Conclusions

CHAPTER 10

Is it True –
No Food is Good Enough?

In a Nutshell: The genes we inherit are crucial to whether or not we will 'fur' our arteries. Once such an inheritance is in place, we can make 'furring' much more likely by smoking, eating the 'baddies' and ignoring diabetes – and, much less likely, by exercising regularly, controlling our weight, and eating food rich in the 'goodies'.

No one food is good enough to supply all the micronutrients needed to maximize our chances of avoiding the 'furring' process in our arteries. Various food combinations can provide enough, but there is a very limited choice. As it turns out, the healthiest daily diet for us today might not be that unfamiliar to a Stone-Age family. Perhaps we evolved successfully on such a diet and cannot cope as healthily with modern alternatives – simply because we were not designed to.

The artery disease that plagues the western world could be due more to the absence of preventative chemicals, than to the presence of fats, although both will contribute. There are foods that can supply some of the chemicals we need, without too many calories, but they are few in number and are not that popular. Also, the foods that contain the best of the best, like offal, shellfish, nuts, seeds and oily fish, are not everybody's 'cup of tea'!

It has been shown that a Mediterranean diet, rich in the right chemicals (but not low in fat), can reduce second heart attacks by 70% over 4 years: a better result than 'statin' drugs! This is consistent with the theory, that the 'goodies' in food (atheroprotective chemicals), are more powerfully good for us than the 'baddies' (atherogenic fats and lysine) are bad for us.

The reduction in cardiovascular deaths in the last thirty years might have several contributory factors: the general reduction of fat intake, an enormous increase in vitamin and supplement tablets consumed, and a steady change towards the Mediterranean diet.

If you have no high blood pressure or heart attacks in your family, are athletic, not overweight, and are not a diabetic, or a pre-diabetic – you may be able to forget about food and its disease implications. If not, and you are to keep your arteries and heart healthy, it is possible to construct a diet of positive overall cardiac value, but few will enjoy it, day in day out, without variation.

The best cardiovascular protection requires that we first eat the best of diets – low in all 'baddies' – salt, saturated fat, trans-fat, lysine, and calories, as well as rich in all the 'goodies. Thereafter most of us are going to need supplementation with all the 'goodies', in order to boost the cardiac value of our modern diets. A 'balanced diet' is essential for general health but for heart and artery disease prevention a more specific diet is required.

In all of us, the 'furring' process starts in our youth and steadily progresses throughout life, predictably related to our age. The older we get, the thicker the inner lining of our arteries will become.

The average thickness of the inner lining of our neck arteries (the intimal thickness or IMT), is so predictably related to age, that it can be used as a measure of our biological age (see graph in Appendix 4). If your inner arterial thickness is less than predicted for your age – you are aging slower than your contempories and are younger biologically than your actual age would suggest. If your artery inner lining is thicker than predicted for your age, you are aging faster than average and you are biologically older than your actual age would suggest.

Because our arteries supply vital blood and oxygen to all our organs, they are of key importance to our healthy survival. Intimal thickness, as a measure of biological age (and there are many others), could thus be regarded as a crucial test of cardiovascular health, and also as an indicator of long-term survival potential. If you have had a medical check-up without having this measured, you will not have been checked for the commonest cause of our demise – the arterial 'furring' process.

This gradual increase in intimal thickness is due to the 'furring' process, and can be regarded as a 'natural' result of aging – up to a point. When the process progresses faster than predicted, we no longer think of it as 'natural', but as a disease process. It forms mounds of cholesterol-laden bumps within our arteries (plaques of 'furring' or atherosclerosis) which, if large enough, will eventually stop the sufficient flow of blood and lead to conditions such as angina, heart attacks (coronary artery disease) and strokes (cerebro-vascular artery disease).

In other organs, such as the kidney, the 'furring' can cause kidney damage and high blood pressure. In the legs, the same process limits the blood supply to the calf muscles, causing pain on walking (claudication). *High blood pressure and artery 'furring' are the two most important components of cardiovascular disease – the major causes of middle-aged death in the western world.*

What is the cause of this dangerous 'furring' process in arteries that goes beyond the simple thickening we see with age? There can be little doubt that the process is largely inherited – it obviously runs in families but is also associated with diabetes, obesity and smoking. *If* *you have not inherited bad genes, it is possible that nothing you do will cause it to occur. However, at the moment, we cannot prove that.* If you have inherited bad cardiovascular genes, the full analysis of which is eagerly awaited, there are a number of measures you can introduce to help yourself. Almost a century of research has shown that certain food chemicals can, either propagate, or inhibit, the 'furring' process, as well as influence the end results of 'furring', such as strokes and heart attacks. You can choose not to smoke or exercise, but you have to eat something, so you must first choose a diet of consistently high cardiac value if you can get used to it.

The degree to which the 'furring' process can be modified will probably vary from one person to another. Eating a diet rich in all of the 'goodies' and low in all of the 'baddies', together with supplementation, exercise, some alcohol, freedom from stress – can all help in a preventative way. Smoking, obesity, stress, diabetes, and eating too many food 'baddies', with too few 'goodies', can all accelerate the problem.

Because we are faced with an increasingly complex set of directives from both medical and nutritional authorities, walking around a supermarket trying to decide what to choose can present quite a problem – if you want to take all of this seriously that is. As well as reading about the salt, sugar and fat content of food displayed on packet foods, others are now choosing to add yet another factor for us to take into account – **the glycaemic factor** – that is, how much the food will raise our blood sugar (this is included in the calculation of overall cardiac value).

To add to the problem, natural foods don't always come in packets, so where is the information about their chemical contents? All of this is of undeniable importance, but are we not now in danger of getting utterly confused by information overload? Apart from being confused, the public is also liable to be misguided by thinking that salt, fat and glycaemic index are the only important constituents. Almost no account is taken of the 'goodies' in food. *This is where the overall cardiac value of food comes in – just one number to look for – one number that expresses the balance of all of the important factors in food, good versus bad.*

Even if you are a diabetic, have high blood pressure, or have some 'furring' in your arteries, reference to **the cardiac value of food allows you to easily answer some simple, but vital questions** – *which foods are truly good, bad or indifferent for my heart, my blood pressure and my diabetes, and, what should my daily diet be in order to maximise my cardiovascular health?'*

Why has a simple single score never been attempted before? All technology starts complex, and then is gradually simplified – that is its natural history. Is it technically valid? The score, as it is, is certainly valid for consumers to use now, but the technical details will need upgrading over time as the results of further scientific experiments become available. Questions such as the variation of food composition, and the actually relevance of each chemical component, are the major issues to be addressed by further research. Answers to questions such as: how much more powerful is trans-fat than saturated fat in causing 'furring' and, how much more important is selenium than omega-3 fatty acid, in preventing the 'furring' process, will need to be answered before the cardiac value can be further refined. This is not for consumers, but for food scientists and cardiologists to work out over the coming decades.

As I have presented it, the cardiac value is a starting point, not an end-point. It will need modification and development over time. For the moment, it provides the only single overall cardiovascular food value score available.

To get a good cardiac value score, food has to be really good for the circulation, and to get a bad score the food has to contain an awful lot of what is bad for the circulation. At a practical level, a good score means that the food will be acceptable for:

- all those who wish to prevent artery 'furring',

- all those who want to halt the 'furring' they already have,

- all those with maturity onset (Type 2) diabetics, and

- all those with salt-sensitive high blood pressure (not everyone is helped by a low salt, high potassium diet).

There would be no point in introducing a score that ignores any of these conditions, simply because they are all inextricably linked to the heart disease processes that cause the majority of our middle-aged deaths.

For those of us over thirty-five years old, guidance about what to eat is needed now – we simply don't have enough time left in life to wait for the research and development. That is not to say that it shouldn't be done! My guess is that the results of genetic engineering will come on-stream long before such answers are available. We will have to wait and see!

ERRORS IN CARDIAC VALUE SCORES

There is one major technical problem with calculating the cardiac value as I have done it – the variability of one type of food with another. I am not sure how accurate the quoted data is from the various reference works available to me, but I have assumed the usual laboratory error of ±10%. To make cardiac value testing more reliable we would have to introduce standardised techniques – have one reputable laboratory measure the chemical concentrations of different samples of food on sale in a particular store, and use that data to do the calculations. That would lead to results that could be relied upon.

Stating my results to two decimal places (implying great accuracy) is contentious since I cannot really know the true accuracy of the data used in my calculations. For this reason, foods that are *truly* different must have extreme differences in their cardiac value. For instance, a food with a cardiac value score of 2 (turkey breast), is likely to be truly different to a food with double (cod = 4.37), or half (water = 1), of that score. There is likely to be no real difference when cardiac values are close to one another, as with cardiac values of 2.6 (brussel sprouts) and 2.8 (lobster).

The only way to achieve improved reliability is to introduce the standardisation of food testing for cardiac value.

HEART DISEASE IS REALLY NOTHING NEW

John Hunter, a famous Scottish surgeon and anatomist, died of coronary artery disease. He was previously reported to have said: 'my life is in the hands of anyone who cares to annoy me!' John Hunter died after getting irate at a St George's Hospital board meeting in London. At a post-mortem examination, his coronary arteries were found to have 'turned to stone'. Any idea that coronary artery disease is simply a modern phenomenon is, therefore, wrong. In those days, fewer people made it to adulthood and middle-age than they do now, and since heart disease mostly occurs in middle-aged people, two hundred years ago you had to be lucky to get it!

Has heart disease changed much in the last 200 years? The standard teaching is, that it increased up to the 1960's, and then decreased. This belief is not based on the very best of evidence – autopsy data, but on the surmise of doctors issuing death certificates. The surmise is, that when older people die suddenly, or in an unexplained way, they must have had heart disease! Perhaps we should forget the years before the 1960's, since it is now truly impossible to verify what was going on. Coronary death, as reported on death certificates, means little if the actual 'furring' in the coronary arteries, or the actual heart damage from a heart attack, was not verified by autopsy.

> *A bit of personal biography:* Mention of St George's Hospital London reminds me of two old friends who taught me a lot.
>
> When I was a British Heart Foundation research fellow, I worked at St George's Hospital, Hyde Park Corner, London – just down the road from Harrod's, and across the square from the first Hard Rock Café. We were there the day after it opened: Paul Kilgfield (an inspired New Yorker and Cardiologist), Alan Gelson (a gifted physician and teacher), and myself.

The very latest research has looked at the occurrence of heart disease in middle-aged men (aged 40 to 59 years old) between the years 1978 and 2000; a period when saturated fat consumption decreased significantly. Major coronary events like heart attacks decreased by 3.6%, but new diagnoses of angina increased by 2.6%. (Lampe, F.C. BMJ.May 2005). Could it be that eating a low fat diet reduces heart attacks, while leaving the 'furring' process in arteries (the cause of angina) unaffected?

THE ELECTRIC LIGHT BULB AS A CAUSE OF HEART DISEASE?

The light bulb, as we know it today, was invented around 1920 and soon after, slowly came into general use. Before that, the gas mantle and candles, were used for lighting. At the time, candles made from animal fat used up much of the animal fat available. After the introduction of the light bulb, and the gradual phasing out of the gas mantle and candles, a surplus of fat had nowhere to go but down a drain, or into the human food chain. This fat, added to manufactured pastries, pies, chocolates and other food products, is atherogenic – it 'furs' arteries. Could this have caused a rise in heart disease between 1920 and 1960, after which, fat consumption and cardiovascular mortality, both started to reduce? Well that is the theory. If it is correct, the electric light bulb had its part to play in the heart disease pandemic!

IS IT A SOCIAL DISEASE?

Heart disease is so much more common in the less well-off, our best efforts should be concentrated there. Depending on how you measure it, **cardiovascular disease (along with cancer), is 3 to 5 times more common in the deprived than in the rich.** The greatest need, then, is to introduce risk-lowering strategies and health advice to children at primary schools in deprived areas, and to introduce the right messages into soap operas, while constantly harping on about them in those newspapers more frequently read by those at risk.

Despite the differences between the rich and the poor, cardio-vascular disease is still a major killer, in all social groups. The two main causes are the cholesterol 'furring' of arteries (atherosclerosis), and high blood pressure. These causes of death can be greatly reduced by controlling blood pressure and by preventing, halting or reversing, the 'furring' and clotting processes within our arteries. By these means, we now know that we can substantially reduce cardio-vascular deaths. The problem is, how to persuade people to get tested early enough – before they develop their first symptoms?

Genes NOT Jeans

> **Anyone for Pie and Mash?**
>
> June Allpress, one of my patients, is famous in London for her East End Pie and Mash shop business. June is a 'go-getter', a once met, never-forgotten character. She has appeared on BBC TV, so she has received some recognition of her talents. I suggested to her jokingly that we should put a range of supplements into one of her pies and name it 'The Heart Pie'. Perhaps, I should ask McDonald's if they would like to co-operate with me in producing a 'HeartBurger'? A bit of fun of course, but come to think of it, not such a bad idea!

There is an undoubted inherited element to both the 'furring' of arteries and high blood pressure. Detecting that inheritance will identify those people most in need of preventative advice. Unfortunately some people inherit such serious forms of these conditions, that there is little we can do for them at present. Others, lucky enough not to have inherited such risks, will probably not get either, whatever they do. Many of us have a risk somewhere between the two. In the longer-term, individual genetic analysis will be available to tell us, who is at risk of heart disease and who is not. In time to come, manipulating the genes that determine our risks should be possible – then it will be the intervention of choice. The current Regius Professor of Clinical Medicine at Oxford University, John Bell, who is directing such studies, expects such practical applications to be available within the next two decades. Until then, we must content ourselves with manipulating our arterial chemistry by less direct means: with drugs that reduce our artery cholesterol formation; dietary change, food supplementation (or the taking of micronutrient supplements), and lifestyle management.

The whole 'furring' process is of chemical origin, from our genes that hold the vital instructions for life, to the abnormal influences on arterial lining metabolism. Because our metabolism is a complex of chemically based processes, chemical treatments are the most likely to work. By contrast, massage and acupuncture are less likely to work because they cannot directly influence artery metabolism. I cannot rule out an indirect effect though, acting through some complicated chemical pathways within the body yet to be discovered. If they want to play by the same rules as medical scientists though, the acupuncturists will have to bear the responsibility of demonstrating that they, too, can affect body chemistry!

NATURE AND NURTURE

Our genes are our blueprints, but does that mean that our destiny is determined at birth? Could our lifestyle influence, if and when, our inheritance will lay down its cards? For instance, exercise, might restrain the effect of those genes which make us fat or which 'fur' our arteries, while smoking might activate those unhealthy genes, which are involved in the origins of cancer and artery 'furring'. How true these statements are, I'm not sure, but they have been the subjects of much discussion for decades. The central question is, which is the more important: nature (our genes), or nurture (our upbringing, lifestyle behaviour, and environmental influence)? The scientific consensus is that both are important, although without blueprints (our genes) we would not exist in the first place, so genes must come first. Having plans for a building is a start, but how the builders interpret those drawings and build the structure, is another.

If nurture does have an effect, then it will have to influence the way in which our blueprints are interpreted. Some people seem unaffected by their surrounding conditions, so could some of us carry genes that determine our sensitivity to environmental factors? This is an important issue because it might explain why some who smoke, or eat the wrong things, never suffer; while others, even though they do all the right things, die prematurely from disease.

IS 'NATURAL' BEST?

If we don't eat we will die, so we all have to eat something, but what? Food is a complex mixture of chemicals with proven 'good' and 'bad' elements for artery 'furring' and blood pressure. Food would seem always to be compromised – it is forever, neither entirely 'good' nor entirely 'bad'. Natural food, and its chemical composition, has evolved through an evolutionary pathway assuring its own survival, independent of human needs. The animals and plants we regard as 'food' have not evolved to benefit us, yet we persist in thinking that their 'natural' quality is somehow best for us. While what occurs 'naturally' will only be best by chance, scientific manipulation such as genetic modification or food chemistry manipulation, offer the prospect of making food predictably better for us.

Must we eat what we are given? The way richer nations eat has changed dramatically in the last century. Many were once underfed, now we are generally overfed. Fast-food outlets often encourage us to 'go large', or 'get extra', at no extra cost, so why not buy what is on special offer? Food experts all agree, that as nations, we in the UK and USA eat too much too often and with little regard to the superfluous calories that contribute to our obesity. If we don't find a way to kerb this trend, it will result in more diabetes and heart disease for the future. On the other hand, lots of athletically fit thin people also consume lots of calories because their exercise demands it – the calorie paradox I mentioned before. **Eating and exercising a lot means a higher turnover of calories and a better chance of acquiring the 'goodies', just like our Stone-Age ancestors.**

The World Health Organisation is, at last, advocating less sugar and salt in manufactured foods, but will those with a vested interest in the food industry try to maintain the status quo? Unfortunately, they can easily afford the expensive TV advertising of their products, and advertising is much more likely to influence public demand than medical opinion.

WHAT ARE WE ACTUALLY EATING?

The UK National Food Survey provides some insight into food consumption changes over the ten-year period: 1990 to the year 2000. The atherogenic, or artery 'furring' foodstuffs, are represented by meat and dairy produce. By 2000 there was less beef (-17%), less pork (-19%), and less lamb (-34%), but more poultry (+1.4%) being eaten. Less full fat (- 47%) and skimmed milk (-15%), but more semi-skimmed (+88%), was being consumed. **This represents a considerable reduction in the saturated fat intake by the UK population over that 10-year period.**

Fruit, vegetables, fish, and wine represent the cardiovascular protective foodstuffs in the survey. Between 1990 and 2000, more bananas (+57%), more juice (+50%), more potato products (+49%), more mushrooms (+29%), and more leaf salad (+18%), were consumed, but fewer apples (-10%), oranges (-33%), fresh greens (-13%), cabbage (-42%), and carrots (-1.8%) were eaten. There was less white fish (-38%), a little more processed fish and shellfish (+20%), but much more fatty fish (+88%) being eaten. Wine consumption increased by 33% in the shorter period between 1995 and 2000. **In summary, these changes represent a significant increase in omega 3 fatty acid, arginine, potassium, taurine, selenium, and zinc intake in the UK population.**

Older and richer people eat more fish. In general, high earners (earning more than £40,000 pa) ate 21% more fish than low earners (£10,000 pa or less).

The fish and wine data is consistent with the rich / poor differences in cardiovascular disease occurrence. Richer people, who can afford it, and those well informed enough to choose it, eat more 'anti-furring' protective foods, along with fewer 'furring' (atherogenic) foods. How much this strategy contributes to the 3 to 5 fold advantage the rich have over the poor is unknown, since there are other lifestyle issues such as smoking and exercise that must also be taken into account.

My opinion is, that taken together, these differences will explain the socio-economic class differences within populations.

Overall then, between 1990 and 2000, less 'furring' food, and more protective food was eaten in the UK. This combination might do more than just add benefits together, in theory the benefits should multiply, as do all the risks of a disease. *The benefit gained from low fat food, would multiply with the benefit of eating more protective chemicals, making the combination a potentially powerful one.*

THE BIG FIGHT: 'THE GOODIES' VERSUS 'THE BADDIES'

It would seem that nature has provided us with food that contains both potentially harmful substances and their antidotes at the same time. A key question then is:

> could it be that the beneficial effect of 'goodies' in food can overcome the damaging effects of the 'baddies' in food?

This is a very important issue, and one I believe to be correct. Although crucial, it is not proven. My guess is that the 'goodies' fairly easily overcome the 'baddies' simply because the 'baddies' (fats) are not as bad as we have held them to be (a low fat diet does not stop heart attacks that much). Could it be that one unit of a protective substance overcomes the bad effects of one unit of fat? I don't know, but I have assumed this to be true for the sake of my initial research. My guess is that fats, although undoubtedly bad for our arteries, can be neutralised by some, if not all, of the 16 'goodies' I have identified as having some 'anti-furring' effect.

All research starts with the formulation of a theory – that is, a set of assumptions that must be proven by experiment, and these assumptions of mine are no exception.

Could it be that the atheroprotective (anti-furring) effect of some chemicals is two to three times greater than the 'furring', or atherogenic effect of fats? I don't know, but we need to find out as soon as possible, because a rapidly advancing pharmaceutical industry has all but convinced us that drugs are the only way forward – the time for the all-dancing, all-singing, pharmaceutical 'magic bullet' or 'polypill', is upon us (see Wald and Law, 2003). A pill containing six drugs including: a 'statin', a beta-blocker, and aspirin (stops clotting), has been suggested for good evidence-based reasons, but concern over its possible side-effects will detract from its possible introduction.

LOW AND HIGH BLOOD PRESSURE

The same principle of balance (good v bad, antagonist v protagonist, 'goody' v 'baddy') could apply to potassium (from fruit and veg) – overcoming the adverse effects of sodium salt when it comes to blood pressure control. This could be important in treating or avoiding high blood pressure and leads to the question – which of these three options is best?

(1) a high sodium salt, low potassium salt diet,

(2) a diet with equal quantities of potassium and sodium,

or (3) a low-salt diet, high in potassium?

You probably think (3) is the correct answer, and you may well be right. For those unaffected by sodium (I am one of them), they are all the same. In fact, if you have inherited a low blood pressure, like me, you might need salt to prevent yourself from feeling faint at times. In very hot weather, or when drinking alcohol, I have to eat extra salt – it stops me fainting. Quite simply, cutting out salt for those with low blood pressure can lower the threshold to fainting. Because there is now a strong general belief that 'salt is bad for us', many now eat much less salt. As a consequence, those of us with a low blood pressure will more frequently faint.

> On average, we need 2–3 grams (2000 to 3000 milligrams) of sodium salt per day, or, one tenth to one fifteenth, of an ounce per day.

Has a low-salt diet policy reduced the occurrence of high blood pressure, or helped treat those with a high blood pressure (hypertension) I wonder? There are many good scientific reasons for thinking that it should be so, which partly explains why many experts agree on the policy. There are others, however, equally expert, who remain sceptical. A low salt diet (or diuretics – pills that make us pass more salt and water) is worth a try if high blood pressure is proving difficult to control. If it works, stick to it; if it does not, reconsider your treatment with your doctor.

In the early 1970's I spent years studying blackouts and almost every week since then I have had to advise a fainting patient not to adhere to a low salt diet. Ever wondered why our tears are salty? The fact is, that our bodies are largely composed of salty water. We need salt, and without the right amount of it, we would die. If it is hot, or we work hard physically, we need more salt because we lose it in sweat. People who often faint due to low blood pressure may need much more.

For those with a high blood pressure tendency, added salt and alcohol can make it worse by a direct effect on our arteries, although this is not the case for everyone. First, get to know if salt and alcohol adversely affect *your* blood pressure, then take the appropriate action. To find out what is right for you, you will need to get your blood pressure taken frequently. You can either take it yourself, get it done in a pharmacy or let your own doctor, or his nurse, do it – and not just once either, because blood pressure is as variable as the English weather! You will need lots of recordings, done under differing conditions, to define your natural range. My blood pressure ranges between 90/50 and 140/80 at the most, and salt is OK for me. If your blood pressure ranges between 150/90 and 165/95, or higher, salt is more likely to be bad for you so a low-salt, high potassium diet, might be best – but it needs proving. If salt is not good for you, have a maximum of 2 – 3 grams, or one fifteenth of an ounce, per day.

> I shouldn't tell you this really, but my friend, Dr Alan Gardner, used to have some fantastic parties. After drinking his home-made beer, I quite often felt faint, and would have to go home early. That was before he gave me his cure – heavily salted peanuts! By maintaining my blood pressure, the salt in the peanuts made me feel better when drinking alcohol. Because some people's, blood pressure is made worse by salt (and sometimes by alcohol), I cannot recommend salt (or drinking parties) to everyone.

Salt is very much hidden in food and because adding up the number of grams that we eat can present problems, I have converted the amount of salt into units for each food. One hundred units of sodium salt every day is enough, so to find out if salt is hidden in food, refer to the appropriate list – Table C, Appendix 2, at the end of this book.

FOOD AND OTHER COMBO'S

When camembert cheese (saturated fat, in combination with lysine) is eaten in France, it is likely to be accompanied by powerful antidotes – red wine, rich in arginine, polyphenols, and other substances. If my hypothesis is correct – that the beneficial effects of these substances can outweigh the deleterious effects of fat – another question is: to what extent?

> The 'furring' effects of some food CANNOT be easily overcome.

According to my calculations, you would need some 175 litres of average red wine, to act as an effective antidote to one portion of some cheeses! The 'teen' diet, examined previously, would need 442 daily protective supplement doses just to elevate its cardiac value to the minimum healthy level. Because it is neither practicable nor healthy to drink that much wine, or consume that many supplements, the message is simply: *first take control of your diet – cut out the 'baddies' and maximise the 'goodies' as much as you can.*

What about mixing the 'bad' with the 'ugly'? Mixing protein and fat can cause artery 'furring' especially when the protein is derived from dairy products (twice as much lysine as arginine), as opposed to soy products (equal amounts of lysine and arginine)(see Table 7).

In theory, it may be twice as bad for our arteries, to combine fat with protein. Milk, cream and cheese (fat with lysine-rich protein), combined with protein from other sources (fish or meat), has the potential (in animals at least), to more than double the amount of 'furring' that will occur with dietary fat alone. Steak (more lysine than arginine), served with a creamy sauce (lysine and fat), and cheeseburgers (meat and cheese), could be especially harmful (only to those predisposed to 'furring' or atherosclerosis, of course).

This idea, like so many ideas, is not new. Based on Biblical text, the Code of Jewish Law states: *'meat and dairy products may not be eaten or cooked together, nor is it permissible to derive any benefit from such mixed foods.'* Also, *'after eating meat or a dish prepared with meat, we should wait six hours before eating dairy food.'* In chemical terms, Biblical, and therefore Jewish Dietary Law, forbids the combination of lysine with saturated fat in one meal. Divine dietary guidance has thus been available since the time of Moses!

Replacing milk and dairy produce with soy products would fit the bill, since removing lysine from milk might be possible, but the result would no longer be 'milk'. One further important conclusion follows: *that lysine, taken as a supplement, before and after a fatty meal, should be either banned, restricted, or carry a health warning!*

As a matter of good heart protection diet strategy, not only should the bad fats and lysine be separated (no dairy produce with meat or fish), but also saturated fat, where it occurs, should perhaps be eaten with arginine (as in nuts and seeds), or taurine (seafood, and the brown meat of turkey and chicken). Shellfish (mussels, whelks, scallops etc) is protective, because it is low in all fat (including cholesterol), and rich in taurine and many other 'goodies'. It does have lots of lysine, but it also has lots of arginine and taurine as well, so I would expect the 'good' to balance out the 'bad'. Shellfish of all sorts should therefore be promoted and the misinformed argument that it is dangerous because of its high cholesterol content, be forgotten.

More controversially –

> *if you smoke and cannot give up, perhaps you* **should** *drink alcohol!*

Although obviously 'tongue-in-cheek', is this responsible advice for a doctor to be giving? Smoking, because it is the single most dangerous behaviour in the human repertoire, can never be condoned. The facts are that smoking 'furs' arteries, and alcohol can prevent it. To what extent smoking and alcohol might counteract one another, like wine and cheese, nobody knows, but it is a theoretical possibility. Because we are not making fast progress, either with anti-smoking campaigns or moves to cut down alcohol consumption, many people still like to smoke and drink at the same time. That, as it happens, could be to their advantage, given that they are going to continue to smoke anyway.

THE MEDITERRANEAN DIET

The Mediterranean diet has been shown to greatly reduce (by 70%) the risks of a second heart attack (so called secondary prevention). The figures suggest that it is almost twice as effective as any 'statin' drug in achieving this reduction. The constituents of this diet (salads, seafood, fish, nuts, wine, vegetable oils and meat once per week) are full of many 'goodies' (protective substances), in combination with some 'baddies' (cheese and cream sauces). *Could this be indirect evidence that the beneficial effects of the 'goodies' far outweigh the adverse effect of the 'baddies'?* If this is the case, I have probably underestimated the effectiveness of the 'goodies'. Perhaps we don't need even one recommended daily dose of each 'goody' per day (an RNI or RDA), to get some benefit for our arteries? After all, the experts who decide on these recommended doses have not specifically addressed the problem of artery 'furring', but our general health needs.

> ✸ *Technical point*: the food that has the potential to stop heart attacks, need not be the same as that which stops 'furring', although there are likely to be many foods that share roles. Heart attacks are due to clotting on top of the 'furring', so an additional process is involved.

Could it be that supplementation with protective substances might make the Mediterranean diet even more beneficial? A

Mediterranean diet is expensive and not the usual food eaten by the lowest paid – those who have most cardiovascular problems. Even so, the poorest inhabitants of Marseille have far fewer heart attacks than the poor of Glasgow. Could it simply be that the Glaswegian 'pie and a pint' is no match for the Frenchman's, fish soup and red wine? As far as the food chemistry is concerned, there is no contest. The chemicals in seafood and wine are substantially more effective for protection. On balance, the average pie is likely to contain many more 'baddies' than 'goodies' and by volume, Glaswegians would need to drink 5 times more beer (one litre) than red wine (200mls) in order to get the same protection from alcohol for their arteries.

One alternative would be to avoid too many 'baddies' as suggested by most food experts (*remember that some fat is essential to health*) and to get the 'goodies' in pill form, especially for those who hate, respond badly to, or are allergic to, fish, seafood, nuts, seeds and alcohol! My calculations suggest that the 'at risk' Glaswegian cannot carry on with his pie and his pint for lunch and avoid artery 'furring', even if he does take protective substances in pill form every day. *My research clearly shows that the best we can do for cardio-protection is to FIRST eat the very best diet, and then to supplement it.* Time will tell, of course, but for those of us over fifty who have evidence of any arterial 'furring' building up – the time we have left to think about it is running out!

Food supplementation with 'goodies' is actually well underway. Phytosterols are added to Flora Pro-Active (butter substitute), in order to help lower blood cholesterol, while folic acid and other vitamins are being added to breakfast cereals. Because, for some groups of people, the appropriate food choices for cardiovascular protection are not commonplace ones these days, achieving widespread acceptance of the best cardioprotective diet will be a tough challenge. Because the best food is expensive, the cheaper alternative of food supplementation will have to be considered seriously.

THE POLYMEAL

One of the latest ideas, published as a cardioprotective diet, is the Polymeal (see Franco, 2004). In Greek the word 'polloi' means 'many', so I presume the authors named their diet to mean that many preventative purposes would be served.

The suggestion is that wine (150mls/day), fish (114 grams, four times a week), dark chocolate (100 grams/day), fruit and vegetables (400 grams/day), garlic (2.7 grams/day), and almonds (68 grams/day) should lower blood pressure and total blood cholesterol sufficiently to 'reduce cardiovascular disease by 76%' in 50 – 100 year old patients. Interestingly, leaving out the wine reduces the effect by the largest amount (down from 76% to 65% protective). None of this has been tried in reality, but worked out on likelihood, using data derived from the Framingham study I mentioned before.

One criticism I have of the polymeal is that the chocolate it includes (because it lowers blood pressure), detracts a little from its 'anti-furring' potential, although the fish, wine and almonds it includes, are all good for this. It also suffers, like most alternatives to the Mediterranean diet, from the boredom factor. I am also surprised that it is suggested for only the over 50's; after all, by the age of 50, the 'furring' process is usually well on its way. The diet could, however, help stabilise the process. This diet has the potential to lower blood pressure and to reduce 'furring' and, like the Mediterranean diet, may prove of value in reducing heart attacks and strokes. It does have a very high cardiac value, but its beneficial effect has still to be proven in practice.

DESIGNER FOOD

Genetically modified food is a topic of current political interest and when a scientific issue becomes a popular issue, problems of understanding and interpretation are bound to pervert opinion. All scientists have a duty to explain their subject even if lots of half-truths have to be used in order to aid general understanding. Even so, many people will leave the decisions to others, be unable or unwilling to understand the arguments, or not want to be involved.

As far as heart disease is concerned, genetic modification has the potential to make food both more protective, and less harmful – two separate valuable objectives. While such improvements are likely to advantage those with a cardiovascular risk, they may not be in everyone's interest. This promise of advantage is very far from being realised, but if the process of development is stopped, progress in preventative medicine may be held back by ignorance. Mind you, while smoking continues (a 30%–50% risk factor on its own), any such research could be regarded as superfluous.

The concern is that many people, with no competence in scientific matters at all, are well seated on their high horses when it comes to deciding about the dangers of genetically modified food. The culture of scientific ignorance we now embrace would be harmless, if it were not for the fact that some of those in power seem untroubled by their lack of knowledge. As a measure of the likely danger, just how many politicians have law and arts degrees and how many science degrees, I wonder? Margaret Thatcher was one exception: she brought a scientific training in chemistry to the job of Prime Minister. Could that, I wonder, have given her an unforgiving requirement for objectivity, and a weapon with which to affront those of a more romantic disposition?

SCIENCE, THE TRUTH, AND STATISTICS

Science has a big problem – the communication of ideas. With only headlines of interest (such as 'ASPIRIN STOPS HEART ATTACKS', or, 'MMR VACCINE CAUSES AUTISM', or 'MOBILE PHONES CAUSE BRAIN TUMOURS), few will question or want to understand the underlying science.

The great majority of those who campaign against genetically modified food might be able to define the word 'modification', but how many of them could write an essay on 'genes and their functions', I wonder? Because those who do understand science come cheap (teachers, research workers), the majority can afford to ignore science and buy-in their expertise, rather than go to all the trouble of understanding it themselves. On this basis, most politicians have to leave the in-depth understanding of scientific issues to experts, while themselves retaining the responsibility for making major decisions on technical matters! However, should expert scientists make the decisions? Scientists also have a problem – many are so immersed in their subject they cannot see the wood for the trees; they would, therefore, only rarely be the best people to make policy decisions.

> Plato suggested an answer – a philosopher King (he did not suggest a queen!). From our current perspective, he would need a combination of many talents – that of William Shakespeare, with his unrivelled knowledge of life in all its aspects; the wisdom and judgement of Solomon, the artistry and science of Leonardo da Vinci, and the absolute political power and stoic philosophy of Marcus Aurelius! Nice idea, let's start looking for him or her, straight away! We are certainly in need of such a person.

WHO IS AT RISK?

First we need to know how best to detect heart disease risk? My research clearly shows that artery scanning beats individual blood cholesterol level as a test for the presence of artery 'furring'. If the majority of people with artery 'furring' are without symptoms, a pressing question for preventative cardiologists is: 'who should be our patients, and how are we to identify them?'

Because symptoms occur very late in the course of the disease, potential patients (that's you and me), do not know who we are! Come to that, only the very few know that *the 'furring' of arteries can be detected early, and that it can be treated effectively*. By contrast, almost everyone seems to know their blood cholesterol level – and some actually have a number fixation about it! They may be wasting their worry, because blood cholesterol level on its own will not provide them with a very good guide to the amount of cholesterol building up in their arteries. Regardless of this, it is a raised blood cholesterol, and not the presence of 'furred' arteries, which most often prompts doctors to recommend a low fat diet and a blood cholesterol-lowering, 'statin' drug. That is what they are paid to do. We justify this by contending that a high blood cholesterol level is an indicator of future long-term risk and should, therefore, be treated long before trouble ensues.

Because doctors have a collective responsibility for the health of nations, it is correct that they should try to influence population statistics – by trying to lower the average population cholesterol level, since that has been proven to reduce overall heart attack numbers. *In my opinion, doctors should treat the presence of cholesterol in the arteries of individuals with the utmost priority, even if the blood cholesterol is normal (which it quite often is). Raised blood cholesterol, in the absence of artery 'furring', should assume a lesser priority.*

Such a policy needs proving in prospective studies, to see if we can improve on current policy, that is, simply to give high blood cholesterol the only priority. Because artery-scanning data has recently been admitted to the ongoing Framingham study data set, an answer will later be forthcoming. Until then, my advice to patients is to take advantage of every measure available ('statins', diet, supplements and lifestyle measures) if their arteries have been shown to be 'furred' and to have their arteries tested regularly. Patients must always be given the option to be treated as one of a group and to have their blood cholesterol treated with a 'statin', even if they don't have artery 'furring', since this has been shown, in groups, to reduce the occurrence of heart attacks. No such benefits can be claimed for individuals though, simply because statistics relate to large groups only and cannot provide reliable or specific guidance to individuals. The absence of artery 'furring', even in the presence of a high blood cholesterol, could mean that taking a 'statin' is unnecessary. Such a policy, which is quite attractive to many anti-drug patients, would need to be proven before it is advised.

FAT OR THIN?

Everyone knows the truth about obesity – it is dangerous. Fat people have it drummed into them all the time, and thin people quite often feel self-righteous about it. How then do we explain the fact that a significant number of people with 'furred' arteries, heart attacks, high blood cholesterol, or a high blood pressure, are actually quite slim? Again and again, the same problem arises – the stark difference between what experience and statistics tell us. Statistics tell us that being overweight is a significant risk. Experience tells us that it quite often isn't. Because we are all so different, there will always be many exceptions to the rule. One of the arts of medicine is to know when to apply the rules. Unfortunately for medical policymakers, no rule or policy will ever be written that will be in every patient's interest all of the time.

My conclusion, taken from both the facts and my own experience, is that body weight on its own does represent a significant risk, but only at the extremes (50% more, or less, than the desirable weight). When combined with diabetes, high blood pressure, unfitness and 'furred' arteries, however, the risk becomes very significant.

FASHIONABLE NUMBERS

Fashion is everywhere, even amongst scientists and their statistical advisers. In fashion for a long time now is a form of number crunching called meta-analysis (from the Greek word 'meta', meaning 'afterwards'). Suppose there have been ten trials on the effect of aspirin on heart attack prevention. Statisticians will, after all the results are in, take all ten trials and lump the results together, hoping to get greater significance from a larger number of subjects. The only problem is that exceptions are overridden in favour of an overall result. A bit like reducing a newspaper story to a headline. Of necessity, the detail is lost and we end up with: 'Read all about it – aspirin prevents heart attacks'. What you will not learn from the headline is that a small number of people who take aspirin will suffer a stroke from bleeding in the brain or anaemia from bleeding in the stomach.

Since we are all bombarded with so much information these days, few doctors have time to read the details in the many research journals published each week. By and large, we are grateful for clear results that lead to clear directives. As time goes by, we are becoming less ready to accept a multiplicity of detailed views, preferring as in many walks of life, to reduce our knowledge down to bite size averages, headlines and summaries. Since many a scientific discovery has been made through pursuing an exception to a rule, there is a little danger in accepting conclusions without detailed criticism and appraisal.

EATING AND OTHER BEHAVIOUR

The British Heart Foundation statistics, published in 2000, should be of interest to all those who want to know more about heart disease and its origins.

They clearly show:

- that within the last thirty years, both in the UK and in Finland, there have been 45% fewer coronary heart disease deaths.

- Obesity has risen significantly, so weight cannot be contributing to the drop, although it could be holding it back.

- Thirty-two percent of Europeans now take no physical activity, extra to basic living requirements.

- During the period 1974 – 1994, smokers have decreased in number (from 51% down to 28%), in UK men.

- We are now eating less saturated fat (although the percentage number of calories from fat overall, is unchanged).

- We are eating more fruit and vegetables (+18%).

- In the UK and Finland, total alcohol consumption has increased by approximately 30%. Alcohol can be protective (1 –2 units maximum / day), so this change could be important.

The trends associated with the drop in coronary deaths support the conclusion that decreased smoking, an increased alcohol intake (both around the 30% level) and decreased saturated fat intake are likely contributing factors.

If that is true, the opposite should be occurring in countries where coronary deaths are on the increase. Let's see.

In Romania, deaths from coronary artery disease, have increased from 300 to 420 deaths per 100,000 of the population, during the same period. During this period, Romanian fruit and vegetable consumption rose by 25%, alcohol consumption almost doubled, and there was no change in the contribution of dietary fat to calorie intake!

Looking at the difference between the UK and Romania, and assuming all the data to be valid (a big assumption, given that even the UK data is not derived from autopsy), alcohol consumption increased in both, while coronary deaths decreased in the UK but increased in Romania. So alcohol may not be the key factor we thought it was. Fruit and vegetable consumption increased in both, so that is not a key factor either. Information on smoking, body weight and exercise is incomplete, so deductions based on their comparison, is not possible.

Could the differences be related to the quality of life? One non-quantifiable, but obvious difference, is the relative political and social instability of Romanian society. One might speculate (tongue in cheek), that background social stress is of significance. The eminent researcher James Henry, might agree. He has spent much of his life investigating environmental stress and coronary heart disease in animals. When I met him in the 1980's he explained how stressing rats with various environmental challenges applied to their cages (cold, overcrowding, the need to fight for food, and uncertainty), could cause increased 'furring' in their coronary arteries and stress-induced heart attacks. In rats, at least, he was in no doubt that environmental stress was a significant cause of heart attacks.

WEALTH, SOCIAL STATUS, AND HEART DISEASE

A major stressor linked to heart disease is the control factor. Taking on more debt than we can afford; working for a boss who is always looking to reduce staff numbers in order to increase profits; the feeling that your lifestyle is under threat – all are stresses that can induce the feeling of not being in control. These situations are more likely to happen to the poor than the rich (the poor often have fewer resources and, therefore, fewer choices), to those who are followers, rather than leaders by nature (followers are not in command), to those who are not born copers, rather than those who always seem to get out of trouble (copers have to be objective about the situation, the non-copers may prefer fantasy).

By and large, the rich smoke less, exercise more (albeit more intensely, and for a shorter time); have more control over their lives, and are more likely to eat a diet that bears comparison to the Mediterranean diet. The Mediterranean diet is not low in fat, yet it is reported to prevent more secondary coronary events (70%), than any 'statin' drug (40%). Even if it were low in fat, *the surprising and anti-intuitive fact is that low fat diets have never been shown to be that effective in reducing heart attack rates. The benefit of the Mediterranean diet is, therefore, much more likely due to its protective chemical content.* The beneficial effects of various chemicals such as omega 3, oleic, linolenic, and linoleic fatty acids, arginine, selenium and folic acid, could easily outweigh the deleterious effects of the fat it does contain. The problem is – the Mediterranean diet is not cheap. It would not be easy to persuade low-income groups to either eat a Mediterranean diet or to buy supplements.

To succeed and get rich through your own business endeavours, you have to be able to read your market objectively (know what your customers will buy), and it helps to have some luck. To get off the ground in any new business venture in this country, you have to be able to overcome all those forces determined to keep you on the ground. Gravity is not involved but local planning restrictions, taxes and bank charges, multiple building and employment regulations, competitors, various inspectors, and all the daily joys of failing computers and inefficient people; all are involved. All of this consumes an enormous amount of energy and you really have to have a need to succeed and get rich, because success is definitely against the odds. No wonder most people want to win the Lottery!

Those living a deprived existence are much more likely than the advantaged to 'take what comes', regardless of the medical implications. The rich, on the other hand, may feel that they have a lot to lose (their money and their lifestyle), should they die prematurely. This makes them much more likely to ask questions such as: 'what *is* my state of health', and, '*does* anything need to be done to improve it? Depression occurs equally in both camps and, regardless of wealth status, can lead to the view that 'we all have to die of something, so why prolong it?' Depressed people have less energy to cope and are likely to be less motivated to get informed about their future medical risks.

Rich or poor, you can only eat one meal at a time, live in one house at a time, and do one thing at a time. If you are secure and happy in yourself, money is irrelevant – although it does have its uses! What money can do, is to put you in control – you can do almost what you want, when you want to do it. If you are rich in advantages, you can more easily change your environment, fly away from it, buy another one, or sell it. Poverty may reduce your opportunity for control, but it doesn't remove it.

Poverty of spirit can arise from a lack of personal faith or be a matter of collective experience; poverty of imagination and intelligence can be inherited, but is sometimes the result of stress. I suspect that these forms of poverty are just as likely to lead to heart disease as a lack of money. So, should we tackle them? If we don't, we might allow the rich to get even richer and healthier and the gap between the rich and the poor to grow ever wider. Governments need to think why it is that health services seem ever increasingly to supply the needs of the poor, while fewer rich people are to be found in private hospitals having their less frequent heart attacks!

The initiating ritual for smoking addiction may be simple enough, beginning with camaraderie, but why then carry on? Are the reasons any more complex than saying – that's just what they do? I doubt that many would argue that smokers haven't yet got the message about its dangers. Most people simply say that they enjoy it. Others say it helps when they are stressed or when they need to concentrate. The majority say that they would like to give up, if only they could find a way.

Manual workers smoke two (males) to ten (females) times more than their professional and more highly paid colleagues, but why? The less well-off are no more prone to habit-forming or addictive behaviour than the rich, so addiction cannot be the fundamental reason for continuing to smoke. Are the rich more likely to be in touch with the medical dangers and more ready to accept the warnings on the cigarettes packets? I think so.

Camaraderie is a reason to start and it is also a reason to continue. While you are having a drink, being sociable, having a good time with other smokers, the need to give up is well over the horizon and out of sight. Disciplinary or draconian measures would stop it, of course, but that would lose votes and tax revenue. One solution that advantages everyone, rich and poor alike, would be to ban smoking in all indoor public places – with NO exceptions. The most recent suggestion concerns 'Boozers and Brasseries', in the UK. In 'boozers' (serious drinking pubs, where no food is sold) smoking it is suggested, should be allowed; in Brasseries it is to be banned. Good plan, if the aim is to further widen the yawning health inequality between the rich and the poor!

Everyone has the right to eat, drink, and be merry, without the associated risks of passive smoking in the confines of public places. Unfortunately, no choice is available for those unfortunate children and their friends who suffer in silence from tobacco smoke whether they like it or not. Read the recent British Medical Journal if you will: passive smoking has just been shown to be much worse than even we in the medical profession previously thought (BMJ July 2004, and Jamrozik, April 2005).

What we must do is to provide the sort of information for smokers that will allow them an informed choice; at the same time as making sure that help is available for all those who have found the will to give up.

Do the rich or intelligent more often look before they leap? Do the rich have more time on their hands for reconnaissance? Do they more frequently ask: 'is there anything wrong with me?' My experience, working with people from all backgrounds, suggests that the answer to each of these questions is 'yes' (anecdotal evidence only, of course). As a result, the rich are more likely to get checked medically, before they have an obvious need. That affords them the dignity of choice, as to what to do – either to wait for an emergency to happen, or to prevent it (not that all emergencies are preventable). The poor are less likely to be checked, because the resources of the NHS are simply too few and its staff simply too busy dealing with the consequences of established disease. The NHS mainly provides a salvage operation, not a preventative one. The less privileged are therefore less likely to have their health and lifestyle direction adjusted early enough to make a difference. At least, that is the way it is for the moment.

VITAMINS AND SUPPLEMENTS

Since the 1960's, during the same period that saw a 45% reduction in cardiovascular deaths, there was a dramatic upward trend (for which I have so far failed to find figures), in the sales of both vitamins and supplements. Large numbers of people now take supplements, whether there is any scientific evidence for them or not. They are taken because people believe in them, and that belief can lead them to spend £70 ($100 US) per month. Even for the most intelligent and well-informed, belief and fashion, not science and evidence, is what motivates. What a colourless world it would be, though, without fashionable gurus and their devotees – just don't let them design the aeroplanes you fly in, advise you about the food you should eat or formulate the drugs you take!

The gulf between the claims of the vitamin and supplement industry and the world of medical science, could not be greater.

But could it be that for no reason, other than serendipity, some of the minerals, vitamins and amino-acids included in such supplements have reduced cardiovascular death rates in both the UK and the USA over the last thirty years? The undoubted value of a Mediterranean diet, together with the possible value of some vitamins and supplements, makes this a real but contentious, unproven possibility.

If there is truth in this suggestion and if as a nation, we wish to control obesity by limiting the amount of food we eat while reducing heart disease, supplements would be a fairly inexpensive way of obtaining the protective chemicals we need. The current trend is for us to increase our body weight from eating excessive carbohydrate and fat calories, while doing less exercise – rather than eating low calorie protective foods, combined with more exercise. For these reasons, the following statement remains true:

**we are overfed (too many calories for our needs),
but undernourished (too few 'goodies').**

If coronary death rates are falling, despite progressive obesity, perhaps eating more portions of the 'goodies' is acceptable (I have suggested 10 – 15 portions, each of approximately 150 Kcals. per day). To eat too much is not healthy because there are other very important quality of life issues at stake. Infirmities due to arthritis and diabetes are likely to increase in prevalence if our love affair with fats and sugars continues unabated.

DOING OUR HOMEWORK

Reconnaissance need not be restricted to the military; it can be used to achieve success in all walks of life – and that success can include beating disease. No good decision can be made without information and getting medical information about your true state of health should be regarded as essential reconnaissance. Questions such as: 'is *my* blood cholesterol a good predictor of *my* cardiac health?' need to be asked. The answer, as I have explained, is quite often –

'no'; but what about the answer to the question: 'is artery screening a better test of *my* artery health than *my* blood cholesterol?' The answer to this is an almost certain – 'yes', although it does no harm to do both. So, if artery screening is not available to you as a NHS patient, what are you to do as a would-be survivor? Now it's your turn to come up with an answer!

Research (or reconnaissance) tells us that smoking, obesity, exercise and alcohol, significantly affect the occurrence of coronary heart disease. Smoking halves, and athletic exercise doubles, life expectancy up to the age of 65 years. Such simple facts, for those with the right determination, can be more influential in prevention than anything a doctor can do for you!

Obesity is currently held to be a major health risk. While acknowledging a growing problem, many people who are larger than they would like to be are only 'cosmetically' overweight, not medically overweight (that is, 50% more than your predicted body weight for your build, age, and height). However, both can increase your insulin resistance (your insulin then does not work so well), which is a key factor in the 'furring' process. So what can we learn about obesity and heart disease from research or reconnaissance? Eating fat, and being overweight, both have a bad influence, but only one that accounts for zero to 15%, of the total cardiovascular risk. That compares poorly to the 50% influence that smoking and exercise can have.

Eating positively good foods (containing lots of atheroprotective nutrients), exemplified by the Mediterranean Diet, contributes a possible 70% advantage to those who have already had a heart attack – we don't know, at present, how protective it will be for those who have yet to have their first heart attack. My research shows, that the dietary chemicals identified as atheroprotective, taken in equivalent RNI doses (not easily obtained from food, without extra calories), are less expensive and could confer an equally great advantage.

My suggestion is that, the best supplements, for which there is no evidence of danger, have a low cost relative to the financial burden of heart disease and might significantly improve the successful outcome already achieved by the best diets. This contentious suggestion deserves to be further researched, if only because it is too important to ignore.

CHAPTER 11

Where do we go from here?
GETTING ENOUGH MICRONUTRIENTS

My food analysis clearly indicates that many commonly eaten foods and most of our usual daily diets are micronutrient deficient and insufficiently cardioprotective. Only a very carefully chosen, admittedly boring diet, can attain a highly cardioprotective value. Because most of us are unlikely to radically change our eating habits in the short-term to an offal, shellfish, nut and fish diet, food supplementation or the taking of supplement tablets, will have to be considered as an important future strategy for cardiovascular health.

Having concluded that supplementation might be of benefit I looked for, but failed to find, any completely acceptable all-in-one commercial product to recommend. There are three problems: those products that contain unnecessary or potentially adverse supplements; those products that lack some essential supplements and those products with inappropriate doses. Having sent some of my patients with proven arterial 'furring' off to their own pharmacy with a list of supplements they might take, they became confused by a multiplicity of products.

As you will have gathered, I have suggested that lysine, iron, copper, and synthetic vitamin E, could have adverse effects on the 'furring' process and that vitamin D, vitamin A, vitamin C and beta-carotene, are unlikely to have any beneficial effect. Nevertheless, many of these are contained in the preparations that can be purchased in health food and pharmacy outlets. It soon became obvious that I needed to design my own set of supplements, containing all of the necessary ingredients with none of the questionable ones.

We do not know which dose of each supplement is appropriate for cardioprotection. Mega-doses of vitamins, based on Linus Pauling's idea that 'more is best' must be resisted: they remain unsubstantiated as far their benefit to atherosclerosis is concerned. We do need to know which doses of cardioprotective micronutrients might be best but that will take lots of further research. Until then, my guess is that 1 – 4 RNI's daily of each atheroprotective substance are required, although, the latest European directives on dosage may restrict such formulation. One important principle is that the smallest effective dose is best. Another is the Goldilocks principle: the correct dose needs to be 'just right' and not too small or too large.

FURTHER RESEARCH

Serious work now needs to begin. What we need to do is observe the combined effect of all these substances on the growth of 'furring' (atheroma), over many years. This we can do, in both carotid and coronary arteries, using neck ultrasound, EBCT scanning and angiography. If they do show the benefit expected, then clinical trials designed to demonstrate a reduction in heart attacks and strokes might be undertaken.

> The first step, in any cardioprotective eating regime, must be to eat the best food possible (of high cardiac value), and then, and only then, to supplement it.

Unfortunately for those of us over 50 years of age, all this might just take too long!

I will shortly be starting such research, although not without first obtaining charitable funding and finding many suitable volunteers. You can find out more at:

www.cardiaccentres.co.uk.

SOME QUESTIONS YET TO BE ANSWERED

Should we screen the arteries of everyone aged 35 and over, every few years? How are we to rid ourselves of poverty and its associated cardiovascular diseases? How can we achieve a better level of scientific literacy so that protective strategies can be better understood? What do we have to do to encourage more exercise? How are we to get people to eat the 'best' of diets'? How can we put an end to the smoking habit? As far as food is concerned, if we cannot easily or cheaply, get enough of the antidotes to artery 'furring' from food alone, should we be taking the appropriate vitamins and supplements as pills or have them added to our food and water? There is much to discover and much to discuss but answers to these questions would benefit our serious heart disease prevalence.

Whatever we may advise, there will always be many who will never be interested in prevention – that is their right. They are happy to trust to luck or, to wait for some authority to force their compliance.

Having treated heart attack and stroke victims all of my working life I decided many years ago, not just to wait for them to happen or to screen patients after the event, but to try detecting the early signs of artery 'furring' long before any catastrophe. So far, my able technician Noreen Connolly has screened the arteries and hearts of over 2000 of my patients. What we have found mostly confirms the findings of others and adds a few further features. Our results are published on my website: **www.cardiaccentres.co.uk**. If you open the page on '**research results**', the details are in: '**Carotid Artery Atheroma and its Associated Clinical Features**'.

In brief, two extreme groups are obvious from our research: those who have a high blood cholesterol and no artery 'furring' and those with a completely normal cholesterol and very bad artery 'furring'. *One important practical result is that there is no useful relationship between the blood cholesterol of any individual and the degree of artery 'furring' found.* Going back to my old student textbooks, I found that Best and Taylor had accepted this conclusion, when in

1961, they wrote their comprehensive textbook of medicine: The Physiological Basis of Medical Practice!

IS ARTERY SCREENING ESSENTIAL?

I believe that the evidence now supports the view that we should regularly include artery screening in every patient suspected of having coronary heart disease; those with a relevant family history and those without symptoms but abnormally high blood fats, homocysteine and CRP. Whether it should be part of every full examination of those over 35 years of age is another matter. For those who consider their life to be worth more than money, doing it routinely every five to ten years regardless of need, could have its advantages. Any degree of artery 'furring' detected could be treated appropriately and monitored to detect disease progression and the direct effect of management.

Carotid artery ultrasound detects the 'furring' process early on and is superior as a test of heart attack risk in individuals to any blood test, including blood cholesterol (LDL or HDL or both), homocysteine, fibrinogen or CRP. *The presence of significant artery 'furring' in the neck arteries is capable of predicting the worst – a 4 : 1 chance of a heart attack (or some other cardiovascular event) within four years.* That is a good enough reason for all those over 35 years of age to have artery scanning performed every five to ten years. The more difficult questions are: who will pay and who will think it worth paying for.

What to do:

your personal check-list for preventing or modifying heart disease:

This applies especially to those with:

- known heart disease;
- a family history of heart disease;
- a high blood cholesterol;
- high blood pressure;
- diabetes;
- and those who sense a deterioration in their health involving a slowing down in pace, breathlessness, or chest tightness.

First and foremost –

Check your arteries
Check your arteries
Check your arteries

THE BIG QUESTION IS:
ARE YOUR ARTERIES 'FURRED' OR NOT?

Next, check your other risk factors.
(Blood cholesterol, homocysteine etc)

If you have a 'furring' problem –
Stop smoking.
Get fit.
Lose weight.

Lower a high blood cholesterol
with a low animal fat diet, 'statins', or a cholesterol absorption inhibitor (such as ezetimibe).

Replace butter and spreads
with a phytosterol or phytostanol product (Flora Pro-Active or Benecol)

Only some food is good enough – MOST IS NOT

Eat a Mediterranean diet,
and consider supplementing it because . . . .

Allow your doctor to:

- treat obviously 'furred' arteries (and raised LDL cholesterol) with 'statins',

- treat a low HDL with exercise, 'statins' and perhaps long-acting nicotinic acid (beware of side effects).

- Treat a raised homocysteine with folic acid, B6, & B12.

- Treat a clotting tendency with aspirin, natural vitamin E, or clopidrogel.

Ask: 'Am I a diabetic?'
If you are a diabetic, take diabetic control
very, very, seriously.

If you are not a diabetic, but have it in your family, ask: 'am I a pre-diabetic?'
This requires a glucose tolerance test to find out.
If you are a pre-diabetic, strictly limit your carbohydrate from now on.

If you have 'furred' arteries –
get a glucose tolerance test done anyway and
consider having a dietary survey done, cross-checked with a blood test for micro-nutrients.

Consider these questions:

- Do I have heart trouble? It doesn't really matter whether you do or you don't, the same principles apply. I can't say it's never too late to take action: it wouldn't always be true. Get tested early: the earlier in life you begin to assess yourself objectively, the better. Artery 'furring' is a progressive accumulating problem that starts in youth. The sooner you start to combat it, the better – that is, if you want to maximize you chances of survival.

- Is there heart disease in your family?

- Are you a smoker?

- Are you unfit?

- Are you overweight?

- Is your total cholesterol high (LDL high, HDL low)?

- Are your blood lipoprotein A, homocysteine, fibrinogen, or C-reactive protein raised?

- Are you diabetic?

- Are you a pre-diabetic?

- Is your blood pressure raised?

- Do you drink alcohol every day?

If any answer to these questions is YES, read the appropriate chapter in this book, and get tested.

Do you know which foods are best and which foods are potentially bad for your arteries?

Do you know which supplements are good for your arteries?

If your arteries are healthy, these are not questions for you.

If your arteries are 'furring' faster than they should, read the appropriate chapters, and learn all about it.

I recommend that everyone over 35 years has at least one carotid artery scan and an exercise test, if only as baseline reference tests (they make future assessment of progress possible). If you have not developed 'furring' by the age of 50 to 60 years, you will probably not develop it. No X-rays are involved, so it is safe. Have these tests done, every one to three years, depending on the initial findings – the worse the finding, the more often you would need them repeated. The rate of growth of 'furring', although variable, is a good guide to risk.

EBCT scanning involves X-rays, and angiography is not a screening procedure. Both are very useful in the appropriate circumstances, but neither are 'first line' tests.

If you have normal arteries, keep up the good work!

If you have slightly 'furred' arteries (so called Class 2 or 3), do everything you can with lifestyle measures (do more exercise, reduce stress, stop smoking, attempt weight-reduction), get your diet as good as it can get (acquaint yourself with the list of high cardiac value foods), and take the right supplements.

If you definitely have 'furred' arteries (so called Class 4 atheroma, or worse), you must have a 'statin' drug, regardless of your blood cholesterol, together with all the other preventative measures.

ALMOST THE LAST WORD!

Will all this talk of death and disease induce anxiety? Of course it will, so don't be surprised if your doctor doesn't agree with screening. Doctors are trained to diagnose and treat disease, not to create unnecessary anxiety. Is it ethical for a doctor to be interested in you before you are a patient? Some will say 'yes', some will say 'no'. Both are valid – it's for you to decide which sort of doctor you want to discuss your life, and future with. Therefore, why not ascertain your doctor's attitude towards screening and preventative medicine. You will need to know if your attitudes are compatible, before you are aware that you need medical advice.

If you fear that maximizing your length of life might expose you to worse – medical conditions that are not preventable or curable, such as emphysema (severe shortness of breath), cancer (pain), blindness and deafness (risk of isolation), infirmity (immobility), dementia (unable to remember or cope), or a longer agony, then you have a strong reason to simply take what comes. There are people who can adjust to these challenges, and thereby gain honour and self-esteem; there are others who cannot.

Survivable heart attacks are OK; you can recover, and hardly know the difference. Heart failure could make you progressively breathless, and leg artery 'furring' could slow down your walking pace, and limit the distance you can walk. These are but some of the possible consequences of artery 'furring', a condition we can help to prevent. I know that the anxiety of knowing that you have an artery problem may not be good for your composure, but developing these conditions because you couldn't be bothered to avoid them, is worse.

As a preventative physician, I have to accept being wrong – our science is far from perfect – but what I cannot accept is not having tried my best to prevent such conditions. We will never be able to foresee or prevent every medical catastrophe, but it is a worthy motive and simple common sense to want to try – after all, lives are at stake.

Medical politicians may tell you that the cost / benefit ratio of some preventative strategies, like cardiac screening, is too high. What they actually mean by this is, that too much public money would have to be spent in order to save one life. The vital questions are then – 'whose life?' and then, 'what is that one life worth?' The objective of publicly funded policy can thus be legitimately different to that of private policy. My patients are largely self-selected by their own attitude – they think that the life at risk could be theirs, and, they think that the personal expenditure needed to save it, is definitely worthwhile!

A lack of personal finance should not prevent anyone getting tested. There are many ways around this problem, one of which might have to be reverting to Victorian times, when charitable funding was much in evidence. I have set up a non-profit making fund for this purpose at my own clinic, but this is hardly going to be good enough for the population at large.

One strategy in life I am fond of – never knock a hole through a brick wall in order to reach the other side when it would be easier to walk around it! There are those who do have the energy for medical politics, but I prefer to spend my energy on my work, rather than waste it persuading committees of old dogs, that new tricks can be worthwhile. If those in authority cannot justify generalized testing because the net worth of saving one life is too expensive (never forget – they are playing with our tax money, and our lives), we might have to find another way!

CHAPTER 12

Further Topics

TRUTH AND STATISTICS (FOR THOSE NOT INTERESTED IN STATISTICS).

Scientists use statistics in an attempt to get to the truth. They talk about it all the time in order to plan their experiments and then to analyse the results. Outside of the world of science they are used by doctors, pharmaceutical companies, politicians and businessmen to persuade us of their point of view. Statistics have their uses and their abuses, so let me attempt to broaden the view to one useful to the general reader by looking at the topic from different standpoints.

Every time anyone uses the word 'statistically', with reference to only you and me, they are conning you – to be exact, they are committing mathematical heresy. That is because **statistics are the mathematics of a large number** of (randomly chosen) **numbers,** and only a large number of (randomly chosen) numbers.

You are an important number of course, but you are only 'one', and you are not randomly chosen (by 'randomly' I mean purely chosen by chance, with no biases applied). What applies to a group cannot . . . repeat . . . *cannot*, apply to you, however much you work the figures!

Averages have their uses but they might not apply to you and me. When it comes to considering your own personal circumstances beware of opinions that are based on an 'average', that most common of quoted statistics. A measure of what is 'average' has only a remote chance of applying *exactly* to you.

Statistics allow the giving of odds, not the giving of certainties. Statistics are a set of man-made mathematical tools from an illusory land, where only contrived measures, and their chance of representing reality exist. They don't belong to the same world of reality we inhabit. Uncertainty is the only thing both worlds have in common.

If I suggested to you, that statistically, you would be better off with a lower blood cholesterol, what would that mean? It means that the average person in a tested group will be better off, not that everyone will be better off. Practicing doctors have to be double agents: we get our guidance from statistics (derived from research done on large numbers of subjects), yet use the results only ever to guide the treatment of individuals. Because research on an individual is very unlikely to apply to a whole group, this is the best we can do, even if it is not the best for each of us. A bit like asking a committee how best to handle problems with your partner – you might get some good guidance about partners in general, but what use would their advice be if it did not apply specifically to yours?

In medical research we use statistics to help overcome personal beliefs or biases – or put another way, we use statistics to help us see whether or not we are fooling ourselves. This is necessary because our human ego continually fights on behalf of our own selfish will, regardless of the odds. Reason can overcome the force, but it may have to win a battle against arrogance and ambition.

The problem with statistics is that the detail (that is what applies to you and me) has to be lost because numbers have to be lumped together. That is its weakness. Its strength lies in being able to show the difference between two groups of data, such as the average body weight of two groups of people – those who do, and those who do not, have sugar in their tea, for instance! If the average body-weights are different (and statisticians can say how likely they are to be different), then it could be that sugar is an important factor, making one group heavier than the other. The question is, what use are statistics if they are not pertinent to you and me? I don't take sugar in tea and I know a lot of people, thinner than me, who do. Statistics are pertinent to us all, if groups are being considered; you and me, however, are not a group large enough to be considered important by any statistician.

We all have very valuable personal experiences of life, and that experience which leads to anecdote is always valid – but not to the statistician. Our experiences cover life, our family, friends and many acquaintances but, to statisticians, they are too personal. A personal, or anecdotal viewpoint, they will say, is not (they prefer to say –'unlikely to be') representative of general experience. Anecdotal descriptions of experience are now scorned by science, whereas once they were King. Scientists will say that anecdotal description is no longer relevant to modern scientific research. Anecdote remains useful to formulate a theory, but you need statistics to take it further and prove it.

When we dispense with detail we may dispense with insight. For Field Marshall Montgomery, much success came from his attention to detail. He often asked the individual opinions of his front line troops. What, he wondered, did they think of the campaign, and how it was going? On one occasion, he was reported to have asked a disillusioned corporal in the North African desert for his thoughts. He was told, 'it would help Sir, if I had a few more bullets to fire at the enemy!' Rommel was defeated, and the rest is history.

Let me try to illustrate the relevance of statistics with some other examples. Consider the view from an airplane window at 35,000 feet, passing over a country like the UK or Germany: lots of forests and green countryside. From this height a forest might look as if it was made up of the same coloured trees. If you were to walk through that same forest, would every tree have the same coloured leaves? Possibly, if it were planted with all the same fir trees; in a natural forest though, there would be trees of many different colours. Walking through such a forest, would you gamble on which tree you might next encounter? You would be unwise to, because one essential feature of nature is its variety. An average is a mathematical construction that has no reality; that is not to say that it is a useless concept for reality. Because the average cheetah is faster than the average man, the average cheetah will always beat the average man in a race. The average is thus a useful group analysis tool, but from nature's standpoint variety is everything, providing as it does, the spark to both evolution and the survival of the fittest. The problem is, variety can boggle the mind, an average should not.

To the statistician, the average colour of trees in a forest is what counts. This is clearly one view of reality, but only one from a distance. The average colour can be measured accurately and can be used to compare different forests. By comparing the average colour of one forest to another, a statistician can say, with prescribed certainty that the composition of different trees within one forest is different to that of another. And that is useful if, and only if you are in the business of comparing whole forests, not individual trees.

The law of scale applies when you want to discuss either the individual perspective, or the statistical viewpoint. Looking at the Earth from the moon, it would not be possible, with the naked eye at least, to discern towns, let alone cars and people, although oceans and landmasses would be visible. This far-off view is equivalent to the statistical view. Would it be right then, for a newly arrived, long-distance space traveller, with his or her first view of Earth, to conclude – 'this planet is dead!' The answer would be, to have a closer look, when all might be revealed. If he/she/it saw the way we behave towards one another, he/she/it might conclude that we are alive, but brain-dead! Having arrived on Earth, he/she/it would see many individuals smoking, and might then conclude that, while there is life, there is little intelligent life! But to make the point, the individual, anecdotal view is not the same as the far-off, statistical one. Each view has its merits, but they are very different merits.

Statisticians come up with conclusions like this: 'the average Japanese is shorter than the average Norwegian'. Useful, if you are in the clothing industry, but if you made all your jackets and trousers of average size, half would be too small, and half too big. Individuality is lost in the statistics, yet individuality is what makes us who we are.

The following statement would also be typical of a statistician's conclusion:

A large randomly chosen group of overweight people have, on average, a poorer health outlook than a large randomly chosen group of slim people of similar age, sex, race and social status.

For particular individuals, this conclusion is valueless, because the great differences between people ensure that any meaningful distinction disappears. In other words, you cannot predict anything about the person sitting next to you – unless you have assessed him or her as an individual. Of what use then is the above statistical statement? For you and me, there is some value in re-stating it as follows:

because the person I am sitting next to is more obese than me, the odds are that he is more likely to have a poorer health outlook than I have – but that doesn't mean that it would be worth gambling on – not, that is, until we have both been assessed as individuals.

I feel a little sorry for statisticians; they only work with large numbers, and that is a real limitation. In everyday life, most doctors work with individuals in some capacity, and need to make decisions about individual situations. *We can draw guidance from generalisations and averages, but the final decision will rest on our personal knowledge of the individual.* Generalisations might have it otherwise, but statisticians have to live with the fact that many fat people are really healthy and many thin people have a real health problem. I'm afraid that this is a circle that can never be squared. I suppose we all have to make a living, and those concerned with large numbers (Ministry of Health, drug companies undertaking clinical trials), need statistics to make informed decisions about what is best for the majority.

So you think all this is academic? It is, until you intend to seek medical advice. If you are still unsure of what I'm getting at, *consider thinking like this: 'I am not a member of a group called 'fat people', or 'thin people', with whom I share a common fate – I am an individual. If I want to learn about my fate, I'll get examined and assessed as an individual, while bearing in mind the results from group studies!'*

Statistics do aim to overcome individual biases and put theories to the test. They thus provide an invaluable tool for scientists. The problem is, that they have become the only acceptable method of scientific analysis, and *must* be used, in one form or another, to report results. There is now little place for the simple descriptive (anecdotal) experiments that led Galileo, Leonardo da Vinci, Michael Faraday and Charles Darwin to discover what they did. Science has moved on to areas of investigation, beyond the looking glass, where intuition is less reliable, and where we are more likely to fool ourselves. That is why we cling on to statistics – to help bring us back to an overview of reality.

FURTHER CARDIOVASCULAR TOPICS

Atheroma or plaque

This is the name we give to the actual patches of cholesterol that build up in the walls of our arteries. These patches can narrow arteries and, eventually, block them. I have referred to this as the 'fur' in the arteries, not that it is the same as the 'furring' in household water pipes and kettles, but it is similar enough to convey understanding.

Atherosclerosis

This is the word we use to refer to the process by which cholesterol 'furs' the inner lining of our arteries. When blockage does occur in the heart and brain arteries, big trouble is sure to follow in the form of heart attacks and strokes. Surely we can detect the process early enough in patients to stop it developing? We shall see. At the moment though, few doctors seem motivated to look before symptoms arise. We mostly content ourselves with blood cholesterol measurements, which are now known to be a poor indicator of the presence of artery 'furring'. Is the artery scanning used to detect 'furring' more expensive? Yes, it is! Is it a much better test? Yes it is. Should accountants or doctors control medicine? What do you think?

A lot of research has been done on atherosclerosis, but only medical scientists ever seem to talk about it. Why is this, when it is the major cause of death in the western world? I guess it is not very newsworthy. Like so many important subjects 'it doesn't sell newspapers', so we the public, remain ignorant of knowledge that could help us avoid heart attacks – if we want to, that is! All we are told is that 'fatty food is bad for us' or that 'obesity kills'. There is an element of truth in both of these statements of course, but the statements might mislead us into thinking that they are the only factors, or even the most important factors. They are not. There is much more to it.

Footballs and golf-balls: 'Good' (HDL) and 'Bad' (LDL) Cholesterol.

Sorry to disappoint all of you sporting enthusiasts, but I am referring here, by way of analogy, to the fats in your blood. Not as challenging as golf and football I must admit, but arguably a touch more important when it comes to life and death.

The cholesterol in the blood has several separate components, each of which, have been thought to be better predictors of heart attacks than total cholesterol. Imagine footballs with golf balls stuck to them, and these, small enough to float around in your blood. The footballs are the 'good' cholesterol (**HDL, or high density lipoprotein**), and the golf balls are the 'bad' cholesterol (**LDL, or low density lipoprotein**). The idea is, that without the footballs, the golf balls (small LDL particles) could seep through small holes in the inner artery lining (**the intima**) and cause cholesterol accumulation – the 'furring' or atherosclerosis, I have been describing. Golf balls stuck to footballs make a molecule too big to seep through the small holes in the inner membrane of the artery. The smaller particles (the LDL cholesterol or golf balls) can get through, so we think of them as potentially dangerous. Because the large particles (HDL cholesterol or footballs) mop up some of the LDL, we think of them as protective. For this reason we have been measuring total cholesterol, LDL, and HDL, in the blood of patients, for over twenty-five years, in order to assess individual 'furring' risk.

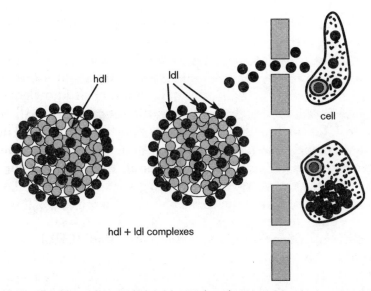

Fig 13 Theory: LDL (bad cholesterol) sticks to HDL (good) cholesterol and so cannot get through the holes in the inner artery lining. LDL alone can get through. Therefore if you have a lot of good (HDL) cholesterol, you might not develop artery 'furring'.

There are, therefore, two danger signs in the blood:

(1) Too much LDL (bad cholesterol, equivalent to the golf balls),

(2) Too little HDL (too few footballs for the bad LDL to stick to).

If everyone were able to get their blood cholesterol below 5.00 (mmols/l), our population would suffer fewer heart attacks. This is because the lower the total blood cholesterol, the lower the LDL (bad). Therefore, a matter of concern for public health doctors is how to reduce the average levels in the blood. Both exercise and taking 'statin' drugs alter our metabolism. Cutting out fatty food, although it may lower the blood level, does so without altering our metabolism and is therefore unlikely to effect a reduction in heart attacks. Surprised? With more than 20 trials of low fat diet showing this, why are we lead to believe that a low fat diet is so healthy?

What are we to believe? For an excellent and sceptical review of the subject, I recommend to you Dr James Le Fanu's book 'Eat Your Heart Out', in which he poses the serious question: is there a conspiracy afoot? If low-fat diets are not that good for us, might it be that those with a vested interest in low-fat foods, are motivated to keep the idea alive? Remember, though, such generalisations may not apply to you and me. What might help you, might not help me.

Having believed in the dangers of fatty food and a high blood cholesterol for so long many doctors have been disappointed to observe that total blood cholesterol and LDL do not reliably predict the presence of artery 'furring' in any individual. Blood levels do however predict the occurrence of heart attacks in populations, but not in individuals. Out of the tests I have just mentioned, a low HDL is perhaps the better predictor of high risk. As it happens, I have only twice in the last 25 years seen someone with a high HDL have a heart attack. By contrast, I have seen very many patients with normal blood cholesterol (and a low LDL) have heart attacks; so for me, the significance of blood cholesterol is not what I was led to believe. My view is, that having too few footballs (HDL cholesterol), is worse than having too many golf balls (LDL cholesterol)!

WHAT LEVEL OF HDL SHOULD YOU HAVE?

The answer is, probably in excess of 1.5 mmols/l. Less than 1.0 mmols/l starts to present a potential problem. A ratio of total cholesterol to HDL of over 7 has been found to be associated with 'furring' in the coronary arteries. So, if you have a blood cholesterol of 4.0 mmols (very good), but an HDL of only 0.5 mmols, your ratio of 8 (4 / 0.5 = 8), is not so good. Alternatively, if your total blood cholesterol is 8.00 mmols (anything above 5.0 mmols is thought to be an 'at-risk' level), and your HDL = 2.0 mmols, your ratio of 4 is very good.

We used to think that these figures would predict the presence of artery disease in individuals (that, after all, is the problem we practical doctors face every day). I now know, having spent 3 years actually measuring what goes on in arteries, that the relationship between the two is not very good at all. In fact, none of the standard risk factors (weight, smoking, family history, blood cholesterol etc) taken together, predict more than 60% of all heart attacks.

This issue about blood fats and their significance is something we doctors will continue to discuss for a long time. Like every subject, it has its ardent supporters and detractors. While that discussion continues in the wings, medical science has moved on. We can now visualise the actual cholesterol in our arteries, so we don't have to guess whether or not it's there, from an indirect blood test like cholesterol level. What point is there then in doing blood tests? The answer is: we still prefer to do them, just to back ourselves each way! It may prove to hold some value in long-term risk prediction for individuals. In any case, screening arteries with ultrasound is not done routinely to assess risk at the moment, although nearly all doctors will do one after a stroke, if not a heart attack. A case of letting the stallion bolt, when checking and locking his stable door beforehand would have saved a lot of trouble! Catching loose stallions, and trying to reverse the effects of a stroke are not equivalent, but they do both require a lot of work.

THE ANTI-OXIDANT THEORY

In a test tube, in a laboratory, anti-oxidants are chemicals that stop oxygen combining with other atoms. That does not mean that they will do the same in the human body. When oxygen combines with the golf ball particles (LDL), it forms oxidized LDL. By reducing the amount of oxidized LDL cholesterol generated (an irritant substance in the artery wall), anti-oxidants are thought to be able to reduce the 'furring' process. Well, that's the theory at least.

Lots of people take anti-oxidants, believing that they will prevent cancer and heart disease. But will they?

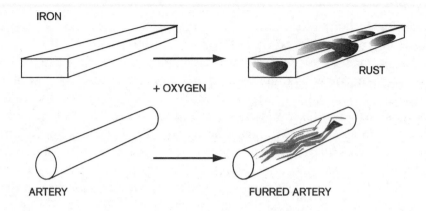

Fig 14 Oxygen rusts iron and helps 'fur' our arteries

Everyone will know that iron, left out in the rain, will rust. You can see it on old cars where they have been damaged. What is actually going on is oxygen combining with the metal, to form iron oxides or rust. The process is called **oxidation**. As it happens, something similar happens to cholesterol in the artery wall. When cholesterol meets oxygen in the arteries, it 'oxidises' – by roughly the same process as the rusting of iron. However, it is only the bad cholesterol (LDL) that is involved. It causes a problem because when it becomes oxidized, LDL creates an irritant or inflammatory reaction within the inner artery lining. It is thought that this soreness, or inflammation in the arteries, attracts large numbers of scavenger cells, whose function it is to gobble up the 'rusty', or oxidised LDL cholesterol.

In theory, anti-oxidants should stop both the rusting of iron, and the production of oxidized LDL cholesterol in our artery walls. Hence the idea that, if we eat lots of anti-oxidants, they might stop the oxidization process and put a stop to the 'furring' of our arteries. Like many good ideas, they do not always work in practice. In fact, the latest evidence from the Heart Protection Study, a very large research study that compared beta-carotene, vitamin C, and synthetic vitamin E (all anti-oxidants) to a 'statin' drug, showed that anti-oxidants did not stop heart attacks in those already at risk.

There are some reasons why they might not have worked. Perhaps some of the patients had arteries that had gone too far and were too 'furred' to benefit. Perhaps the anti-oxidants were not given for long enough? Both are possibilities.

Other evidence also shows no beneficial effect from either vitamin C or beta-carotene, whereas there can be a very significant effect from 'natural', rather than synthetic, vitamin E (the CHAOS Study). Unfortunately, the researchers of the Heart Protection Study chose to use synthetic vitamin E, and lost the opportunity to verify or refute the effect of 'natural' vitamin E!

CARDIOVASCULAR DISEASE

This refers to all diseases of the heart and circulation (the arteries which carry oxygen in the blood around the body, and the veins which return the blood back to the heart). These diseases are mostly caused by atherosclerosis and high blood pressure. They are both killers, and the commonest causes of death in the western world.

THE CIRCULATION - WHAT DOES IT DO?

Oxygen is the fuel we live on and, to live, we must get that oxygen from the air that surrounds us into our lungs and onward to all our organs. From the lungs it must get into the blood and be transported to all our tissues, where it is burned for energy, much like petrol is burned in the engine of a car.

Our organs, like the brain and heart, need oxygen by the bucket full. The arteries are tubes made of muscle that take our blood, rich in oxygen, from the lungs to our tissues. When you feel your pulse at the wrist, you are feeling one of your arteries carrying blood and oxygen to your hand. The blood is pumped by the heart at a certain pressure (the blood pressure), and at a certain rate (pulse rate), depending on circumstances. Blood and oxygen are not delivered at a constant rate, but at a rate that will vary with demand. Emotion, physical activity, even digesting food, and thinking, will all increase the amount of blood pumped, and the amount of oxygen delivered. But how does your body do this? There are two major mechanisms. Firstly, the heart can pump faster and harder, and secondly, the arteries can open up, and let more blood through.

HIGH BLOOD PRESSURE OR HYPERTENSION

Anyone who knows how to blow up a party balloon can understand blood pressure. What happens is this: first, you blow hard into the balloon (high pressure phase); then you hold the end, to retain the air, while you take another breath (the balloon now holds a certain passive pressure of air – the lower pressure phase). Then you blow and hold, blow and hold, until the balloon is fully inflated. There are two phases – the blowing, high-pressure phase, and the passive, or low-pressure phase, between blows. In essence, the heart does the same thing – it pumps blood out into the circulation (the higher pressure or systolic phase), then rests (the low pressure or diastolic phase), in order to prepare for the next beat. As with the balloon blowing, the blood pressure consists of two pressures. For instance, 110/60 means that while the heart pumps it produces a maximum pressure of 110, while in between beats, the resting pressure in the system is 60. The analogy works quite well because the circulation is actually a branching tree of tubes – in effect, a balloon filled with your blood.

> **☯ Technical Point:**
> Actual blood pressures are measured in millimeters of mercury ('Hg' for short). If you fill a tube with mercury – a heavy liquid metal, the column would press down with a certain pressure. The 110 and 60, refer to a pressure equal to columns of 110 and 60 millimetres of mercury (abbreviated as 'mms Hg') (= 4½ and 2½ inches of mercury). So doctors say you have a blood pressure of 110/60 mms Hg.

WHAT IS A NORMAL BLOOD PRESSURE?

It is becoming increasingly accepted that a pressure of 110/60 is ideal, and that pressure above this is a potential risk. This is an extreme view, because the tangible risks of a high blood pressure do not really start until the pressure is consistently above 150/90. Almost nobody will disagree that a consistent blood pressure above 160/95 would be wise to treat. The problem is that blood pressure changes like the British weather. One minute it rains, then the next it shines. So which blood pressure should we take as significant – the one when you are asleep, or the one on peak exercise? Because blood pressure is so variable, we can be sure only of two types of blood pressure – that which is always raised, and that which is always normal. Those 'in-between' people are a problem to us.

THE PROBLEM OF HIGH BLOOD PRESSURE

Now let's take a look at what high blood pressure can do to you. High blood pressure affects your arteries, but in a different way to cholesterol. Cholesterol mainly affects the larger arteries, and blood pressure the very small ones. The arteries are tubes made of muscle, and high blood pressure can make that muscle thicker. Your heart is also made of muscle and it too can get thicker and bulkier, simply because it works harder when you have a consistently high blood pressure. When this thickening is present, you can be sure that you need

> This process of muscular thickening in high blood pressure is called arteriosclerosis, and is not to be confused with atherosclerosis, which refers only to cholesterol formation.

treatment for your high blood pressure, implying that detecting this change as soon as possible is of great importance. This is why everyone with high blood pressure should have a regular heart echo-sound (echocardiogram) every 1 – 2 years. Firstly, we need to detect the presence of muscle thickening (called hypertrophy), then, we need to stop it getting worse. If hypertrophy (thickened heart muscle) is seen to develop, and that can take one year or more, you might conclude that you are not on the best of treatments. **Two objectives of blood pressure treatment are to stop the development of muscle thickening (hypertrophy), and the other is to consistently lower the blood pressure in all situations. Many, but not all, modern drug therapies are thought to do both.**

Blood pressure affects the small arteries in your body differently to those in your brain. High blood pressure thickens the walls of bodily arteries, but thins those in the brain. This thinning can lead to a 'blow-out' (or aneurysm), the bursting of a brain blood vessel, haemorrhage, and subsequent brain damage. This can result in what is called a **haemorrhagic stroke.** Some of these aneurysms are, however, there from birth, and do not always burst. Alternatively, if a brain artery blocks with cholesterol and then clots, what may follow is **an ischaemic stroke.** The word ischaemia means – an insufficient amount of blood getting to a tissue – usually because of a narrowed artery.

Here is an illustration of what high blood pressure does to the artery tubes in your body and brain:

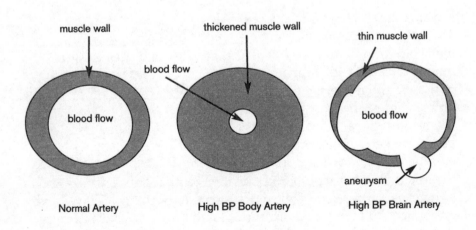

muscle wall

thickened muscle wall

thin muscle wall

blood flow

blood flow

blood flow

blood flow

aneurysm

Normal Artery

High BP Body Artery

High BP Brain Artery

Fig 15

In high blood pressure, the small arteries get more muscular, and the internal bore (or internal cross sectional diameter) gets smaller, a process which makes it harder for the heart to pump blood through them. The result is pressure that rises further. A further rise in pressure causes further artery muscle growth, more resistance to blood flow, and more blood pressure – in other words – a vicious circle.

Epilogue

> The least I could hope for is to help you live for one more day –
> although which day, I could not say.
>
> If all those special people, who once gave us their unconditional love
> and support, could have been given one extra day, we would have a
> second chance to tell them just how much we owed them.

To consider the western way of death, while millions continue to die
of starvation, is poignant at best, and obscene at worst. The very
least each of us should do, is to try and influence major world
organizations to use our money, not just to pay themselves, but also
to help eradicate starvation. I may be a child of the West and I may
have benefited from its nurture, but that doesn't mean that I have to
agree with its priorities. As many poorer nations strive to join our
frenetic capitalist system, they should not ignore some facts about
our collective cultural values. Wealth can distance some of us from
the needs of the less fortunate, and reduce our incentive to be that
Good Samaritan. We will use a hand to write a cheque, but are
reluctant to use it to pull a starving person to his feet, and feed him
with our own spoon. Ignoring the starving altogether, is however,
worse.

From a doctor's chair, life appears neither just nor fair. Like
lightning, disease seems to strike at random. This is an illusion, of
course, created by our lack of understanding, aided and abetted by
arrogance and apathy – in fact, many diseases are present years
before we become aware of them. An improved knowledge of
medical matters might help, but that would take a lot of doing! If
vigilance and reconnaissance could also be taught they would pay

preventative medical dividends, since both are essential strategies for any would-be survivor.

Patients and doctors are sometimes guilty of arrogant egocentric traits. These can result in an attitude that sometimes opposes the spirit of enquiry and may block the path to early diagnosis. Other attitudes are also counterproductive. All scientists, including doctors, should be ruled by altruism – in practice, some are ruled by malice, especially when they have personal reasons to disagree with their patients or colleagues. Many patients, unaware of these traits, may wonder why they feel incompatible with their doctor.

In contrast to the salvage operation of daily medical work, the main mission of preventative medicine is to maximize our chances of survival in any way we can. Genetic engineering offers more hope than any other previous development, but it is far from being realised. Until the fruits of this research are available, we must continue to detect disease processes as early as we can and start managing them, even before they generate their first symptoms. To advantage the majority, foresight, imagination and financial commitment would all be required – unfortunately these are all in very short supply. It would seem that we have the tools for the job, but none of the right priorities.

Science has advanced beyond all belief, while human nature has remained largely unchanged. We are still programmed for a short life, driven by the same old hang-ups that motivated our pre-historic ancestors. The biggest advance we could hope for ourselves is an advance in our psychosocial outlook to one another, to the same level of sophistication as our science. We might then benefit from our scientific power. While ego, self-interest and the satiation of all our desires motivate us, we will all have to struggle to preserve life beyond its selfish or commercial value.

You don't need a lot of common sense to appreciate that it is preferable to predict and avoid catastrophe, rather than face it unprepared. Even though there are no guaranties of success, and no good proof of improved outcomes, I still think that heart disease avoidance is worthy of great effort; after all, the more we try, the more we are likely to improve our treatment and predictive techniques. I will never understand why so few share this view, except to say that, for the general public, health resources always seem limited, however much tax we pay.

Without anyone noticing it, the life of the system we call civilized society, has become more valuable than the lives of those it was born to protect. Because of a lack of awareness and a growing feeling of powerlessness, apathetic inertia will, I am sure, ensure the survival of the status quo!

About the Author

Dr David H. Dighton was a graduate of the London Hospital Medical School, and is a member of both the Royal College of Physicians, and the Royal Society of Medicine, UK, although he has no fondness for clubs or societies in general. He cannot imagine why anyone would want to be anything else in life but a doctor. Given the chance, he would go right back to the beginning, and do it all over again!

He is a full-time private cardiologist and physician, with a 5 figure patient list and a word-processing-induced waist measurement, needing urgent attention. He has been the Medical Director of The Cardiac Centre at Loughton Clinic, Loughton, Essex, UK, since he started it with Noreen Connolly, his physiological technician, in 2001. He is Medical Director of the Loughton Clinic, which he conceived with his London Hospital contemporary, Dr David Baxter, in 1973.

From David Baxter he learned about the world of business and money. Unfortunately, he did not learn his lessons well. He has exposed himself to radiation for 35 years, and continues to irradiate himself regularly as an investigatory cardiologist at the Wellington Hospital, London.

He probably owes his acceptance into the medical profession to the late, and much respected, Dr John Ellis, the Dean of the London Hospital Medical School in 1961. He gave him the chance to use what talents he had, when others would never have dared.

David was introduced to objective thinking at a very young age. His neighbour, a pharmacist, John Powell, was his first and, perhaps, most exacting mentor. With unforgiving rigor, he was further schooled by his schoolboy friend Mike, now the late Prof Michael Stock, at the then South West Essex Technical College. Even then, Mike had the mind of a scientist, and was clearly destined to make a significant contribution. Further development occurred at medical school, now the Royal London, where his tutor Dr John Wright, introduced him to wisdom in medical thinking. Balanced thinking was introduced later on at Whipp's Cross Hospital, in East London, where he came under the considerable influence of a special mate (Cockney for 'friend), Dr Dick ('no bullshit tolerated under any circumstances') Barrett.

He was elevated by the intellectual rigors of working with Dr's Alan Harris, Aubrey Leatham, Paul Kligfield and Alan Gelson, while working at what was then a cardiac research hot-house, St George's Hospital at Hyde Park Corner, London; often frequenting the first Hard Rock Café – just across the road. His research into Aubrey Leatham's initial question: 'why does the heart go slow?', allowed him to separate those who did, from those who did not, need a pacemaker for their blackouts. At St George's, he was privileged to befriend Jeff Davies, the inventor of pacemakers, and Graham Leech, a gifted engineer and member of that St George's team, who were first in the UK to work on cardiac ultrasound.

At Charing Cross Hospital he worked on the interactions between behaviour, stress, and heart disease, with Dr Peter Nixon, a lateral-thinking man of both genius and charisma, wit and insight; but a man before his time. From Peter he learned to unlearn, and to question every dogma, regardless of the political consequences. Unfortunately, Peter fell foul of medical politics and was robbed of the recognition he deserved. From his background as an officer in what became the SAS, Peter's view of David was that he was 'too secure', and therefore, potentially dangerous! An insightful view few have come to appreciate. After working with Peter, and as Chef de Clinique at the Vrije Universiteit, Amsterdam, David worked with Pim de Feyter and learned how earnestness pays dividends.

His intellectual development was further developed on Greek

beaches (aided by Laphroig), and in Greek tavernas (aided by Retsina), by Dr Roderick Storring – Anglophile, Francophile, Grecophile, chest physician, philosopher, pretty good tennis player and golfer, but unaccomplished linguist. As a philosopher, Rod intuitively knows what life is all about, without being able to answer that crucial intellectual question: 'what is life all about?' Unlike Rod, David likes to think that he can get by in many different languages – it's true he can get by in Cockney!

David also likes to think that he can equal the musical talents of another life-long friend, Dr Alan Gardner, but he is mistaken. Both would like to match Ken's talent. Alan has provided constant inspiration for a cherished belief they both share: 'if you can dream it, you can do it'. Alan has never failed to realize his own dreams, and to inspire those of many others.

David's non-professional influences owe everything to his father's sense of humour, and to the security of being, that was his legacy. From his mother he gets whatever other talents he has. God only knows where his looks come from – few want to know either!

He has had enormous support and encouragement in life from many wonderful people, too numerous to mention (he fears not to mention . . . You, perhaps!), who have steadfastly taken almost everything he says, with a laugh and a pinch of salt. That's how he likes it. He distrusts forever serious, (and therefore usually) insecure people.

Apart from Watson and Crick's remark – 'the significance of what we have discovered has not escaped us', and virtually the whole of Shakespeare; nearly all his favourite remarks are of Jewish origin.

John Bard is a friend who used to own a hospital in New Orleans. To sum up his own, bottom-line attitude to life, David often quotes John's father (a proclamation, he originally used to placate the workers in his East-End, smoked salmon factory):

'Why worry?

You're only here for a lifetime . . . you're not here for ever!'

Glossary

ACE inhibitors: Drugs that lower blood pressure and improve heart failure. Side effects: cough and impotence.

Adrenaline: a chemical in the blood that can make the heart beat with more force.

AGI: Atherogenic Index. Potential of a food to cause artery 'furring'.

Alpha-blocker: a drug to open arteries. Used for angina and high blood pressure.

Amino-acid: Chemical sub-units of all proteins.

Aneurysm: Occurs in arteries. Equivalent to a 'blow out' in a tyre. A thin bubble appears which can rupture. Aneurysms occur in the aorta and in brain arteries (cerebral aneurysm).

Angina: Pain or more commonly, tightness in the chest on walking. Due to 'furring' of the heart or coronary arteries.

Angiogram: An X-ray picture taken by injecting an iodine-based dye into the heart cavities or coronary arteries.

Angioplasty: A method of opening narrowed coronary arteries using a balloon catheter inserted into the heart.

Aorta: The main artery leading from the heart to the body.

Aortic valve: The main outlet valve. It gets leaky (incompetence), and constricted (stenosis).

API: Atheroprotective Index. The potential of food to prevent artery 'furring'.

Arcus senilis: A faint white ring around the outer iris of the eye.

Arginine: An amino-acid component of vegetable protein.

Artery: The tubes or blood vessels that carry oxygenated blood from the heart to the tissues.

Atherogenic: Likely to cause the 'furring' of arteries.

Atheroprotective: Likely to prevent the 'furring' of arteries.

Atheroma or atherosclerosis: Cholesterol formation beneath the inner lining of the arteries.

Atrium: The priming or top chambers of the heart. Plural: atria.

Atrial fibrillation: A chaotic, irregular heart rhythm, arising from the atria. There is an attendant risk of clot formation within the heart. It can be a cause of strokes.

Beta-blocker: A drug that blocks the effects of adrenaline. This is used in some forms of high blood pressure and tachycardia.

Blood pressure: The pressure of the pulse within an artery. The maximum pressure reached is called the systolic pressure. The pressure between beats is called the diastolic pressure.

Bradycardia: A slow heart rate (less than 50 beats/min). Found in athletes and those with heart block.

Bruce Protocol: A standardized treadmill exercise test. An international standard for ECG exercise testing.

CABG: Coronary Artery By-pass Graft (sometimes pronounced 'cabbage').

Cardiomegaly: An enlarged heart. Found in heart failure, high blood pressure, and heart valve problems.

Cardiomyopathy: Heart muscle disease.

Cardioprotective: Protects against heart disease – artery 'furring', and high blood pressure especially.

Cardiovascular disease: Diseases of the heart and circulation.

Carotid arteries: Arteries in the neck that supply the brain with blood and oxygen.

Catecholamine: A collective term for adrenaline and nor-adrenaline etc

Catheterisation: A method of examining the heart from the inside. A plastic tube is inserted into an artery and advanced under X-ray control to the heart. Angiography is then performed.

Chromosome: A lump of inherited genetic material, exact copies of which are kept in the nucleus of each of our cells. Twenty-three pairs of chromosomes make a complete set.

Claudication: Pain in the calf muscles on walking. Due to narrowed arteries supplying the legs.

Cor pulmonale: Heart failure from severe lung disease.

Coronary: A common term for heart attack. The name of the heart arteries.

Costochondritis: Painful inflammation of the cartilage attached to ribs.

CVA: A Cerebro-Vascular Accident or stroke.

De-fibrillation: Any method that stops the heart fibrillating. Drug and electrical methods can be used.

Delta-wave (δ-wave): An unusual electrical ECG wave found in people with a particular type of tachycardia or fast heartbeat.

Diabetes: A condition that causes an abnormally raised blood sugar, sugar in the urine (this is actually what the word 'diabetes' means), and an abnormal fat metabolism – hence more artery disease. In pre-diabetes blood glucose is mostly normal but eating takes the level up higher than the normal limits. Such people may eventually become diabetic.

Diastolic: The resting phase of the heart beat, after the main pumping chamber has contracted. In this period the heart is 'primed' by the contracting atria.

Digoxin: drug derived from foxglove. This is used to slow down the rate of the heart. It is also thought to improve the strength of heart contraction.

Diuretic: A tablet that makes your kidney's pass more salt and water.

EBCT: (Electron Beam Computed Tomogram). A fast X-ray of the heart. Shows chalk in the coronary arteries. A normal result means a low risk of current coronary artery disease.

ECG: Electrocardiogram or recording of the heart's electrical activity.

Echocardiogram: (echo-sounding) or ultrasound. A picture of ultrasonic reflections from the heart valves, chambers and heart muscle.

Ectopic: An extra heart beat.

EEG: An electrical brain tracing.

Endemic: A medical condition found among a specified group of people.

Endothelium: The intima or inner lining of all arteries.

Enzyme: A protein that accelerates the way a chemical process works within the body – enzymes help digestion for instance.

Epidemic: A medical condition that occurs at certain times only.

Exercise test: An ECG during exercise on a treadmill or bicycle. Often used to diagnose narrowed heart arteries and rhythm problems.

Electrophysiology: Study of the heart's electrical activity using a catheter inside the heart.

Extra beats: Ventricular (main pumping chamber) or atrial (priming chamber) early or premature electrical impulses that give the feeling of a 'missed' or extra beat. They are usually innocent.

Fibrillation: Fast irregular electrical heart activity. Fatal if not corrected when arising from the main pumping chambers (ventricular fibrillation); a potentially dangerous issue when atrial fibrillation.

Fibrinogen: A blood clotting factor.

Glycaemia: Refers to blood glucose, hyperglycaemia is the raised blood glucose that occurs in diabetics. A substance is glycaemic if it is capable of raising the blood glucose. Table sugar, glucose and starch are all glycaemic, fruit sugar or fructose, is not.

Glycaemic index: The potential of any food to raise our blood sugar. The gold standard is glucose itself. This raises the blood level most, so its glycaemic index is said to = 1. Pasta raises blood glucose half as much (weight for weight) so its glycaemic index is said to = 0.5. The higher the glycaemic index the worse the food is for diabetics and pre-diabetics.

Gene: That section of a chromosome that determines a specific biological process or trait for the whole person.

HDL: High density lipoprotein. Large protective elements of blood fat.

Heart attack: See infarct.

Heart block: Delayed electrical transmission through heart tissue, which can cause blackouts (syncope).

Heart Failure: A weak heart failing to pump enough blood results in breathlessness and / or swollen legs and fatigue.

Hypertension: High blood pressure. 'Re-active', or 'labile', means it goes up and down all the time. 'Consistent', if over 160 (systolic or top figure) or over 95 (diastolic or lower figure).

Hyperventilation: Over-breathing.

Infarct: Death of heart tissue i.e. cardiac infarct = heart attack. They can be anterior – in the front of the heart; inferior – underneath, or posterior – behind the heart.

Intima: The inner lining of all arteries. Its thickness is called the IMT.

Ischaemia: Less blood than needed reaching any part of the body.

IVUS: An Intra-vascular Ultrasound Scan.

J-point: A specific point on the main or QRS wave of the ECG.

JVP: Jugular venous pulse. The fluid level of the heart. Raised in right heart failure.

LDL: Low density lipoprotein – very small bits of blood fat that contribute to artery 'furring' or atherosclerosis.

Lysine: An amino-acid component of animal protein.

Micronutrient: A chemical in food, essential to health, but which exists in very small (micro) amounts (magnesium, selenium etc).

Mitral valve: One of the 4 main heart valves. Mitral stenosis is when it is constricted. This used to follow rheumatic fever.

Murmur: A noise due to a defective heart valve or hole in the heart.

Myocardium: The heart muscle.

Node: The sino-atrial and A-V nodes are part of the heart's electrical system.

PAI-1: A blood clotting factor.

Pandemic: A condition that exists everywhere, all over the world.

Perfusion Scan: A scan showing blood flow to an internal organ.

Pericardium: A sac in which the heart sits. Pericarditis occurs when it is inflamed. Pericardial effusion is when it becomes filled with fluid.

PET: Positron Emission Tomography: a type of radioactive scan used to observe the metabolism of a tissue in action.

Placebo: A harmless, inactive tablet or procedure, used in research to contrast with the effects of an active tablet or procedure.

Pre-diabetes: See diabetes

Pulmonary: Pertaining to the lungs.

Pulmonary hypertension: High artery pressure in the lungs.

Pulmonary oedema: Fluid in the lungs. Often from raised left heart pressures or valve blockage – mitral stenosis.

q-wave: A sign of previous heart attack or infarct on the ECG.

r-wave: Part of the main wave of the ECG.

Reversion: (or cardioversion). Conversion of the heart rhythm back to normal.

Rheumatic Fever: Throat infection that leads to an immune reaction leading to fever and arthritis, as well as heart and kidney inflammation. Common in UK, up to 1950's: now rare. Still present in 3rd World.

s-wave: Follows the r-wave.

'Sartan' drug: Used for hypertension. This has been proven to prevent strokes and heart attacks.

Stenosis: Partial blockage of an artery or valve. A significant stenosis is one where flow of blood is reduced.

Stent: A very small tubular wire mesh inserted in a blood vessel to keep it open.

Syncope: A blackout.

t-wave: Recovery wave of the ECG.

Tachycardia: Fast heart beating. Comes in various forms: supraventricular, when it arises from the top chambers or atria; ventricular, when it comes from the pumping chambers. Nodal or junctional, when it comes from the middle part of the heart.

Thrombosis: A blood clot.

TIA: Transient Ischaemic Attack. A transient stroke.

Tietze's Syndrome: Chest pain from inflamed chest wall cartilages.

Tricuspid: A valve on the right side of the heart.

Trinitrin: A tablet under the tongue to dilate the coronary arteries. Used for angina.

Troponin: A chemical released by the heart during a heart attack.

u-wave: Follows the t-wave.

Ventricular: Pertaining to the main pumping chambers.

Vasodilatation: Blood vessels opening up.

Wenckebach phenomenon: A type of electrical delay in the heart.

WPW: (Wolff-Parkinson-White Syndrome) a type of fast beating of the heart caused by an extra or by-pass electrical pathway in the heart.

X: Syndrome X: Chest pain identical to angina but with no coronary artery disease.

Xanthelasma: Yellowish skin patch denoting the collection of cholesterol.

Further reading and References

Albert, C.M., Hennekens, C.H., O'Donnell, C.J. et al. *Fish Consumption and Risk of Sudden Death*. JAMA. 1998; **279**: 23-28.

Dr Atkins' New Diet Revolution, first published in 1992 in the UK by Vermillion.

Bolles, Edmund B. *Galileo's Commandment*. An anthology of great science writing. Abacus Books. 2000.

Brewer, Sarah. *The Daily Telegraph Encyclopaedia of Vitamins, Minerals and Herbal Supplements*. Robinson. London. 2002.

CLAS Study: Azen. S.P., Mack, W.J., Cashin-Hemphill, L. *et al.* Progression of coronary artery disease predicts coronary artery events: long-term follow-up from the Cholesterol Lowering Atherosclerosis Study (CLAS). Circulation. 1996; 93: 34-41.

CHAOS Study.
Stephens, N.G., Parsons, A., Schonfield, P.M., *et al.* Randomised controlled trial of vitamin E in patients with coronary disease: Cambridge Heart Antioxidant Study (CHAOS). Lancet. 1996; 347: 781-786.

Code of Jewish Law. Rabbi S. Ganzfield and H.E. Goldin. 1961. Hebrew Publishing Company. New York. Vol 1: Pages 146-7.

da Luz, P.L., et al. This paper was published in the *Journal of Experimental Pathology* in 1999. Volume 65, pages 150-9.

DART Study: Burr, M.L., Fehily, A.M., Gilbert, J.F., *et al.* Effects of changes in fat, fish and fibre intakes on death and myocardial re-infarction: diet and re-infarction trial (DART). Lancet. 1989; ii: 757–61.

De Lorgeril, M., Salen P., *et al*. European Journal of Clinical Nutrition. 1997. Volume 51(2). 116-22.

De Lorgeril, M., Salen, P. *et al*. Archives of Internal Medicine. 1998. Volume 158(11), 1181-7.

De Lorgeril, M. *et al. The Lyon Diet*. Circulation.1999, vol 99(6), p 779-85.

Dighton, D. H. (1980). *Sleep Therapy*. General Practitioner 25.1.1980.

Efendy, J.L., *et al*. Atherosclerosis. July 1997, volume 132 (1), pages 37 – 42.

Fairhurst, K. BMJ.1998, vol 317, p 1130-4.

Framingham Study: American Heart Journal (1975): 90; 322–8.

Franco, O.H., Bonneux, L., de Laet, C., et al. The Polymeal: a more natural, safer, and probably tastier (than the Polypill) strategy to reduce cardiovascular disease by more than 75%.

Gaetano, G., et al, published in 'Nutrition, Metabolism, and Cardiovascular Diseases, 2001, volume 11 (4 supplement) pages 47-50).

Galileo Galilæi Lynceo. 1632. *Dialogus de Systemate Mundi*.

GISSI Study: Gruppo Italiano per lo Studio della Sopravivenza nell'infarto miocardico. Dietary supplementation with n-3 polyunstaurated fatty acids and vitamin E after myocardial infarction: results of the GISSI-Prevenzione trial. Lancet. 1999; 354: 447–455.

Hands, E. S. Nutrients in Food. Lippincott, Williams and Wilkins, 2000.

Hankey, G. Current opinion in lipidology. 2002. Vol 13, p 645-51.

Heart Protection Study. International Journal of Clinical Practice. 2002, vol 56, p53-56.

Herrnstein and Murray, *The Bell Curve*. Free Press, NY USA, 1994.

HERS: Heart and Estrogen-Progestin Replacement Study (HERS). Neurology (2004): 62; 968-970.

Hooper et al. Cochrane Database of Systematic Reviews, 2003, Issue 2, Update software, Oxford, ISSN:1469-493X

Ito, M., Toda, T., Kummerow, F.A., Nishimori, I. Effect of magnesium deficiency on ultrastructural changes in coronary arteries of swine. Acta Pathologica Japonica. 1986; 36:225-34.

Jamrozik, Konrad (2005). Estimate of deaths attributable to passive smoking among UK adults: database analysis. BMJ; 330: 812 – 815.

Kaprio, J., et al Atherosclerosis. 2000: 150; 193-200

Keil, U., and colleagues. 1997. Epidemiology. Volume 8: p 150–156.

Kritchevsky, D., Tepper, S.A., Klurfield, D.M. (1985) J.A.O.C.S. Volume 64:1167-71.

Kritchevsky, S.B., Shimakawa, T., Tell, G.S., Dennis, B. *et al.* Dietary antioxidants and carotid artery wall thickness: the ARIC study. Circulation. 1995; 92: 2132-2150.

Lakka, T.A.. et al Atherosclerosis. 2001: 154; 497-504.

Lampe, F.C., Morris, R.W., Walker, M. et al. Trends in rates of different forms of diagnosed coronary heart disease, 1978 to 2000: prospective, population based study of British men. BMJ.(2005); 330: 1046-9.

Law, Malcolm (2000). British Medical Journal):320; 861-864. Plant Sterol and Stanol Margarines and Health.

Law, M., Wald, D.S., Morris, J.K. (2000) Homocysteine and cardiovascular disease: evidence on causality from meta-analysis. BMJ. 2002; 325: 1202-6.

Le Fanu, James. (1987). Eat Your Heart Out. Macmillan.

Leng, G.C., et al., Atherosclerosis. 2000:152; 167-174.

Leonardo da Vinci's Notebooks. (1923).pp 78-79. Edward McCurdy. Empire State Book Company. New York.

Lewis, G. R. 1001 Chemicals in Everyday Products.

Liao, F., Folsom, A.R., Brancati, F.L. Is low magnesium level a risk factor for coronary artery disease? The Atherosclerosis Risk in Communities (ARIC) Study. American Heart Journal. 1998; 136: 480-90.

McCance, R. A., Widdowson, E.M. The Composition of Foods. 2002. Food Standards Agency and Institute of Food Research. Crown Copyright.

Morrells, M.J., Shahidi, F., Chi-Tang Ho. Free Radicals in Food Chemistry. Nutrition and Health Effects. American Chemical Society (2002).

Myeong-Ki, H., Mintz, G., Cheol Wahn, L., et al. Comparisons of coronary plaque rupture between stable angina and acute myocardial infarction. Circulation (2004): 110; 928 – 933.

National Heart and Lung Family Study: Djoussé, Pankow, J.S., Eckfeldt, J.H. et al. Relation between dietary linolenic acid and coronary artery disease in the National Heart, Lung, and Blood Institute Family Heart Study. The American Journal of Clinical

Nutrition.2001; 74(5): 612-9.

Niebauer and Hambrecht, 1995

Orekhov, A.N., and colleagues, Annals of Medicine (1995), volume 27, pages 63-65.

Oxford Dictionary of Quotations. 1999. Oxford University Press.

Pignone, M., BMJ. 2000, vol 321, p983-6.

Reunanen, A., Knekt, P., Marniemi, J. et al. Serum calcium, magnesium, copper, and zinc and risk of cardiovascular death. European Journal of Clinical Nutrition. 1996; 50: 431-7.

Sabaté, J., 1999. The American Journal of Clinical Nutrition. Volume 70(3 suppl), p500S-503S.

Salonen, J.T., Ylä-Herttuala, S., Yamamoto, R., Butler, S. *et al.* Auto-antibody against oxidized LDL and progression of carotid atherosclerosis. Lancet. 1992; 339: 883-6.

Singh, R.B., Shinde, S.N., Chopra, R.K., et al. Effect of co-enzyme-10 on experimental atherosclerosis and chemical composition and quality of atheroma in rabbits. Atherosclerosis. 2000; 148/2:275-282.

Smith, George, D. Lifestyle, health, and health promotion in Nazi Germany. BMJ (2004); 329: 1424-5.

Souci, Fachmann, Kraut. Food Composition and Nutritional Tables. 2000. Medpharm Scientific Publishers.

Steiner, R.M., and colleagues, The American Journal of Clinical Nutrition, 1996, volume 64(6), pages 866-70.

Taylor, A.J.,Watkins, T., Medicine and Science in Sports and Exercise 2002: 34; 228-233.

Thorogood, M., Mann, J. et al. British Medical Journal. 1994. Volume 308(6945) p 1667-70.

Vinson, J.A. et al. In the journal: Atherosclerosis in 2001, volume 156, pages 62 to 72.

Wald, N.J., Law, M.R. A strategy to reduce cardiovascular disease by more than 80%. BMJ 2003; 326:1419-23.

Wannamethee, S.G. 1988. International Journal of Epidemiology. Volume 17: p 307-316.

WHI Study: Women's Health initiative Study. The SOGC Statement. Journal of Obstetrics and Gynaecology Canada (2002): 24; 783-90, 793-802.

Wilde, Oscar. The Importance of Being Ernest.

WHO Technical Report Series. 916. 5.4. (2003). Diet, Nutrition and the Prevention of Chronic Diseases.

Cardiac Value
Food 'Goodies' and 'Baddies'

CVo – means **overall cardiac value.** CVo16 is based on all the 16 cardioprotective chemicals that I believe to be important. CVo7 is based on the WHO recommended cardioprotective foods containing 7 of these 16 beneficial or protective chemicals.

The food 'goodies': Foods with a cardiac value (CVo16 score) of 3.0, and over; or a CVo7 score of 1.6 and over.

The food 'baddies': Foods with a cardiac value (CVo16 & CVo7 score) less than that of pure water. Water scores '1'.

Foods that are 'neutral', that is, they are neither 'good', nor 'bad' for the heart and circulation, have a cardiac value score (CVo 16) of between '1' and 3.0 or a score between '1' and 1.6 for CVo7.

Table 1

Food List in order of Cardiac Value (CVo16)
OVERALL CARDIAC VALUE (CVo WHO & CVo 16)

Portion Analysis Food	Portion Wt (grams)	Portion Wt (ozs)	Kcals/ Portion	Cardiac Values CVo7	CVo16 Indexed
LIVER (PIG)	54	1.6	102	0.77	**30.85**
LIVER (BEEF)	85	2.6	144	0.76	**28.53**
WALNUTS	28	0.8	193	**17.41**	**21.24**
KIDNEY (BEEF)	85	2.6	117	1.52	**16.43**
WHELK	85	2.6	77	0.95	**13.94**
OYSTERS	70	2.1	96	0.54	**12.44**
MUSSEL	85	2.6	88	1.13	**11.74**

Portion Analysis Food	Portion Wt (grams)	Portion Wt (ozs)	Kcals/ Portion	Cardiac Values CVo7	CVo16
SESAME SEEDS	28	0.8	167	8.91	9.83
CUTTLE FISH	85	2.6	90	1.13	9.72
HAZELNUTS	28	0.8	182	7.55	8.89
CRAB (STEAMED)	118	3.6	151	1.16	8.29
LIVER (CHICKEN)	85	2.6	133	2.03	7.38
ALMONDS	28	0.8	171	6.22	7.37
LENTILS	100	3.0	105	1.88	7.21
SOYBEANS (DRY-ROASTED)	50	1.5	318	2.47	7.12
SUNFLOWER SEEDS	28	0.8	160	5.45	6.75
OIL (WALNUT)	14	0.4	126	6.33	6.33
SALMON (pink)	150	4.5	323	4.62	6.06
SUNFLOWER OIL	14	0.4	126	5.28	5.99
SHRIMP	50	1.5	47	0.92	5.36
BLACKEYED PEAS	80	2.4	93	1.88	5.20
HADDOCK	150	4.5	134	1.27	4.98
OCTOPUS	85	2.6	60	0.93	4.91
TUNA	150	4.5	150	3.62	4.85
SCOLLOP	120	3.6	90	1.17	4.77
HALIBUT	150	4.5	182	1.59	4.65
SOLE	127	3.8	116	1.32	4.38
COD	180	5.5	171	1.13	4.37
OIL (WHEATGERM)	14	0.4	126	3.55	4.27
OIL (CORN)	14	0.4	126	4.19	4.27
HEART (BEEF)	85	2.6	192	0.52	3.74
HERRING	143	4.3	259	1.54	3.62
MACKEREL	88	2.7	210	0.88	3.50
POTATO (FLESH)	100	3.0	77	2.88	3.50
SARDINES (in oil)	50	1.5	110	1.04	3.49
SUNFLOWER FLOUR	28	0.8	163	1.63	3.46
PEANUT BUTTER	32	1.0	194	2.87	3.46
AVOCADO	100	3.0	190	3.62	3.43
PEANUTS	28	0.8	158	2.63	3.31
BRAN FLAKES	50	1.5	135	1.03	3.10
LIMA BEANS	78	2.4	264	1.54	3.06
SWORDFISH	106	3.2	147	1.57	2.91
SPINACH	100	3.0	19	1.70	2.90
LOBSTER	145	4.4	149	0.42	2.75
BRUSSEL SPROUTS	78	2.4	27	1.74	2.62
PEAS (GARDEN)	80	2.4	67	1.19	2.54
MILKSHAKE	200	6.1	39	1.03	2.54
OATMEAL	234	7.1	878	2.27	2.51
TOFU	100	3.0	73	0.81	2.41
OVALTINE	200	6.1	35	1.36	2.40
POTATO (FLESH & SKIN)	200	6.1	270	1.14	2.39

Portion Analysis Food	Portion Wt (grams)	Portion Wt (ozs)	Kcals/ Portion	Cardiac Values CVo7	Cardiac Values CVo16
BEANS (BAKED)	100	3.0	84	0.87	2.22
RICE (BROWN)	100	3.0	357	1.03	2.13
CORN	100	3.0	111	**1.64**	2.13
ASPARAGUS	60	1.8	15	**1.65**	2.08
PEPPER (GREEN)	74	2.2	39	1.29	2.03
TURKEY (BREAST ROASTED)	85	2.6	130	0.55	2.01
COTTAGE CHEESE	100	3.0	101	1.22	2.01
LETTUCE	55	1.7	7	**1.65**	1.98
BRAZIL NUTS	28	0.8	191	1.28	1.97
PASTA	57	1.7	164	1.02	1.93
CHICKEN (DARK MEAT)	114	3.5	211	1.42	1.89
EGG (WHITE)	33	1.0	12	0.98	1.89
BEER (average)	500	15.2	145	1.29	1.88
EGG (YOLK)	17	0.5	58	1.42	1.88
CHICKEN BREAST (ROASTED)	196	5.9	300	1.38	1.83
RED WINE	100	3.0	68	1.03	1.81
RICE KRISPIES	25	0.8	70	0.92	1.79
EEL	136	4.1	147	1.98	1.75
SHREDDED WHEAT	50	1.5	189	0.83	1.72
TOMATO	100	3.0	17	1.34	1.70
STRAWBERRY	83	2.5	22	1.45	1.67
MAGARINE	5	0.2	37	**1.60**	1.62
WHITE WINE	100	3.0	66	1.03	1.61
TURKEY (DARK MEAT)	85	2.6	150	0.68	1.60
POTATO (SWEET)	100	3.0	87	1.05	1.58
BROCCOLI	44	1.3	24	1.22	1.56
BANANA	75	2.3	87	0.99	1.54
CAULIFLOWER	50	1.5	14	1.24	1.54
ONION	50	1.5	18	1.12	1.53
TEA	200	6.1	0	1.03	1.50
APPLE	138	4.2	65	1.38	1.48
CABBAGE	75	2.3	12	1.20	1.47
FLORA PRO-ACTIVE	5	0.2	68	1.13	1.46
MANGO	100	3.0	68	1.11	1.42
OIL (HAZELNUT)	14	0.4	126	0.88	1.41
SAUSAGES (PORK)	100	3.0	230	1.41	1.40
PINE NUTS	28	0.8	193	0.27	1.40
MILK (1% FAT)	245	7.4	113	0.88	1.39
PAPAYA	100	3.0	39	1.23	1.34
ORANGE JUICE	124	3.8	56	1.05	1.33
BEVERAGES: COFFEE	200	6.1	0	1.01	1.29
CARROTS	50	1.5	12	1.08	1.24
RICE (LONG-GRAIN WHITE)	100	3.0	359	0.83	1.21
CORNFLAKES	100	3.0	376	0.55	1.20

Portion Analysis Food	Portion Wt (grams)	Portion Wt (ozs)	Kcals/ Portion	Cardiac Values CVo7	CVo16
PEAS (PROCESSED)	80	2.4	79	0.86	1.20
BREAD (WHOLEWHEAT)	28	0.8	61	0.70	1.17
DUCK (ROASTED)	85	2.6	166	1.02	1.16
BREAD (WHITE AVERAGE)	30	0.9	66	0.77	1.14
YOGURT	100	3.0	56	0.77	1.08
HONEY	33	1.0	109	1.00	1.05
COLA	250	7.6	10	1.00	1.01
DIET COLA	250	7.6	0	1.00	1.01
WATER	**1000**	**30.3**	**0**	**1.00**	**1.00**
PORK (LEG ROASTED)	85	2.6	155	0.32	0.95
BEEF (RUMP) COOKED	100	3.0	177	0.27	0.94
OIL (COD LIVER)	14 0.	4	126	0.86	0.93
OIL (OLIVE)	14	0.4	126	0.82	0.82
ANCHOVY (in oil)	85	2.6	162	0.41	0.80
LAMB (LEG ROASTED)	85	2.6	187	0.29	0.79
PARMESAN	6	0.2	27	0.63	0.75
ALMOND OIL	14	0.4	126	0.48	0.74
PALM OIL	14	0.4	126	0.62	0.66
BUTTER	5	0.2	37	0.55	0.56
CHEDDAR	28	0.8	116	0.39	0.43
CRISPS (POTATO)	30	0.9	137	0.25	0.39
CAMEMBERT	62	1.9	180	0.38	0.3
ICE CREAM	66	2.0	117	0.18	0.26
HAMBURGER	250	7.6	608	0.05	0.25
COCONUT	23	0.7	139	0.14	0.19
CHOCOLATE: MILK	44	1.3	229	0.09	0.16
PLAIN CHOCOLATE	44	1.3	224	0.10	0.13
CHEESEBURGER (triple meat)	400	12.1	1036	0.02	0.11
WHITE CHOCOLATE	44	1.3	260	0.07	0.08

Table 2

Alphabetic Food List and Cardiac Value

The food 'goodies': Foods with a cardiac value (CVo16 score) of over 3.0, and CVo7 of 1.6 and over.

The food 'baddies': Foods with a cardiac value (CVo 16 score) less than that of water (CVo16 & CVo7 = 1)

Food that is 'neutral' has neither a good, nor a bad score of between '1' and 3.0 (CVo16) and '1' and 1.6 (CVo7).

OVERALL CARDIAC VALUE (CVo7 WHO based & CVo16)
Of foods in alphabetical order

Portion Analysis Food	Portion Wt (grams)	Portion Wt (ozs)	Kcals/ Portion	Cardiac Values CVo7	CVo16
ALMONDS	**28**	**0.8**	**171**	**6.22**	**7.37**
ANCHOVY (in oil)	85	2.6	162	0.41	0.80
APPLE	138	4.2	65	1.38	1.48
ASPARAGUS	60	1.8	15	**1.65**	2.08
AVOCADO	**100**	**3.0**	**190**	**3.62**	**3.43**
BANANA	75	2.3	87	0.99	1.54
BEANS (BAKED)	100	3.0	84	0.87	2.22
BEEF (RUMP) COOKED	100	3.0	177	0.27	0.94
BEER (average)	500	15.2	145	1.29	1.88
BEVERAGES: COFFEE	200	6.1	0	1.01	1.29
BLACKEYED PEAS	**80**	**2.4**	**93**	**1.88**	**5.20**
BRAN FLAKES	**50**	**1.5**	**135**	**1.03**	**3.10**
BRAZIL NUTS	28	0.8	191	1.28	1.97
BREAD (WHITE AVERAGE)	30	0.9	66	0.77	1.14
BREAD (WHOLEWHEAT)	28	0.8	61	0.70	1.17
BROCCOLI	44	1.3	24	1.22	1.56
BRUSSEL SPROUTS	78	2.4	27	1.74	2.62
BUTTER	5	0.2	37	0.55	0.56
CABBAGE	75	2.3	12	1.20	1.47
CAMEMBERT	62	1.9	180	0.38	0.30
CARROTS	50	1.5	12	1.08	1.24
CAULIFLOWER	50	1.5	14	1.24	1.54
CHEDDAR	28	0.8	116	0.39	0.43
CHEESEBURGER (triple meat)	400	12.1	1036	0.02	0.10
CHICKEN (DARK MEAT)	114	3.5	211	1.42	1.89
CHICKEN BREAST (ROASTED)	196	5.9	300	1.38	1.83
CHOCOLATE: MILK	44	1.3	229	0.09	0.16
COCONUT	23	0.7	139	0.14	0.19
COD	**180**	**5.5**	**171**	**1.13**	**4.37**
COLA	250	7.6	10	1.00	1.01
CORN	100	3.0	111	**1.64**	2.13
CORNFLAKES	100	3.0	376	0.55	1.20
COTTAGE CHEESE	100	3.0	101	1.22	2.01
CRAB (STEAMED)	**118**	**3.6**	**151**	**1.16**	**8.29**
CRISPS (POTATO)	30	0.9	137	0.25	0.39
CUTTLE FISH	**85**	**2.6**	**90**	**1.13**	**9.72**

Portion Analysis Food	Portion Wt (grams)	Portion Wt (ozs)	Kcals/ Portion	Cardiac Values	
				CVo7	CVo16
DIET COLA	250	7.6	0	1.00	1.01
DUCK (ROASTED)	85	2.6	166	1.02	1.16
EEL	136	4.1	147	**1.98**	1.75
EGG (WHITE)	33	1.0	12	0.98	1.89
EGG (YOLK)	17	0.5	58	1.42	1.88
FLORA PRO-ACTIVE	5	0.2	68	1.13	1.46
HADDOCK	**150**	**4.5**	**134**	1.27	**4.98**
HALIBUT	**150**	**4.5**	**182**	1.59	**4.65**
HAMBURGER	250	7.6	608	0.05	0.25
HAZELNUTS	**28**	**0.8**	**182**	**7.55**	**8.89**
HEART (BEEF)	**85**	**2.6**	**192**	0.52	**3.74**
HERRING	**143**	**4.3**	**259**	1.54	**3.62**
HONEY	33	1.0	109	1.00	1.05
ICE CREAM	66	2.0	117	0.18	0.26
KIDNEY (BEEF)	**85**	**2.6**	**117**	1.52	**16.43**
LAMB (LEG ROASTED)	85	2.6	187	0.29	0.79
LENTILS	**100**	**3.0**	**105**	**1.88**	**7.21**
LETTUCE	55	1.7	7	1.65	1.98
LIMA BEANS	**78**	**2.4**	**264**	1.54	**3.06**
LIVER (BEEF)	**85**	**2.6**	**144**	0.76	**28.53**
LIVER (CHICKEN)	**85**	**2.6**	**133**	**2.03**	**7.38**
LIVER (PIG)	**54**	**1.6**	**102**	0.77	**30.85**
LOBSTER	**145**	**4.4**	**149**	0.42	**2.75**
MACKEREL	**88**	**2.7**	**210**	0.88	**3.50**
MAGARINE	5	0.2	37	**1.60**	1.62
MANGO	100	3.0	68	1.11	1.42
MILK (1% FAT)	245	7.4	113	0.88	1.39
MILKSHAKE	200	6.1	39	1.03	2.54
MUSSEL	**85**	**2.6**	**88**	1.13	**11.74**
OATMEAL	234	7.1	878	2.27	2.51
OCTOPUS	**85**	**2.6**	**60**	0.93	**4.91**
OIL (ALMOND)	14	0.4	126	0.48	0.74
OIL (COD LIVER)	14	0.4	126	0.85	0.92
OIL (CORN)	**14**	**0.4**	**126**	**4.19**	**4.27**
OIL (HAZELNUT)	14	0.4	126	0.88	1.41
OIL (OLIVE)	14	0.4	126	0.82	0.82
OIL (PALM)	14	0.4	126	0.62	0.66
OIL (SUNFLOWER)	**14**	**0.4**	**126**	**5.28**	**5.99**
OIL (WALNUT)	**14**	**0.4**	**126**	**6.33**	**6.33**
OIL (WHEATGERM)	**14**	**0.4**	**126**	**3.55**	**4.27**
ONION	50	1.5	18	1.12	1.53
ORANGE JUICE	124	3.8	56	1.05	1.33
OVALTINE	200	6.1	35	1.36	2.4
OYSTERS	**70**	**2.1**	**96**	0.54	**12.44**

Portion Analysis Food	Portion Wt (grams)	Portion Wt (ozs)	Kcals/ Portion	Cardiac Values CVo7	CVo16
PAPAYA	100	3.0	39	1.23	1.34
PARMESAN	6	0.2	27	0.63	0.75
PASTA	57	1.7	164	1.02	1.93
PEANUT BUTTER	**32**	**1.0**	**194**	**2.87**	**3.46**
PEANUTS	**28**	**0.8**	**158**	**2.63**	**3.31**
PEAS (GARDEN)	80	2.4	67	1.19	2.54
PEAS (PROCESSED)	80	2.4	79	0.86	1.20
PEPPER (GREEN)	74	2.2	39	1.29	2.03
PINE NUTS	28	0.8	193	0.27	1.40
PLAIN CHOCOLATE	44	1.3	224	0.10	0.13
PORK (LEG ROASTED)	85	2.6	155	0.32	0.95
POTATO (FLESH & SKIN)	200	6.1	270	1.14	2.39
POTATO (FLESH)	**100**	**3.0**	**77**	**2.88**	**3.50**
POTATO (SWEET)	100	3.0	87	1.05	1.58
RED WINE	100	3.0	68	1.03	1.81
RICE (BROWN)	100	3.0	357	1.03	2.13
RICE (LONG-GRAIN WHITE)	100	3.0	359	0.83	1.21
RICE KRISPIES	25	0.8	70	0.92	1.79
SALMON (PINK/BAKED)	**150**	**4.5**	**323**	**4.62**	**6.06**
SARDINES (in oil)	**50**	**1.5**	**110**	1.04	**3.49**
SAUSAGES (PORK)	100	3.0	230	1.41	1.40
SCOLLOP	**120**	**3.6**	**90**	1.17	**4.77**
SESAME SEEDS	**28**	**0.8**	**167**	**8.91**	**9.83**
SHREDDED WHEAT	50	1.5	189	0.83	1.72
SHRIMP	**50**	**1.5**	**47**	0.92	**5.36**
SOLE	**127**	**3.8**	**116**	1.32	**4.38**
SOYBEANS (DRY-ROASTED)	**50**	**1.5**	**318**	**2.47**	**7.12**
SPINACH	100	3.0	19	1.70	2.90
STRAWBERRY	83	2.5	22	1.45	1.67
SUNFLOWER FLOUR	**28**	**0.8**	**163**	**1.63**	**3.46**
SUNFLOWER SEEDS	**28**	**0.8**	**160**	**5.45**	**6.75**
SWORDFISH	106	3.2	147	1.57	2.91
TEA	200	6.1	0	1.03	1.50
TOFU	100	3.0	73	0.81	2.41
TOMATO	100	3.0	17	1.34	1.70
TUNA	**150**	**4.5**	**150**	**3.62**	**4.85**
TURKEY (BREAST ROASTED)	85	2.6	130	0.55	2.01
TURKEY (DARK MEAT)	85	2.6	150	0.68	1.60
WALNUTS	**28**	**0.8**	**193**	**17.41**	**21.24**
WATER	1000	30.3	0	1.00	1.00
WHELK	**85**	**2.6**	**77**	**0.95**	**13.94**
WHITE CHOCOLATE	44	1.3	260	0.07	0.08
WHITE WINE	100	3.0	66	1.03	1.61
YOGURT	100	3.0	56	0.77	1.08

Food Units

Table A

Daily Units of Carbohydrate & Saturated Fat
100 Calorie Units = 1000KCals/day; 100 Diabetic units= 50g carbohydrate
/day; 100 Saturated fat units = 7.78 grams of fat/day

Portion Analysis Food	Portion Wt (grams)	Portion Wt (ozs)	CVo16 Cardiac Value	Calorie Units	Diabetic Units	Sat. Fat Units
ALMONDS	28	0.8	7.37	17	1	18
ANCHOVY (in oil)	85	2.6	0.80	16	0	14
APPLE	138	4.2	1.48	6	6	1
ASPARAGUS	60	1.8	2.08	2	1	1
AVOCADO	100	3.0	3.43	19	0	53
BANANA	75	2.3	1.54	9	17	1
BEANS (BAKED)	100	3.0	2.22	8	11	1
BEEF (RUMP) COOKED	100	3.0	0.94	18	0	100
BEER (average)	500	15.2	1.88	15	2	0
BEVERAGES: COFFEE	200	6.1	1.29	0	0	0
BLACKEYED PEAS	80	2.4	5.20	9	27	2
BRAN FLAKES	50	1.5	3.10	14	35	3
BRAZIL NUTS	28	0.8	1.97	19	0	58
BREAD (WHITE AVERAGE)	30	0.9	1.14	7	18	3
BREAD (WHOLEWHEAT)	28	0.8	1.17	6	16	4
BROCCOLI	44	1.3	1.56	2	1	1
BRUSSEL SPROUTS	78	2.4	2.62	3	2	0
BUTTER	5	0.2	0.56	4	0	32
CABBAGE	75	2.3	1.47	1	3	1
CAMEMBERT	62	1.9	0.30	18	0	122
CARROTS	50	1.5	1.24	1	2	1
CAULIFLOWER	50	1.5	1.54	1	1	3
CHEDDAR	28	0.8	0.43	12	0	76
CHEESEBURGER (triple meat)	400	12.1	0.10	104	98	319
CHICKEN (DARK MEAT)	114	3.5	1.89	21	0	54
CHICKEN BREAST (ROASTED)	196	5.9	1.83	30	0	55

Portion Analysis Food	Portion Wt (grams)	Portion Wt (ozs)	CVo16 Cardiac Value	Calorie Units	Diabetic Units	Sat. Fat Units
CHOCOLATE: MILK	44	1.3	0.16	23	28	103
COCONUT	23	0.7	0.19	14	0	158
COD	180	5.5	4.37	17	0	4
COLA	250	7.6	1.01	1	0	0
CORN	100	3.0	2.13	11	22	3
CORNFLAKES	100	3.0	1.20	38	139	3
COTTAGE CHEESE	100	3.0	2.01	10	0	8
CRAB (STEAMED)	118	3.6	8.29	15	0	4
CRISPS (POTATO)	30	0.9	0.39	14	16	36
CUTTLE FISH	85	2.6	9.72	0	0	0
DIET COLA	250	7.6	1.01	0	0	0
DUCK (ROASTED)	33	1.0	1.89	1	0	0
EEL	85	2.6	1.16	17	0	105
EGG (WHITE)	136	4.1	1.75	15	0	46
EGG (YOLK)	17	0.5	1.88	6	0	21
FLORA PRO-ACTIVE	5	0.2	1.46	7	0	0
HADDOCK	150	4.5	4.98	13	0	4
HALIBUT	150	4.5	4.65	18	0	8
HAMBURGER	250	7.6	0.25	61	57	129
HAZELNUTS	28	0.8	8.89	18	0	17
HEART (BEEF)	85	2.6	3.74	19	0	32
HERRING	143	4.3	3.62	26	0	48
HONEY	33	1.0	1.05	11	0	0
ICE CREAM	66	2.0	0.26	12	6	58
KIDNEY (BEEF)	85	2.6	16.43	12	0	12
LAMB (LEG ROASTED)	85	2.6	0.79	19	0	90
LENTILS	100	3.0	7.21	11	9	1
LETTUCE	55	1.7	1.98	1	1	0
LIMA BEANS	78	2.4	3.06	26	36	3
LIVER (BEEF)	85	2.6	28.53	14	0	17
LIVER (CHICKEN)	85	2.6	7.38	13	1	21
LIVER (PIG)	54	1.6	30.85	10	3	17
LOBSTER	145	4.4	2.75	15	0	31
MACKEREL	88	2.7	3.50	21	0	48
MAGARINE	5	0.2	1.62	4	0	9
MANGO	100	3.0	1.42	7	17	1
MILK (1% FAT)	245	7.4	1.39	11	0	19
MILKSHAKE	200	6.1	2.54	4	0	0
MUSSEL	85	2.6	11.74	9	0	9
OATMEAL	234	7.1	2.51	88	151	6
OCTOPUS	85	2.6	4.91	6	0	8
OIL (ALMOND)	14	0.4	0.74	13	0	14
OIL (COD LIVER)	14	0.4	0.92	13	0	41

Portion Analysis Food	Portion Wt (grams)	Portion Wt (ozs)	CVo16 Cardiac Value	Calorie Units	Diabetic Units	Sat. Fat Units
OIL (CORN)	14	0.4	**4.27**	13	0	26
OIL (HAZELNUT)	14	0.4	1.41	13	0	2
OIL (OLIVE)	14	0.4	0.82	13	0	24
OIL (PALM)	14	0.4	0.66	13	0	147
OIL (SUNFLOWER)	14	0.4	**5.99**	13	0	18
OIL (WALNUT)	14	0.4	**6.33**	13	0	17
OIL (WHEATGERM)	14	0.4	**4.27**	13	0	33
ONION	50	1.5	1.53	2	**3**	0
ORANGE JUICE	124	3.8	1.33	6	**12**	0
OVALTINE	200	6.1	2.40	4	0	0
OYSTERS	70	2.1	**12.44**	10	**11**	14
PAPAYA	100	3.0	1.34	4	**10**	0
PARMESAN	6	0.2	0.75	3	0	14
PASTA	57	1.7	1.93	16	**31**	3
PEANUT BUTTER	32	1.0	**3.46**	19	1	40
PEANUTS	28	0.8	**3.31**	16	1	46
PEAS (GARDEN)	80	2.4	2.54	7	**16**	0
PEAS (PROCESSED)	80	2.4	1.20	8	**15**	1
PEPPER (GREEN)	74	2.2	2.03	4	**9**	0
PINE NUTS	28	0.8	1.40	19	0	51
PLAIN CHOCOLATE	44	1.3	0.13	22	**38**	95
PORK (ROAST LEG)	85	2.6	0.95	15	0	71
POTATO (FLESH)	100	3.0	**3.50**	8	**23**	0
POTATO (SWEET)	100	3.0	1.58	9	**11**	1
RED WINE	100	3.0	1.81	7	0	0
RICE (BROWN)	100	3.0	2.13	36	**107**	3
RICE (LONG-GRAIN WHITE)	100	3.0	1.21	36	**115**	0
RICE KRISPIES	25	0.8	1.79	7	**29**	1
SALMON (PINK/BAKED)	150	4.5	**6.06**	32	0	11
SARDINES (in oil)	50	1.5	**3.49**	11	0	11
SAUSAGES (PORK)	100	3.0	1.40	23	6	63
SCOLLOP	120	3.6	**4.77**	0	0	9
SESAME SEEDS	28	0.8	**9.83**	17	0	24
SHREDDED WHEAT	50	1.5	1.72	19	**48**	2
SHRIMP	50	1.5	**5.36**	5	0	3
SOLE	127	3.8	**4.38**	12	0	6
SOYBEANS (DRY-ROASTED)	50	1.5	**7.12**	32	3	14
SPINACH	100	3.0	2.90	2	1	0
STRAWBERRY	83	2.5	1.67	2	2	0
SUNFLOWER FLOUR	28	0.8	**3.46**	16	1	16
SUNFLOWER SEEDS	28	0.8	**6.75**	16	0	19
SWORDFISH	106	3.2	2.91	15	0	19
TEA	200	6.1	1.50	0	0	0

Portion Analysis Food	Portion Wt (grams)	Portion Wt (ozs)	CVo16 Cardiac Value	Calorie Units	Diabetic Units	Sat. Fat Units
TOFU	100	3.0	2.41	7	0	4
TOMATO	100	3.0	1.70	2	2	0
TUNA	150	4.5	4.85	15	0	5
TURKEY (BREAST ROASTED)	85	2.6	2.01	13	0	23
TURKEY (DARK MEAT)	85	2.6	1.60	15	0	33
WALNUTS	28	0.8	21.24	19	0	0
WATER	1000	30.3	1.00	0	0	0
WHELK	85	2.6	13.94	8	0	0
WHITE CHOCOLATE	44	1.3	0.08	26	65	104
WHITE WINE	100	3.0	1.61	7	1	0
YOGURT	100	3.0	1.08	6	4	13

Table B

Food Good for both Diabetes and the Heart:

That is Carbohydrate Units less than 10, & a Cardiac Value more than 3.0.

Daily Units of Carbohydrate & Saturated Fat
100 Calorie Units = 1000KCals/day; 100 Diabetic units = 50g carbohydrate /day; 100 Saturated fat units = 7.78 grams of fat/day

Portion Analysis Food	Portion Wt (grams)	Portion Wt (ozs)	CVo16 Cardiac Value	Calorie Units	Diabetic Units	Sat. Fat Units
ANCHOVY (in oil)	85	2.6	0.80	16	0	14
AVOCADO	100	3.0	3.43	19	0	53
BEEF (RUMP) COOKED	100	3.0	0.94	18	0	100
BEVERAGES: COFFEE	200	6.1	1.29	0	0	0
BUTTER	5	0.2	0.56	4	0	32
CAMEMBERT	62	1.9	0.30	18	0	122
CHEDDAR	28	0.8	0.43	12	0	76
CHICKEN (DARK MEAT)	114	3.5	1.89	21	0	54
CHICKEN BREAST (ROASTED)	196	5.9	1.83	30	0	55
COD	180	5.5	4.37	17	0	4
COLA	250	7.6	1.01	1	0	0
COTTAGE CHEESE	100	3.0	2.01	10	0	8
CRAB (STEAMED)	118	3.6	8.29	15	0	4
CUTTLE FISH	85	2.6	9.72	0	0	0

Portion Analysis Food	Portion Wt (grams)	Portion Wt (ozs)	CVo16 Cardiac Value	Calorie Units	Diabetic Units	Sat. Fat Units
DIET COLA	250	7.6	1.01	0	0	0
DUCK (ROASTED)	85	2.6	1.16	17	0	105
EEL	136	4.1	1.75	15	0	46
HADDOCK	150	4.5	4.98	13	0	4
HALIBUT	150	4.5	4.65	18	0	8
HEART (BEEF)	85	2.6	3.74	19	0	32
HERRING	143	4.3	3.62	26	0	48
HONEY	33	1.0	1.05	11	0	0
KIDNEY (BEEF)	85	2.6	16.43	12	0	12
LAMB (LEG ROASTED)	85	2.6	0.79	19	0	90
LIVER (BEEF)	85	2.6	28.53	14	0	17
LOBSTER	145	4.4	2.75	15	0	31
MACKEREL	88	2.7	3.50	21	0	48
MAGARINE	5	0.2	1.62	4	0	9
MILK (1% FAT)	245	7.4	1.39	11	0	19
MILKSHAKE	200	6.1	2.54	4	0	0
MUSSEL	85	2.6	11.74	9	0	9
OCTOPUS	85	2.6	4.91	6	0	8
OIL (ALMOND)	14	0.4	0.74	13	0	14
OIL (COD LIVER)	14	0.4	0.92	13	0	41
OIL (CORN)	14	0.4	4.27	13	0	26
OIL (HAZELNUT)	14	0.4	1.41	13	0	2
OIL (OLIVE)	14	0.4	0.82	13	0	24
OIL (PALM)	14	0.4	0.66	13	0	147
OIL (SUNFLOWER)	14	0.4	5.99	13	0	18
OIL (WALNUT)	14	0.4	6.33	13	0	17
OIL (WHEATGERM)	14	0.4	4.27	13	0	33
OVALTINE	200	6.1	2.40	4	0	0
PORK (LEG ROASTED)	85	2.6	0.95	15	0	71
SALMON (PINK/BAKED)	150	4.5	6.06	32	0	11
SARDINES (in oil)	50	1.5	3.49	11	0	11
SCOLLOP	120	3.6	4.77	0	0	9
SHRIMP	50	1.5	5.36	5	0	3
SOLE	127	3.8	4.38	12	0	6
SWORDFISH	106	3.2	2.91	15	0	19
TEA	200	6.1	1.50	0	0	0
TOFU	100	3.0	2.41	7	0	4
TUNA	150	4.5	4.85	15	0	5
TURKEY (BREAST ROASTED)	85	2.6	2.01	13	0	23
TURKEY (DARK MEAT)	85	2.6	1.60	15	0	33
WATER	1000	30.3	1.00	0	0	0
WHELK	85	2.6	13.94	8	0	0
EGG (WHITE)	33	1.0	1.89	1	0	0

Portion Analysis Food	Portion Wt (grams)	Portion Wt (ozs)	CVo16 Cardiac Value	Calorie Units	Diabetic Units	Sat. Fat Units
EGG (YOLK)	17	0.5	1.88	6	0	21
FLORA PRO-ACTIVE	5	0.2	1.46	7	0	0
RED WINE	100	3.0	1.81	7	0	0
SESAME SEEDS	**28**	**0.8**	**9.83**	**17**	**0**	**24**
PARMESAN	6	0.2	0.75	3	0	14
BRAZIL NUTS	28	0.8	1.97	19	0	58
WALNUTS	**28**	**0.8**	**21.24**	**19**	**0**	**0**
SUNFLOWER SEEDS	28	0.8	6.75	16	0	19
PINE NUTS	28	0.8	1.40	19	0	51
COCONUT	23	0.7	0.19	14	0	158
HAZELNUTS	**28**	**0.8**	**8.89**	**18**	**0**	**17**
ALMONDS	**28**	**0.8**	**7.37**	**17**	**1**	**18**
BROCCOLI	44	1.3	1.56	2	1	1
ASPARAGUS	60	1.8	2.08	2	1	1
LETTUCE	55	1.7	1.98	1	1	0
CAULIFLOWER	50	1.5	1.54	1	1	3
PEANUTS	**28**	**0.8**	**3.31**	**16**	**1**	**46**
PEANUT BUTTER	**32**	**1.0**	**3.46**	**19**	**1**	**40**
LIVER (CHICKEN)	**85**	**2.6**	**7.38**	**13**	**1**	**21**
WHITE WINE	100	3.0	1.61	7	1	0
SUNFLOWER FLOUR	**28**	**0.8**	**3.46**	**16**	**1**	**16**
SPINACH	100	3.0	2.90	2	1	0
TOMATO	100	3.0	1.70	2	2	0
BEER (average)	500	15.2	1.88	15	2	0
BRUSSEL SPROUTS	78	2.4	2.62	3	2	0
STRAWBERRY	83	2.5	1.67	2	2	0
CARROTS	50	1.5	1.24	1	2	1
SOYBEANS (DRY-ROASTED)	**50**	**1.5**	**7.12**	**32**	**3**	**14**
ONION	50	1.5	1.53	2	3	0
CABBAGE	75	2.3	1.47	1	3	1
LIVER (PIG)	**54**	**1.6**	**30.85**	**10**	**3**	**17**
YOGURT	100	3.0	1.08	6	4	13
SAUSAGES (PORK)	100	3.0	1.40	23	6	63
PEPPER (GREEN)	74	2.2	2.03	4	9	0
LENTILS	**100**	**3.0**	**7.21**	**11**	**9**	**1**
PAPAYA	100	3.0	1.34	4	10	0
OYSTERS	**70**	**2.1**	**12.44**	**10**	**11**	**14**
POTATO (SWEET)	100	3.0	1.58	9	11	1
BEANS (BAKED)	100	3.0	2.22	8	11	1
ORANGE JUICE	124	3.8	1.33	6	12	0
PEAS (PROCESSED)	80	2.4	1.20	8	15	1
BREAD (WHOLEWHEAT)	28	0.8	1.17	6	16	4
PEAS (GARDEN)	80	2.4	2.54	7	16	0

Portion Analysis Food	Portion Wt (grams)	Portion Wt (ozs)	CVo16 Cardiac Value	Calorie Units	Diabetic Units	Sat. Fat Units
CRISPS (POTATO)	30	0.9	0.39	14	16	36
BANANA	75	2.3	1.54	9	17	1
MANGO	100	3.0	1.42	7	17	1
BREAD (WHITE AVERAGE)	30	0.9	1.14	7	18	3
CORN	100	3.0	2.13	11	22	3
POTATO (FLESH)	100	3.0	3.50	8	23	0
BLACKEYED PEAS	80	2.4	5.20	9	27	2
CHOCOLATE: MILK	44	1.3	0.16	23	28	103
RICE KRISPIES	25	0.8	1.79	7	29	1
PASTA	57	1.7	1.93	16	31	3
BRAN FLAKES	50	1.5	3.10	14	35	3
LIMA BEANS	78	2.4	3.06	26	36	3
PLAIN CHOCOLATE	44	1.3	0.13	22	38	95
SHREDDED WHEAT	50	1.5	1.72	19	48	2
HAMBURGER	250	7.6	0.25	61	57	129
WHITE CHOCOLATE	44	1.3	0.08	26	65	104
POTATO (FLESH & SKIN)	200	6.1	2.39	27	80	0
CHEESEBURGER (triple meat)	400	12.1	0.10	104	109	319
RICE (BROWN)	100	3.0	2.13	36	107	3
RICE (LONG-GRAIN WHITE)	100	3.0	1.21	36	115	0
CORNFLAKES	100	3.0	1.20	38	139	3
OATMEAL	234	7.1	2.51	88	151	6

Table C

Daily Units of Sodium & Potassium Salts

100 Calorie Units = 1000KCals/day; 100 sodium salt units =1600mgs sodium (Na) /day, 100 potassium units = 3200mgs potassium (K)/day

Portion Analysis Food	Portion Wt (grams)	Portion Wt (ozs)	CVo16 Cardiac Value	Calorie Units	Salt Units	Potassium Units
ANCHOVY (in oil)	85	2.6	0.80	16	209	7
AVOCADO	100	3.0	3.43	19	0	0
BEEF (RUMP) COOKED	100	3.0	0.94	18	5	14
BEVERAGES: COFFEE	200	6.1	1.29	0	0	0
BUTTER	5	0.2	0.56	4	2	0
CAMEMBERT	62	1.9	0.30	18	23	2
CHEDDAR	28	0.8	0.43	12	13	1
CHICKEN (DARK MEAT)	114	3.5	1.89	21	4	14
CHICKEN BREAST (ROASTED)	196	5.9	1.83	30	10	22

Portion Analysis Food	Portion Wt (grams)	Portion Wt (ozs)	CVo16 Cardiac Value	Calorie Units	Salt Units	Potassium Units
COD	180	5.5	**4.37**	17	18	17
COLA	250	7.6	1.01	1	0	0
COTTAGE CHEESE	100	3.0	2.01	10	19	5
CRAB (STEAMED)	118	3.6	**8.29**	15	31	10
CUTTLE FISH	85	2.6	**9.72**	0	5	7
DIET COLA	250	7.6	1.01	0	0	0
DUCK (ROASTED)	85	2.6	1.16	17	5	8
EEL	136	4.1	1.75	15	56	2
HADDOCK	150	4.5	**4.98**	13	7	19
HALIBUT	150	4.5	**4.65**	18	7	25
HEART (BEEF)	85	2.6	**3.74**	19	4	6
HERRING	143	4.3	**3.62**	26	14	20
HONEY	33	1.0	1.05	11	0	0
KIDNEY (BEEF)	85	2.6	**16.43**	12	8	6
LAMB (LEG ROASTED)	85	2.6	0.79	19	3	10
LIVER (BEEF)	85	2.6	**28.53**	14	8	6
LOBSTER	145	4.4	2.75	15	30	13
MACKEREL	88	2.7	**3.50**	21	3	11
MAGARINE	5	0.2	1.62	4	3	0
MILK (1% FAT)	245	7.4	1.39	11	7	13
MILKSHAKE	200	6.1	2.54	4	0	0
MUSSEL	85	2.6	**11.74**	9	19	4
OCTOPUS	85	2.6	**4.91**	6	10	4
OIL (ALMOND)	14	0.4	0.74	13	0	0
OIL (COD LIVER)	14	0.4	0.92	13	0	1
OIL (CORN)	14	0.4	**4.27**	13	0	0
OIL (HAZELNUT)	14	0.4	1.41	13	0	0
OIL (OLIVE)	14	0.4	0.82	13	0	0
OIL (PALM)	14	0.4	0.66	13	0	0
OIL (SUNFLOWER)	14	0.4	**5.99**	13	0	0
OIL (WALNUT)	14	0.4	**6.33**	13	0	0
OIL (WHEATGERM)	14	0.4	**4.27**	13	0	0
OVALTINE	200	6.1	2.40	4	0	0
PORK (LEG ROASTED)	85	2.6	0.95	15	4	11
SALMON (pink/baked)	150	4.5	**6.06**	32	5	20
SARDINES (in oil)	50	1.5	**3.49**	11	14	7
SCOLLOP	120	3.6	**4.77**	0	0	0
SHRIMP	50	1.5	**5.36**	5	12	1
SOLE	127	3.8	**4.38**	12	10	12
SWORDFISH	106	3.2	2.91	15	11	16
TEA	200	6.1	1.50	0	0	0
TOFU	100	3.0	2.41	7	0	0
TUNA	150	4.5	**4.85**	15	27	13

Portion Analysis Food	Portion Wt (grams)	Portion Wt (ozs)	CVo16 Cardiac Value	Calorie Units	Salt Units	Potassium Units
TURKEY (BREAST ROASTED)	85	2.6	2.01	13	3	11
TURKEY (DARK MEAT)	85	2.6	1.60	15	6	9
WATER	1000	30.3	1.00	0	0	0
WHELK	85	2.6	13.94	8	15	5
EGG (WHITE)	33	1.0	1.89	1	4	2
EGG (YOLK)	17	0.5	1.88	6	1	1
FLORA PRO-ACTIVE	5	0.2	1.46	7	0	0
RED WINE	100	3.0	1.81	7	0	4
SESAME SEEDS	28	0.8	9.83	17	0	5
PARMESAN	6	0.2	0.75	3	3	0
BRAZIL NUTS	28	0.8	1.97	19	0	7
WALNUTS	28	0.8	21.24	19	0	4
SUNFLOWER SEEDS	28	0.8	6.75	16	0	7
PINE NUTS	28	0.8	1.40	19	0	6
COCONUT	23	0.7	0.19	14	0	5
HAZELNUTS	28	0.8	8.89	18	0	7
ALMONDS	28	0.8	7.37	17	0	7
BROCCOLI	44	1.3	1.56	2	0	2
ASPARAGUS	60	1.8	2.08	2	0	5
LETTUCE	55	1.7	1.98	1	0	3
CAULIFLOWER	50	1.5	1.54	1	0	2
PEANUTS	28	0.8	3.31	16	0	6
PEANUT BUTTER	32	1.0	3.46	19	7	7
LIVER (CHICKEN)	85	2.6	7.38	13	4	9
WHITE WINE	100	3.0	1.61	7	0	2
SUNFLOWER FLOUR	28	0.8	3.46	16	0	6
SPINACH	100	3.0	2.90	2	8	8
TOMATO	100	3.0	1.70	2	1	8
BEER (average)	500	15.2	1.88	15	2	7
BRUSSEL SPROUTS	78	2.4	2.62	3	0	8
STRAWBERRY	83	2.5	1.67	2	0	4
CARROTS	50	1.5	1.24	1	2	2
SOYBEANS (DRY-ROASTED)	50	1.5	7.12	32	0	29
ONION	50	1.5	1.53	2	0	3
CABBAGE	75	2.3	1.47	1	0	3
LIVER (PIG)	54	1.6	30.85	10	4	5
YOGURT	100	3.0	1.08	6	5	9
SAUSAGES (PORK)	100	3.0	1.40	23	75	6
APPLE	138	4.2	1.48	6	0	6
ICE CREAM	66	2.0	0.26	12	2	4
PEPPER (GREEN)	74	2.2	2.03	4	0	5
LENTILS	100	3.0	7.21	11	0	10
PAPAYA	100	3.0	1.34	4	0	7

Portion Analysis Food	Portion Wt (grams)	Portion Wt (ozs)	CVo16 Cardiac Value	Calorie Units	Salt Units	Potassium Units
OYSTERS	70	2.1	12.44	10	0	0
POTATO (sweet)	100	3.0	1.58	9	2	10
BEANS (baked)	100	3.0	2.22	8	33	10
ORANGE JUICE	124	3.8	1.33	6	1	6
PEAS (PROCESSED)	80	2.4	1.20	8	19	4
BREAD (WHOLEWHEAT)	28	0.8	1.17	6	10	3
PEAS (GARDEN)	80	2.4	2.54	7	0	4
CRISPS (POTATO)	30	0.9	0.39	14	14	10
BANANA	75	2.3	1.54	9	0	10
MANGO	100	3.0	1.42	7	0	6
BREAD (WHITE AVERAGE)	30	0.9	1.14	7	9	1
CORN	100	3.0	2.13	11	0	8
POTATO (FLESH)	100	3.0	3.50	8	0	12
BLACKEYED PEAS	80	2.4	5.20	9	1	31
CHOCOLATE: MILK	44	1.3	0.16	23	2	6
RICE KRISPIES	25	0.8	1.79	7	10	1
PASTA	57	1.7	1.93	16	1	1
BRAN FLAKES	50	1.5	3.10	14	25	10
LIMA BEANS	78	2.4	3.06	26	20	8
PLAIN CHOCOLATE	44	1.3	0.13	22	0	4
SHREDDED WHEAT	50	1.5	1.72	19	0	6
HAMBURGER	250	7.6	0.25	61	97	18
WHITE CHOCOLATE	44	1.3	0.08	26	3	5
POTATO (FLESH & SKIN)	200	6.1	2.39	27	2	42
CHEESEBURGER (triple meat)	400	12.1	0.10	104	170	28
RICE (BROWN)	100	3.0	2.13	36	0	3
RICE (LONG-GRAIN WHITE)	100	3.0	1.21	36	0	2
CORNFLAKES	100	3.0	1.20	38	63	3
OATMEAL	234	7.1	2.51	88	83	3

Table D

Low to High Sodium (in ascending order)
The choice for those with high blood pressure
(ie low sodium and cardiac value (CVo16) greater than 3)

Daily Units of Sodium & Potassium Salts
100 Calorie Units = 1000KCals/day; 100 sodium salt units =1600mgs
sodium (Na) /day, 100 potassium units = 3200mgs potassium (K)/day

Portion Analysis Food	Portion Wt (grams)	Portion Wt (ozs)	CVo16 Cardiac Value	Calorie Units	Salt Units	Potassium Units
AVOCADO	100	3.0	3.43	19	0	0
BEVERAGES: COFFEE	200	6.1	1.29	0	0	0
COLA	250	7.6	1.01	1	0	0
DIET COLA	250	7.6	1.01	0	0	0
HONEY	33	1.0	1.05	11	0	0
MILKSHAKE	200	6.1	2.54	4	0	0
OIL (ALMOND)	14	0.4	0.74	13	0	0
OIL (COD LIVER)	14	0.4	0.91	13	0	0
OIL (CORN)	14	0.4	4.27	13	0	0
OIL (HAZELNUT)	14	0.4	1.41	13	0	0
OIL (OLIVE)	14	0.4	0.82	13	0	0
OIL (PALM)	14	0.4	0.66	13	0	0
OIL (SUNFLOWER)	14	0.4	5.99	13	0	0
OIL (WALNUT)	14	0.4	6.33	13	0	0
OIL (WHEATGERM)	14	0.4	4.27	13	0	0
OVALTINE	200	6.1	2.40	4	0	0
SCOLLOP	120	3.6	4.77	0	0	0
TEA	200	6.1	1.50	0	0	0
TOFU	100	3.0	2.41	7	0	0
WATER	1000	30.3	1.00	0	0	0
FLORA PRO-ACTIVE	5	0.2	1.46	7	0	0
SUNFLOWER FLOUR	28	0.8	3.46	16	0	6
OYSTERS	70	2.1	12.44	10	0	0
PINE NUTS	28	0.8	1.40	19	0	6
PEANUTS (unsalted)	28	0.8	3.31	16	0	6
ASPARAGUS	60	1.8	2.08	2	0	5
BANANA	75	2.3	1.54	9	0	10
BRAZIL NUTS	28	0.8	1.97	19	0	7
SUNFLOWER SEEDS	28	0.8	6.75	16	0	7
CORN	100	3.0	2.13	11	0	8
RICE (BROWN)	100	3.0	2.13	36	0	3

Portion Analysis Food	Portion Wt (grams)	Portion Wt (ozs)	CVo16 Cardiac Value	Calorie Units	Salt Units	Potassium Units
RICE (LONG-GRAIN WHITE)	100	3.0	1.21	36	0	2
LETTUCE	55	1.7	1.98	1	0	3
ONION	50	1.5	1.53	2	0	3
BRUSSEL SPROUTS	78	2.4	2.62	3	0	8
PEAS (GARDEN)	80	2.4	2.54	7	0	4
HAZELNUTS	**28**	**0.8**	**8.89**	**18**	**0**	**7**
WALNUTS	**28**	**0.8**	**21.24**	**19**	**0**	**4**
MANGO	100	3.0	1.42	7	0	6
CAULIFLOWER	50	1.5	1.54	1	0	2
PLAIN CHOCOLATE	44	1.3	0.13	22	0	4
LENTILS	**100**	**3.0**	**7.21**	**11**	**0**	**10**
ALMONDS	**28**	**0.8**	**7.37**	**17**	**0**	**7**
WHITE WINE	100	3.0	1.61	7	0	2
SHREDDED WHEAT	50	1.5	1.72	19	0	6
APPLE	138	4.2	1.48	6	0	6
SOYBEANS (DRY-ROASTED)	**50**	**1.5**	**7.12**	**32**	**0**	**29**
STRAWBERRY	83	2.5	1.67	2	0	4
PAPAYA	100	3.0	1.34	4	0	7
PEPPER (GREEN)	74	2.2	2.03	4	0	5
SESAME SEEDS	**28**	**0.8**	**9.83**	**17**	**0**	**5**
BROCCOLI	44	1.3	1.56	2	0	2
CABBAGE	75	2.3	1.47	1	0	3
COCONUT	23	0.7	0.19	14	0	5
RED WINE	100	3.0	1.81	7	0	4
POTATO (FLESH)	**100**	**3.0**	**3.50**	**8**	**0**	**12**
EGG (YOLK)	17	0.5	1.88	6	1	1
TOMATO	100	3.0	1.70	2	1	8
PASTA	57	1.7	1.93	16	1	1
ORANGE JUICE	124	3.8	1.33	6	1	6
BLACKEYED PEAS	**80**	**2.4**	**5.20**	**9**	**1**	**31**
POTATO (FLESH & SKIN)	200	6.1	2.39	27	2	42
CARROTS	50	1.5	1.24	1	2	2
BUTTER	5	0.2	0.56	4	2	0
POTATO (SWEET)	100	3.0	1.58	9	2	10
BEER (average)	500	15.2	1.88	15	2	7
CHOCOLATE: MILK	44	1.3	0.16	23	2	6
ICE CREAM	66	2.0	0.26	12	2	4
TURKEY (BREAST ROASTED)	85	2.6	2.01	13	3	11
PARMESAN	6	0.2	0.75	3	3	0
MAGARINE	5	0.2	1.62	4	3	0
WHITE CHOCOLATE	44	1.3	0.08	26	3	5
LAMB (LEG ROASTED)	85	2.6	0.79	19	3	10
MACKEREL	**88**	**2.7**	**3.50**	**21**	**3**	**11**

Portion Analysis Food	Portion Wt (grams)	Portion Wt (ozs)	CVo16 Cardiac Value	Calorie Units	Salt Units	Potassium Units	
PORK (LEG ROASTED)	85	2.6	0.95	15	4	11	
EGG (WHITE)	33	1.0	1.89	1	4	2	
LIVER (CHICKEN)	**85**	**2.6**	**7.38**	**13**	**4**	**9**	
CHICKEN (DARK MEAT)	114	3.5	1.89	21	4	14	
LIVER (PIG)	**54**	**1.6**	**30.85**	**10**	**4**	**5**	
HEART (BEEF)	**85**	**2.6**	**3.74**	**19**	**4**	**6**	
SALMON (PINK/BAKED)	150	4.5	6.06	32	5	20	
BEEF (RUMP) COOKED	100	3.0	0.94	18	5	14	
CUTTLE FISH	**85**	**2.6**	**9.72**	**0**	**5**	**7**	
YOGURT	100	3.0	1.08	6	5	9	
DUCK (ROASTED)	85	2.6	1.16	17	5	8	
TURKEY (DARK MEAT)	85	2.6	1.60	15	6	9	
HALIBUT	**150**	**4.5**	**4.65**	**18**	**7**	**25**	
MILK (1% FAT)	245	7.4	1.39	11	7	13	
HADDOCK	**150**	**4.5**	**4.98**	**13**	**7**	**19**	
PEANUT BUTTER	**32**	**1.0**	**3.46**	**19**	**7**	**7**	
SPINACH	100	3.0	2.9	2	8	18	
KIDNEY (beef)	85	2.6	**16.43**		12	8	6
LIVER (beef)	85	2.6	**28.53**	14	8	6	
BREAD (WHITE AVERAGE)	30	0.9	1.14	7	9	1	
SOLE	127	3.8	**4.38**	12	10	12	
CHICKEN BREAST (ROASTED)	196	5.9	1.83	30	10	22	
OCTOPUS	85	2.6	**4.91**	6	10	4	
BREAD (WHOLEWHEAT)	28	0.8	1.17	6	10	3	
RICE KRISPIES	25	0.8	1.79	7	10	1	
SWORDFISH	106	3.2	**2.91**	15	11	16	
SHRIMP	50	1.5	**5.36**	5	12	1	
CHEDDAR	28	0.8	0.43	12	13	1	
CRISPS (POTATO)	30	0.9	0.39	14	14	10	
SARDINES (in oil)	50	1.5	**3.49**	11	14	7	
HERRING	143	4.3	**3.62**	26	14	20	
WHELK	85	2.6	**13.94**	8	15	5	
COD	180	5.5	**4.37**	17	18	17	
COTTAGE CHEESE	100	3.0	2.01	10	19	5	
PEAS (PROCESSED)	80	2.4	1.20	8	19	4	
MUSSEL	85	2.6	**11.74**	9	19	4	
LIMA BEANS	78	2.4	3.06	26	20	8	
CAMEMBERT	62	1.9	0.30	18	23	2	
BRAN FLAKES	50	1.5	**3.10**	14	25	10	
TUNA	150	4.5	**4.85**	15	27	13	
LOBSTER	145	4.4	2.75	15	30	13	
CRAB (STEAMED)	118	3.6	**8.29**	15	31	10	
BEANS (BAKED)	100	3.0	2.22	8	33	10	

Portion Analysis Food	Portion Wt (grams)	Portion Wt (ozs)	CVo16 Cardiac Value	Calorie Units	Salt Units	Potassium Units
EEL	136	4.1	1.75	15	56	2
CORNFLAKES	100	3.0	1.20	38	63	3
SAUSAGES (PORK)	100	3.0	1.40	23	75	6
OATMEAL	234	7.1	2.51	88	83	3
HAMBURGER	250	7.6	0.25	61	97	18
CHEESEBURGER (triple meat)	400	12.1	0.10	104	170	28
ANCHOVY (in oil)	85	2.6	0.80	16	209	7

Table E

Fatty Acid and Vitamin Units

NB: Om-3 = omega 3 oil, Llenic = linolenic acid, Lleic = Linoleic acid

Atheroprotective substance Units (Anti-Furring) in Food & their CARDIAC VALUE (CVo16)

100 Units = Folate 230mgs/day; Fibre 20g/day; Phytosterols 3g/day. All fatty acids= 1g/day

Portion Analysis Food Index	Portion Wt (grams)	CVo16 Cardiac Value	Kcal Units	Om-3 Units	Oleic Units	Llenic Units	Lleic Units	Folate Units	B6 Units	B12 Units	Vit E Units
ALMONDS	28	7.37	17	11	913	7	353	6	3	0	67
ANCHOVY (in oil)	85	0.80	16	124	22	3	4	3	8	53	0
APPLE	138	1.48	6	2	2	6	28	2	5	0	0
ASPARAGUS	60	2.08	2	1	0	0	4	57	5	0	3
AVOCADO	100	3.43	19	9	1510	17	166	27	19	0	14
BANANA	75	1.54	9	2	1	2	3	4	35	1	0
BEANS (baked)	100	2.22	8	0	0	0	0	10	9	0	4
BEEF (rump) COOKED	100	0.94	18	19	92	3	8	2	43	300	1
BEER (average)	500	1.88	15	0	0	0	0	26	20	1	0
BEVERAGES: COFFEE	200	1.29	0	0	0	0	0	1	0	8	0
BLACKEYED PEAS	80	5.20	9	7	0	0	0	73	5	0	?
BRAN FLAKES	50	3.10	14	0	0	0	0	27	77	85	42
BRAZIL NUTS	28	1.97	19	2	549	0	0	1	12	0	50
BREAD (white average)	30	1.14	7	1	0	0	0	12	1	1	0
BREAD (wholewheat)	28	1.17	6	1	0	0	0	6	3	0	0
BROCCOLI	44	1.56	2	6	0	0	0	12	4	0	2
BRUSSEL SPROUTS	78	2.62	3	4	4	12	3	29	15	0	8
BUTTER	5	0.56	4	6	93	2	6	0	0	2	1
CABBAGE	75	1.47	1	8	0	3	4	7	7	0	1
CAMEMBERT	62	0.30	18	17	322	10	23	17	9	81	0
CARROTS	50	1.24	1	1	0	1	5	3	5	0	0
CAULIFLOWER	50	1.54	1	16	0	11	3	12	7	0	0

Portion Analysis / Food Index	Portion Wt (grams)	CVo16 Cardiac Value	Kcal Units	Om-3 Units	Oleic Units	Llenic Units	Lleic Units	Folate Units	B6 Units	B12 Units	Vit E Units
CHEDDAR	28	0.43	12	10	185	7	14	2	1	24	0
CHEESEBURGER (triple meat)	400	0.10	104	71	0	0	0	40	51	800	10
CHICKEN (dark meat)	114	1.89	21	21	323	9	232	3	25	32	0
CHICKEN BREAST (roasted)	196	1.83	30	20	332	12	214	3	73	63	0
CHOCOLATE: MILK	44	0.16	23	0	0	0	0	2	1	44	2
COCONUT	23	0.19	14	0	48	0	16	1	1	0	3
COD	180	4.37	17	29	13	8	3	6	34	189	0
COLA	250	1.01	1	0	0	0	0	0	0	0	0
CORN	100	2.13	11	1	87	3	0	20	4	0	0
CORNFLAKES	100	1.20	38	0	0	0	0	145	113	90	4
COTTAGE CHEESE	100	2.01	10	1	101	4	10	5	5	64	0
CRAB (steamed)	118	8.29	15	58	0	0	0	22	13	807	0
CRISPS (potato)	30	0.39	14	0	0	0	0	6	9	0	10
CUTTLE FISH	85	9.72	0	0	0	0	0	11	35	356	0
DIET COLA	250	1.01	0	0	0	0	0	0	0	0	0
DUCK (roasted)	85	1.16	17	25	622	15	174	2	10	26	0
EEL	136	1.75	15	118	938	90	167	10	7	393	0
EGG (white)	33	1.89	1	0	0	0	0	0	0	6	0
EGG (yolk)	17	1.88	6	4	199	4	80	8	4	45	5
FLORA PRO-ACTIVE	5	1.46	7	0	0	0	0	0	0	0	33
HADDOCK	150	4.98	13	36	9	1	1	9	35	209	0
HALIBUT	150	4.65	18	82	31	4	3	9	40	206	0
HAMBURGER	250	0.25	61	19	0	0	0	26	30	250	6
HAZELNUTS	28	8.89	18	4	1282	3	238	9	11	0	70
HEART (beef)	85	3.74	19	55	0	0	28	1	12	1216	0
HERRING	143	3.62	26	308	248	9	22	7	33	1873	13
HONEY	33	1.05	11	0	0	0	0	0	0	0	0
ICE CREAM	66	0.26	12	11	0	0	0	1	2	26	0
KIDNEY (beef)	85	16.43	12	1	218	5	5	36	29	4360	0
LAMB (leg roasted)	85	0.79	19	24	92	4	8	6	8	216	0
LENTILS	100	7.21	11	9	0	0	0	78	12	0	0
LETTUCE	55	1.98	1	4	0	39	3	13	13	0	2
LIMA BEANS	78	3.06	26	22	10	19	44	4	3	0	3
LIVER (beef)	85	28.53	14	18	0	0	0	81	83	9520	5
LIVER (chicken)	85	7.38	13	9	86	1	42	335	33	1900	17
LIVER (pig)	54	30.85	10	4	29	1	25	38	21	0	
LOBSTER	145	2.75	15	10	36	11	8	7	7	435	0
MACKEREL	88	3.50	21	116	135	22	15	1	27	1672	17
MAGARINE	5	1.62	4	2	134	10	88	0	0	0	5
MANGO	100	1.42	7	4	9	7	1	0	9	0	11
MILK (1% fat)	245	1.39	11	0	93	7	3	5	7	91	0

Portion Analysis Food Index	Portion Wt (grams)	CVo16 Cardiac Value	Kcal Units	Om-3 Units	Oleic Units	Llenic Units	Lleic Units	Folate Units	B6 Units	B12 Units	Vit E Units
MILKSHAKE	200	2.54	4	0	0	0	0	3	4	100	0
MUSSEL	85	11.74	9	70	11	2	5	28	6	2040	0
OATMEAL	234	2.51	88	5	608	19	686	4	3	0	0
OCTOPUS	85	4.91	6	58	0	0	0	3	6	209	0
OIL (almond)	14	0.74	13	0	0	0	0	0	0	0	55
OIL (cod liver)	14	0.92	13	263	0	0	0	0	0	0	28
OIL (corn)	14	4.27	13	10	361	13	774	0	0	0	24
OIL (hazelnut)	14	1.41	13	0	0	0	0	0	0	0	60
OIL (olive)	14	0.82	138	1	12	116	0	0	0	0	
OIL (palm)	14	0.66	13	0	519	7	141	0	0	0	46
OIL (sunflower)	14	5.99	13	0	279	7	882	0	0	0	170
OIL (walnut)	14	6.33	13	146	256	181	771	0	0	0	1
OIL (wheatgerm)	14	4.27	13	97	189	109	780	0	0	0	260
ONION	50	1.53	2	0	0	1	5	4	7	0	2
ORANGE JUICE	124	1.33	6	1	0	0	0	10	6	0	2
OVALTINE	200	2.40	4	0	0	0	0	35	27	0	40
OYSTERS	70	12.44	10	19	4	2	1	5	4	1960	0
PAPAYA	100	1.34	4	3	1	2	0	17	1	0	0
PARMESAN	6	0.75	3	2	35	1	2	0	1	8	0
PASTA	57	1.93	16	5	0	0	0	44	3	18	0
PEANUT BUTTER	32	3.46	19	2	822	0	330	7	12	0	16
PEANUTS	28	3.31	16	0	619	15	389	13	11	0	28
PEAS (garden)	80	2.54	7	2	0	0	0	9	5	0	2
PEAS (processed)	80	1.20	8	0	0	0	0	4	5	0	2
PEPPER (green)	74	2.03	4	2	1	4	6	9	3	0	0
PINE NUTS	28	1.40	19	18	0	0	0	7	2	0	0
PLAIN CHOCOLATE	44	0.13	22	0	0	0	0	2	1	0	6
PORK (leg roasted)	85	0.95	15	4	71	2	9	4	23	60	0
POTATO (flesh & skin)	200	2.39	27	2	0	0	0	30	56	0	2
POTATO (flesh)	100	3.50	8	8	180	2	3	11	21	0	1
POTATO (sweet)	100	1.58	9	2	0	0	0	3	3	0	3
RED WINE	100	1.81	7	0	0	0	0	0	7	1	0
RICE (BROWN)	100	2.13	36	1	54	3	78	2	10	0	2
SALMON (pink/baked)	150	6.06	32	156	408	53	65	3	26	577	5
SARDINES (in oil)	50	3.49	11	75	28	2	4	3	6	446	0
SAUSAGES (pork)	100	1.40	23	0	1150	49	246	1	21	177	0
SCOLLOP	120	4.77	0	93	0	0	0	6	11	159	?
SESAME SEEDS	28	9.83	17	11	1128	0	1196	12	15	0	0
SHREDDED WHEAT	50	1.72	19	0	0	0	0	9	8	0	6
SHRIMP	50	5.36	5	16	6	0	3	1	5	75	0
SOLE	127	4.38	12	66	27	1	6	5	20	319	0
SOYBEANS (dry-roasted)	50	7.12	32	51	0	0	0	138	22	0	25

Portion Analysis Food Index	Portion Wt (grams)	CVo16 Cardiac Value	Kcal Units	Om-3 Units	Oleic Units	Llenic Units	Lleic Units	Folate Units	B6 Units	B12 Units	Vit E Units
SPINACH	100	2.90	2	9	1	13	3	35	6	0	17
STRAWBERRY	83	1.67	2	6	5	9	11	7	3	0	2
SUNFLOWER FLOUR	28	3.46	16	0	64	1	176	0	0	0	0
SUNFLOWER SEEDS	28	6.75	16	2	375	3	781	0	0	0	106
SWORDFISH	106	2.91	15	112	143	24	4	1	27	214	0
TEA	200	1.50	0	0	0	0	0	3	0	40	0
TOFU	100	2.41	7	0	0	0	0	7	5	0	10
TOMATO	100	1.70	2	0	2	1	9	10	9	0	12
TUNA	150	4.85	15	42	392	32	35	1	22	175	0
TURKEY (breast roasted)	85	2.01	13	9	18	0	15	2	27	31	0
TURKEY (dark meat)	85	1.60	15	14	64	0	68	3	19	31	1
WALNUTS	28	21.24	19	93	302	210	958	8	11	0	11
WATER	1000	1.00	0	0	0	0	0	0	0	0	0
WHELK	85	13.94	8	10	0	0	0	2	19	771	0
WHITE CHOCOLATE	44	0.08	26	0	0	0	0	2	2	0	5
WHITE WINE	100	1.61	7	0	0	0	0	2	10	0	0
YOGURT	100	1.08	6	2	35	1	4	13	1	49	0

Table F

Daily Units of Fibre and Phytosterol in Food

100 Units = Fibre 20g/day; Phytosterols 3g/day

Portion Analysis Alphabetical Food Index	Portion Wt (grams)	Portion Wt (ozs)	CVo16 Cardiac Value	Calories Units	Fibre Units	Phytosterol Units
ALMONDS	28	0.8	7.37	17	10	1
ANCHOVY (in oil)	85	2.6	0.80	16	0	0
APPLE	138	4.2	1.48	6	12	1
ASPARAGUS	60	1.8	2.08	2	5	0
AVOCADO	100	3.0	3.43	19	17	0
BANANA	75	2.3	1.54	9	4	0
BEANS (baked)	100	3.0	2.22	8	19	0
BEEF (rump) COOKED	100	3.0	0.94	18	0	3
BEER (average)	500	15.2	1.88	15	0	0
BEVERAGES: COFFEE	200	6.1	1.29	0	0	0
BLACKEYED PEAS	80	2.4	5.20	9	33	0
BRAN FLAKES	50	1.5	3.10	14	61	0
BRAZIL NUTS	28	0.8	1.97	19	6	0
BREAD (white average)	30	0.9	1.14	7	3	0

Portion Analysis Alphabetical Food Index	Portion Wt (grams)	Portion Wt (ozs)	CVo16 Cardiac Value	Calories Units	Fibre Units	Phytosterol Units
BREAD (wholewheat)	28	0.8	1.17	6	7	0
BROCCOLI	44	1.3	1.56	2	13	0
BRUSSEL SPROUTS	78	2.4	2.62	3	12	0
BUTTER	5	0.2	0.56	4	0	0
CABBAGE	75	2.3	1.47	1	7	0
CAMEMBERT	62	1.9	0.30	18	0	0
CARROTS	50	1.5	1.24	1	6	0
CAULIFLOWER	50	1.5	1.54	1	4	0
CHEDDAR	28	0.8	0.43	12	0	0
CHEESEBURGER (triple meat)	400	12.1	0.10	104	?	0
CHICKEN (dark meat)	114	3.5	1.89	21	0	14
CHICKEN BREAST (roasted)	196	5.9	1.83	30	0	2
CHOCOLATE: MILK	44	1.3	0.16	23	2	0
COCONUT	23	0.7	0.19	14	16	0
COD	180	5.5	4.37	17	0	0
COLA	250	7.6	1.01	1	0	0
CORN	100	3.0	2.13	11	11	0
CORNFLAKES	100	3.0	1.20	38	5	0
COTTAGE CHEESE	100	3.0	2.01	10	0	0
CRAB (steamed)	118	3.6	8.29	15	0	11
CRISPS (potato)	30	0.9	0.39	14	9	0
CUTTLE FISH	85	2.6	9.72	0	0	0
DIET COLA	250	7.6	1.01	0	0	0
DUCK (roasted)	85	2.6	1.16	17	0	0
EEL	136	4.1	1.75	15	0	0
EGG (white)	33	1.0	1.89	1	0	0
EGG (yolk)	17	0.5	1.88	6	0	0
FLORA PRO-ACTIVE	5	0.2	1.46	7	0	13
HADDOCK	150	4.5	4.98	13	0	0
HALIBUT	150	4.5	4.65	18	0	0
HAMBURGER	250	7.6	0.25	61	10	0
HAZELNUTS	28	0.8	8.89	18	9	0
HEART (beef)	85	2.6	3.74	19	0	6
HERRING	143	4.3	3.62	26	0	0
HONEY	33	1.0	1.05	11	0	0
ICE CREAM	66	2.0	0.26	12	0	0
KIDNEY (beef)	85	2.6	16.43	12	0	3
LAMB (leg roasted)	85	2.6	0.79	19	0	6
LENTILS	100	3.0	7.21	11	19	0
LETTUCE	55	1.7	1.98	1	2	0
LIMA BEANS	78	2.4	3.06	26	81	0
LIVER (beef)	85	2.6	28.53	14	0	0

Portion Analysis Alphabetical Food Index	Portion Wt (grams)	Portion Wt (ozs)	CVo16 Cardiac Value	Calories Units	Fibre Units	Phytosterol Units
LIVER (chicken)	85	2.6	**7.38**	13	0	0
LIVER (pig)	54	1.6	**30.85**	10	0	1
LOBSTER	145	4.4	2.75	15	0	0
MACKEREL	88	2.7	**3.50**	21	0	0
MAGARINE	5	0.2	1.62	4	0	1
MANGO	100	3.0	1.42	7	9	0
MILK (1% fat)	245	7.4	1.39	11	0	0
MILKSHAKE	200	6.1	2.54	4	0	0
MUSSEL	85	2.6	**11.74**	9	0	10
OATMEAL	234	7.1	2.51	88	83	0
OCTOPUS	85	2.6	**4.91**	6	0	11
OIL (almond)	14	0.4	0.74	13	0	1
OIL (cod liver)	14	0.4	0.92	13	0	0
OIL (corn)	14	0.4	**4.27**	13	0	5
OIL (hazelnut)	14	0.4	1.41	13	0	1
OIL (olive)	14	0.4	0.82	13	0	1
OIL (palm)	14	0.4	0.66	13	0	0
OIL (sunflower)	14	0.4	**5.99**	13	0	0
OIL (walnut)	14	0.4	**6.33**	13	0	1
OIL (wheatgerm)	14	0.4	**4.27**	13	0	3
ONION	50	1.5	1.53	2	4	0
ORANGE JUICE	124	3.8	1.33	6	1	0
OVALTINE	200	6.1	2.40	4	1	0
OYSTERS	70	2.1	**12.44**	10	0	0
PAPAYA	100	3.0	1.34	4	9	0
PARMESAN	6	0.2	0.75	3	0	0
PASTA	57	1.7	1.93	16	11	0
PEANUT BUTTER	32	1.0	**3.46**	19	9	1
PEANUTS	28	0.8	**3.31**	16	9	2
PEAS (garden)	80	2.4	**2.54**	7	22	0
PEAS (processed)	80	2.4	1.20	8	19	0
PEPPER (green)	74	2.2	2.03	4	12	0
PINE NUTS	28	0.8	1.40	19	3	1
PLAIN CHOCOLATE	44	1.3	0.13	22	6	0
PORK (leg roasted)	85	2.6	0.95	15	0	3
POTATO (flesh & skin)	200	6.1	2.39	27	14	0
POTATO (flesh)	100	3.0	**3.50**	8	14	0
POTATO (sweet)	100	3.0	1.58	9	12	0
RED WINE	100	3.0	1.81	7	0	0
RICE (brown)	100	3.0	2.13	36	10	0
RICE (long-grain white)	100	3.0	1.21	36	1	0
SARDINES (in oil)	50	1.5	**3.49**	11	0	0
SAUSAGES (pork)	100	3.0	1.40	23	8	0

Portion Analysis Alphabetical Food Index	Portion Wt (grams)	Portion Wt (ozs)	CVo16 Cardiac Value	Calories Units	Fibre Units	Phytosterol Units
SCOLLOP	120	3.6	4.77	0	0	0
SESAME SEEDS	28	0.8	9.83	17	11	7
SHREDDED WHEAT	50	1.5	1.72	19	25	0
SHRIMP	50	1.5	5.36	5	0	5
SOLE	127	3.8	4.38	12	0	0
SOYBEANS (dry-roasted)	50	1.5	7.12	32	68	0
SPINACH	100	3.0	2.90	2	11	0
STRAWBERRY	83	2.5	1.67	2	4	0
SUNFLOWER FLOUR	28	0.8	3.46	16	8	0
SUNFLOWER SEEDS	28	0.8	6.75	16	15	5
SWORDFISH	106	3.2	2.91	15	0	0
TEA	200	6.1	1.50	0	0	0
TOFU	100	3.0	2.41	7	?	0
TOMATO	100	3.0	1.70	2	5	0
TUNA	150	4.5	4.85	15	0	0
TURKEY (breast roasted)	85	2.6	2.01	13	0	0
TURKEY (dark meat)	85	2.6	1.60	15	0	0
WALNUTS	28	0.8	21.24	19	5	1
WATER	1000	30.3	1.00	0	0	0
WHELK	85	2.6	13.94	8	0	0
WHITE CHOCOLATE	44	1.3	0.08	26	6	0
WHITE WINE	100	3.0	1.61	7	0	0
YOGURT	100	3.0	1.08	6	0	0

Table G
Minerals & Amino Acid Units

NB: Mg = Magnesium, Mn = Manganese, Se = Selenium, Zn = Zinc

Daily Units of Minerals & Amino-acids + CARDIAC VALUE (CVo16)

100 Units = 230mgs Mg; 5mgs Mn; 70mcgs Se; 12mgs Zn; 250mgs Amino-acid/day

Portion Analysis Food Index	Portion Wt (g)	Portion Wt (ozs)	CVo16 Cardiac Value	Kcal Units	Mg Units	Mn Units	Se Units	Zn Units	Arginine Units	Taurine Units
ALMONDS	28	0.8	7.37	17	30	10	1	7	196	0
ANCHOVY (in oil)	85	2.6	0.80	16	14	2	44	12	416	0
APPLE	138	4.2	1.48	6	2	0	0	1	4	0
ASPARAGUS	60	1.8	2.08	2	3	2	1	4	29	0
AVOCADO	100	3.0	3.43	19	10	4	0	3	24	0
BANANA	75	2.3	1.54	9	9	2	1	1	16	0
beans (baked)	100	3.0	2.22	8	12	6	3	4	215	0
BEEF (rump) COOKED	100	3.0	0.94	18	12	0	14	46	711	30

Portion Analysis Food Index	Portion Wt (g)	Portion Wt (ozs)	CVo16 Cardiac Value	Kcal Units	Mg Units	Mn Units	Se Units	Zn Units	Arginine Units	Taurine Units
BEER (average)	500	15.2	1.88	15	14	1	0	0	24	0
BEVERAGES:										
COFFEE	200	6.1	1.29	0	13	4	1	1	0	0
BLACKEYED PEAS	80	2.4	**5.20**	9	14	8	3	7	**522**	0
BRAN FLAKES	50	1.5	**3.10**	14	24	0	3	10	**176**	0
BRAZIL NUTS	28	0.8	1.97	19	46	10	14	13	**237**	0
BREAD (white average)	30	0.9	1.14	7	3	2	12	2	38	0
BREAD (wholewheat)	28	0.8	1.17	6	10	12	15	5	34	0
BROCCOLI	44	1.3	1.56	2	4	2	2	2	24	0
BRUSSEL SPROUTS	78	2.4	2.62	3	9	4	2	3	48	0
BUTTER	5	0.2	0.56	4	0	0	0	0	1	0
CABBAGE	75	2.3	1.47	1	1	3	2	1	16	0
CAMEMBERT	62	1.9	0.30	18	5	0	13	12	16	0
CARROTS	50	1.5	1.24	1	1	1	1	0	9	0
CAULIFLOWER	50	1.5	1.54	1	4	4	0	3	19	0
CHEDDAR	28	0.8	0.43	12	3	0	6	7	96	0
CHEESEBURGER (triple meat)	400	12.1	0.10	104	43	18	86	**100**	**1400**	0
CHICKEN (dark meat)	114	3.5	1.89	21	10	0	38	25	**720**	152
CHICKEN BREAST (roasted)	196	5.9	1.83	30	21	0	62	17	**1444**	10
CHOCOLATE: MILK	44	1.3	0.16	23	9	2	3	4	36	0
COCONUT	23	0.7	0.19	14	8	8	4	2	40	0
COD	180	5.5	**4.37**	17	30	0	97	9	**988**	0
COLA	250	7.6	1.01	1	1	0	0	0	0	0
CORN	100	3.0	2.13	11	14	4	0	3	52	0
CORNFLAKES	100	3.0	1.20	38	4	2	7	2	96	0
COTTAGE CHEESE	100	3.0	2.01	10	2	0	13	3	**202**	0
CRAB (steamed)	118	3.6	**8.29**	15	16	4	68	42	**796**	112
CRISPS (potato)	30	0.9	0.39	14	6	2	0	2	40	0
CUTTLE FISH	85	2.6	**9.72**	0	20	4	**109**	25	804	0
DIET COLA	250	7.6	1.01	0	1	0	0	0	0	0
DUCK (roasted)	85	2.6	1.16	17	6	0	24	13	**432**	0
EEL	136	4.1	1.75	15	18	2	21	30	**773**	0
EGG (white)	33	1.0	1.89	1	2	0	8	0	90	0
EGG (yolk)	17	0.5	1.88	6	1	0	11	4	87	0
FLORA PRO-ACTIVE	5	0.2	1.46	7	0	1	**0**	0	**0**	0

Portion Analysis Food Index	Portion Wt (g)	Portion Wt (ozs)	CVo16 Cardiac Value	Kcal Units	Mg Units	Mn Units	Se Units	Zn Units	Arginine Units	Taurine Units
HADDOCK	150	4.5	**4.98**	13	30	0	**87**	6	**960**	0
HALIBUT	150	4.5	**4.65**	18	64	1	**100**	7	**960**	0
HAMBURGER	250	7.6	0.25	61	28	13	57	63	**788**	0
HAZELNUTS	28	0.8	8.89	18	18	27	1	5	**208**	0
HEART (BEEF)	85	2.6	**3.74**	19	8	0	23	26	**656**	80
HERRING	143	4.3	**3.62**	26	24	2	96	15	**788**	0
HONEY	33	1.0	1.05	11	0	2	0	2	0	0
ICE CREAM	66	2.0	0.26	12	4	0	2	4	32	0
KIDNEY (beef)	85	2.6	**16.43**	12	6	4	**255**	30	**512**	48
LAMB (leg roasted)	85	2.6	0.79	19	8	0	5	30	**504**	80
LENTILS	100	3.0	7.21	11	41	28	11	29	**832**	0
LETTUCE	55	1.7	1.98	1	1	3	1	0	14	0
LIMA BEANS	78	2.4	**3.06**	26	18	20	2	5	**393**	0
LIVER (beef)	85	2.6	**28.53**	14	7	8	?	43	**520**	0
LIVER (chicken)	85	2.6	**7.38**	13	8	6	0	27	**508**	0
LIVER (pig)	54	1.6	**30.85**	10	3	4	0	30	**344**	17
LOBSTER	145	4.4	2.75	15	20	2	**160**	34	**1004**	0
MACKEREL	88	2.7	**3.50**	21	34	0	65	0	**504**	0
MAGARINE	5	0.2	1.62	4	0	0	0	0	0	0
MANGO	100	3.0	1.42	7	5	6	0	1	8	0
MILK (1% fat)	245	7.4	1.39	11	12	0	4	9	**137**	0
MILKSHAKE	200	6.1	2.54	4	10	0	6	2	**120**	0
MUSSEL	85	2.6	**11.74**	9	12	**116**	**109**	19	**592**	140
OATMEAL	234	7.1	2.51	88	22	28	27	10	**172**	0
OCTOPUS	85	2.6	**4.91**	6	10	0	54	12	**740**	152
OIL (almond)	14	0.4	0.74	13	0	0	0	0	0	0
OIL (cod liver)	14	0.4	0.92	13	0	0	0	0	0	0
OIL (corn)	14	0.4	**4.27**	13	0	0	0	0	0	0
OIL (hazelnut)	14	0.4	1.41	13	0	0	0	0	0	0
OIL (olive)	14	0.4	0.82	13	0	0	0	0	0	0
OIL (palm)	14	0.4	0.66	13	0	0	0	0	0	0
OIL (sunflower)	14	0.4	**5.99**	13	0	0	0	0	0	0
OIL (walnut)	14	0.4	**6.33**	13	0	0	0 0	0	0	
OIL (wheatgerm)	14	0.4	**4.27**	13	0	0	0	0	0	0
ONION	50	1.5	1.53	2	1	1	1	1	30	0
ORANGE JUICE	124	3.8	1.33	6	6	0	0	1	16	0
OVALTINE	200	6.1	2.40	4	6	0	0	0	**116**	0
OYSTERS	70	2.1	**12.44**	10	26	10	72	**1064**	288	0
PAPAYA	100	3.0	1.34	4	4	2	0	2	4	0
PARMESAN	6	0.2	0.75	3	2	0	3	2	32	0
PASTA	57	1.7	1.93	16	10	6	17	6	92	0
PEANUT BUTTER	32	1.0	**3.46**	19	20	12	3	7	**271**	0
PEANUTS	28	0.8	**3.31**	16	12	6	2	4	**316**	0

Portion Analysis Food Index	Portion Wt (g)	Portion Wt (ozs)	CVo16 Cardiac Value	Kcal Units	Mg Units	Mn Units	Se Units	Zn Units	Arginine Units	Taurine Units
PEAS (garden)	80	2.4	2.54	7	12	8	2	8	128	0
PEAS (processed)	80	2.4	1.20	8	8	5	0	5	24	0
PEPPER (GREEN)	74	2.2	2.03	4	3	1	0	1	76	0
PINE NUTS	28	0.8	1.40	19	26	24	7	10	504	0
PLAIN CHOCOLATE	44	1.3	0.13	22	16	6	3	5	0	0
PORK (leg roasted)	85	2.6	0.95	15	8	0	55	21	584	48
POTATO (flesh & skin)	200	6.1	2.39	27	26	8	6	8	84	0
POTATO (flesh)	100	3.0	3.50	8	7	2	1	3	48	0
POTATO (sweet)	100	3.0	1.58	9	18	8	1	3	26	0
RED WINE	100	3.0	1.81	7	22	10	0	0	35	0
RICE (brown)	100	3.0	2.13	36	17	22	10	5	240	0
RICE (long-grain)	100	3.0	1.21	7	4	5	1	2	68	0
RICE KRISPIES	25	0.8	1.79	7	4	5	1	2	48	0
SALMON (pink/baked)	150	4.5	6.06	32	16	0	96	0	917	0
SARDINES (in oil)	50	1.5	3.49	11	8	0	38	6	300	0
SAUSAGES (pork)	100	3.0	1.40	23	8	5	10	14	582	0
SCOLLOP	120	3.6	4.77	0	26	2	140	9	568	0
SESAME SEEDS	28	0.8	9.83	17	39	14	2	18	260	0
SHREDDED WHEAT	50	1.5	1.72	19	26	0	2	10	104	0
SHRIMP	50	1.5	5.36	5	31	0	41	7	364	130
SOLE	127	3.8	4.38	12	30	0	106	7	736	0
SOYBEANS (dry-roasted)	50	1.5	7.12	32	78	38	24	34	1000	0
SPINACH	100	3.0	2.90	2	35	18	2	6	52	0
STRAWBERRY	83	2.5	1.67	2	3	5	0	1	8	0
SUNFLOWER FLOUR	28	0.8	3.46	16	0	0	0	43	427	0
SUNFLOWER SEEDS	28	0.8	6.75	16	44	12	20	12	208	0
SWORDFISH	106	3.2	2.91	15	14	0	93	13	644	0
TEA	200	6.1	1.50	0	2	6	0	0	0	0
TOFU	100	3.0	2.41	7	9	8	0	6	213	0
TOMATO	100	3.0	1.70	2	4	2	1	1	7	0
TUNA	150	4.5	4.85	15	17	0	177	10	1046	0
TURKEY (breast roasted)	85	2.6	2.01	13	10	0	12	15	676	0
TURKEY (dark meat)	85	2.6	1.60	15	8	0	4	30	660	0
WALNUTS	28	0.8	21.24	19	19	16	7	8	400	0

Portion Analysis Food Index	Portion Wt (g)	Portion Wt (ozs)	CVo16 Cardiac Value	Kcal Units	Mg Units	Mn Units	Se Units	Zn Units	Arginine Units	Taurine Units
WATER	1000	30.3	1.00	0	0	0	0	0	0	0
WHELK	85	2.6	13.94	8	29	8	54	12	1680	0
WHITE CHOCOLATE	44	1.3	0.08	26	5	0	0	3	0	0
WHITE WINE	100	3.0	1.61	7	16	10	0	0	22	0
YOGURT	100	3.0	1.08	6	6	0	3	5	54	0

Table 1

Combined Sources of Protective Chemicals in Food
of Individual Cardiac Value > 1.20 and Kcals < 150 per portion

Key to abbreviations: g = grams, N = number of atheroprotective chemicals present, Wt = weight. arg = arginine, Se = selenium, Zn = zinc, B12 = vitamin B12, oleic = oleic acid, linoleic = linoleic acid, linolenic = linolenic acid

Portion Analysis Food	Number of chemicals	Protective Chemicals Present	Portion Wt grams
TUNA	4	arg + B12 + oleic + Se	150
SCOLLOP	3	arg + B12 + Se	120
OYSTERS	3	arg + B12 + Zn	70
LIVER (chicken)	3	arg + B12 + folic	85
KIDNEY (beef)	3	arg + B12 + Se	85
SESAME SEEDS	3	arg + linoleic + oleic	28
SUNFLOWER SEEDS	3	arg + linoleic + oleic	28
OIL (walnut)	3	linoleic + linolenic + oleic	14
HAZELNUTS	3	arg + linoleic + oleic	28
ALMONDS	3	arg + linoleic + oleic	28
CUTTLE FISH	3	arg + B12 + Se	85
SHRIMP	3	arg + B12 + taurine	50
SOLE	3	arg + B12 + Se	127
CRAB (steamed)	3	arg + B12 + taurine	118
SALMON (pink/baked)	3	arg + B12 + oleic	150
OIL (sunflower)	2	linoleic + oleic	14
MUSSEL	2	arg + B12	85
HERRING	2	arg + B12	143
HEART (beef)	2	arg + B12	85

Portion Analysis Food	Number of chemicals	Protective Chemicals Present	Portion Wt grams
LIVER (beef)	2	arg + B12	85
SARDINES (in oil)	2	arg + B12	50
LOBSTER	2	arg + B12	145
MACKEREL	2	arg + B12	88
LIVER (pig)	2	arg + B12	54
OIL (corn)	2	linoleic + oleic	14
OCTOPUS	2	arg + B12	85
HADDOCK	2	arg + B12	150
SWORDFISH	2 arg + B12	106	
MILKSHAKE	2	arg + B12	200
TEA	1	B12	200
AVOCADO	1	oleic	100
CHICKEN BREAST (roasted)	1	arg	196
OIL (wheatgerm)	1	linoleic	14
EEL	1	Arg	136
TURKEY (breast roasted)	1	arg	85
PEANUT BUTTER	1	oleic	32
TURKEY (dark meat)	1	arg	85
CHICKEN (dark meat)	1	arg	114
PEANUTS	1	oleic	28
BRAZIL NUTS	1	oleic	28
PINE NUTS	1	arg	28
EGG (white)	1	arg	33
TOFU	1	arg	100
LIMA BEANS	1	arg	78
BEANS (baked)	1	arg	100
COTTAGE CHEESE	1	arg	100
PEAS (garden)	1	arg	80
BRAN FLAKES	1	arg	50
LETTUCE	1	linolenic	55
RICE (brown)	1	arg	100
PEPPER (green)	1	arg	74
CORN	1	oleic	100

APPENDIX 4

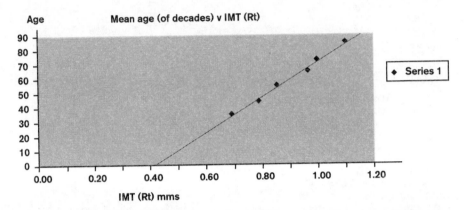

Age   **Mean age (of decades) v IMT (Rt)**

In the graph above the thickness of the inner carotid (neck) artery lining (intimal thickness or IMT) in millimetres, is shown on the bottom, increasing from left to right. On the left is ascending chronological age in years. To find arterial biological age, measure the intimal thickness at any point and find the age at which that particular thickness is expected.

APPENDIX 5

These are the full Tables of the abbreviated versions in the text.

To avoid confusion I have retained the same Table numbers as in the text. Tables 1 & 2 are therefore missing.

Table 3

Atherogenic Index (AGI)
Analysis per portion. In descending order of AGI.
(NB: One ounce = 33 grams)

Food	Portion Size (in grams)	AGI Score
CHEESEBURGER (triple meat)	400	64.81
HAMBURGER	250	20.89
CAMEMBERT	62	17.27
BEEF (rump) COOKED	100	16.08
LAMB (leg roasted)	85	14.70
CHICKEN BREAST (roasted)	196	14.38
COCONUT	23	13.38
DUCK (roasted)	85	12.78
OIL (palm)	14	12.40
PORK (leg roasted)	85	11.23
HERRING	143	10.31
MILK CHOCOLATE	44	10.07
EEL	136	10.01
CHICKEN (dark meat)	114	9.81
SAUSAGES (pork)	100	9.71
CHEDDAR	28	9.46
MACKEREL	88	8.26
ICE CREAM	66	6.59
TURKEY (dark meat)	85	6.46
HEART (beef)	85	5.99
LOBSTER	145	5.78
BRAZIL NUTS	28	5.66
AVOCADO	100	5.59
PINE NUTS	28	5.30
SWORDFISH	106	4.98

Food	Portion Size (in grams)	AGI Score
TURKEY (breast roasted)	85	4.93
PEANUTS	28	4.86
PEANUT BUTTER	32	4.63
SALMON (pink/baked)	150	4.57
LIVER (chicken)	85	4.29
OIL (cod liver)	14	4.28
HALIBUT	150	4.03
CRISPS (potato)	30	3.98
TUNA	150	3.75
BUTTER	**5**	**3.67**
OIL (wheatgerm)	14	3.60
LIVER (beef)	85	3.57
MILK (1% fat)	245	3.56
ANCHOVY (in oil)	85	3.46
COD	180	3.43
LIVER (pig)	54	3.37
KIDNEY (beef)	85	3.35
SOLE	127	3.32
SOYBEANS (dry-roasted)	50	3.22
HADDOCK	150	3.11
OIL (corn)	14	3.02
SESAME SEEDS	28	3.00
EGG (yolk)	17	2.95
OIL (olive)	14	2.90
SARDINES (in oil)	50	2.72
SUNFLOWER SEEDS	28	2.65
OCTOPUS	85	2.62
OYSTERS	70	2.58
YOGURT	100	2.53
SUNFLOWER FLOUR	28	2.48
ALMONDS	28	2.48
PARMESAN	6	2.46
MUSSEL	85	2.42
OIL (sunflower)	14	2.40
HAZELNUTS	28	2.37
SCOLLOP	120	2.34
OIL (walnut)	14	2.30
COTTAGE CHEESE	100	2.25
WALNUTS	28	2.10
OIL (almond)	14	2.10
CRAB (steamed)	118	2.07
MAGARINE	5	2.04
WHELK	85	1.77
LENTILS	100	1.62

Food	Portion Size (in grams)	AGI Score
OATMEAL	234	1.59
LIMA BEANS	78	1.55
CUTTLE FISH	85	1.53
BLACKEYED PEAS	80	1.53
TOFU	100	1.48
FLORA PRO-ACTIVE	5	1.43
MILKSHAKE	200	1.36
OVALTINE	200	1.35
BREAD (wholewheat)	28	1.32
SHRIMP	50	1.32
RICE (brown)	100	1.29
BEANS (baked)	100	1.28
BRAN FLAKES	50	1.27
CORNFLAKES	100	1.26
CORN	100	1.24
PASTA	57	1.24
BREAD (white average)	30	1.22
CAULIFLOWER	50	1.21
SHREDDED WHEAT	50	1.20
OIL (hazelnut)	14	1.14
APPLE	138	1.11
BANANA	75	1.11
BROCCOLI	44	1.10
POTATO (sweet)	100	1.10
POTATO (flesh & skin)	200	1.09
RICE KRISPIES	25	1.09
PEAS (processed)	80	1.09
CABBAGE	75	1.09
ASPARAGUS	60	1.08
MANGO	100	1.07
EGG (white)	33	1.07
CARROTS	50	1.06
PEAS (garden)	80	1.05
PAPAYA	100	1.05
SPINACH	100	1.05
POTATO (flesh)	100	1.04
PEPPER (green)	74	1.04
BRUSSEL SPROUTS	78	1.02
RICE (long-grain white)	100	1.02
TOMATO	100	1.01
LETTUCE	55	1.01
BEER (average)	500	1.01
ONION	50	1.01
STRAWBERRY	83	1.01

Food	Portion Size (in grams)	AGI Score
ORANGE JUICE	124	1.00
TEA	200	1.00
BEVERAGES: COFFEE	200	1.00
WHITE WINE	100	1.00
RED WINE	100	1.00
HONEY	33	1.00
COLA	250	1.00
DIET COLA		1.00
WATER	**1000**	**1.00**

Table 4

The Atherogenic Effect Index (AGI)
per100g of each food in descending order.

Food	AGI Score
OIL (PALM)	82.44
PARMESAN	65.40
COCONUT	56.17
BUTTER	55.79
CHEDDAR	48.20
CAMEMBERT	33.25
OIL (cod liver)	24.43
CHOCOLATE: MILK	23.76
MAGARINE	21.70
OIL (wheatgerm)	19.58
BRAZIL NUTS	18.86
PINE NUTS	18.56
LAMB (leg roasted)	18.23
PEANUTS	16.76
BEEF (rump) COOKED	16.08
DUCK (roasted)	15.48
OIL (corn)	15.41
EGG (yolk)	15.35
OIL (olive)	14.58
PORK (leg roasted)	13.86
PEANUT BUTTER	13.54
CRISPS (potato)	11.86
OIL (sunflower)	11.01
OIL (walnut)	10.29
CHEESEBURGER (triple meat)	10.15
ICE CREAM	9.82

Food	AGI Score
SAUSAGES (pork)	9.71
MACKEREL	9.67
FLORA PRO-ACTIVE	9.50
OIL (almond)	8.86
SESAME SEEDS	8.76
CHICKEN (dark meat)	8.34
TURKEY (dark meat)	7.84
SUNFLOWER SEEDS	7.72
SUNFLOWER FLOUR	7.43
HEART (beef)	7.22
HAMBURGER	7.12
EEL	6.81
ALMONDS	6.70
SOYBEANS (dry-roasted)	6.62
HERRING	6.59
LIVER (PIG)	6.22
HAZELNUTS	6.21
CHICKEN BREAST (roasted)	6.01
TURKEY (breast roasted)	5.91
AVOCADO	5.59
WALNUTS	5.39
SARDINES (in oil)	5.22
LIVER (chicken)	5.06
SWORDFISH	4.67
LIVER (beef)	4.16
ANCHOVY (in oil)	4.04
LOBSTER	3.95
KIDNEY (beef)	3.88
OYSTERS	3.38
SALMON (pink/baked)	3.10
OCTOPUS	2.98
HALIBUT	2.81
MUSSEL	2.73
SOLE	2.72
TUNA	2.67
YOGURT	2.53
HADDOCK	2.30
COTTAGE CHEESE	2.25
COD	2.21
BREAD (wholewheat)	2.20
SCOLLOP	2.08
OIL (hazelnut)	2.01
WHELK	1.91
MILK (1% fat)	1.89
CRAB (steamed)	1.88

Food	AGI Score
BREAD (white average)	1.75
LIMA BEANS	1.73
BLACKEYED PEAS	1.68
SHRIMP	1.66
CUTTLE FISH	1.63
LENTILS	1.62
BRAN FLAKES	1.57
TOFU	1.48
CAULIFLOWER	1.43
PASTA	1.42
SHREDDED WHEAT	1.41
RICE KRISPIES	1.38
RICE (brown)	1.29
BEANS (baked)	1.28
CORNFLAKES	1.26
OATMEAL	1.25
BROCCOLI	1.24
CORN	1.24
EGG (white)	1.21
MILKSHAKE	1.18
OVALTINE	1.18
BANANA	1.15
ASPARAGUS	1.13
CABBAGE	1.11
PEAS (processed)	1.11
CARROTS	1.11
POTATO (sweet)	1.10
APPLE	1.08
MANGO	1.07
PEAS (garden)	1.07
PAPAYA	1.05
SPINACH	1.05
PEPPER (green)	1.05
POTATO (flesh & skin)	1.05
POTATO (flesh)	1.04
BRUSSEL SPROUTS	1.03
LETTUCE	1.02
RICE (long-grain white)	1.02
ONION	1.01
TOMATO	1.01
STRAWBERRY	1.01
BEER (average)	1.00
ORANGE JUICE	1.00
TEA	1.00
BEVERAGES: COFFEE	1.00

Food	AGI Score
WHITE WINE	1.00
RED WINE	1.00
HONEY	1.00
COLA	1.00
DIET COLA	1.00
WATER	1.00

Table 5

Saturated Fat & Cholesterol in Food
Ranked in descending order of saturated fat content

Note: I gram = one thirtieth of an ounce. One milligram (mg) = one thousandth of one gram

100 MILLIGRAMS = ONE THREE HUNDREDTHS OF AN OUNCE

FOOD	WEIGHT of Portion grams	CHOLESTEROL milligrams	SATURATED FAT milligrams
CHEESEBURGER (triple meat)	400	128	24800
HAMBURGER	250	188	10000
CAMEMBERT	62	45	9500
DUCK (roasted)	85	98	8200
CHOCOLATE: WHITE	44	10	8096
CHOCOLATE: MILK	44	10	8052
BEEF (rump) COOKED	100	76	7765
LAMB (leg roasted)	85	85	7000
CHEDDAR	28	27	5900
PORK (leg roasted)	85	85	5500
PANCREAS	85	223	5000
SAUSAGES (pork)	100	55	4900
ICE CREAM	66	16	4500
CHICKEN BREAST (roasted)	196	184	4300
CHICKEN (dark meat)	114	93	4200
HERRING	143	61	3700
MACKEREL	88	48	3700
EEL	136	107	3600
OIL (cod liver)	14	80	3200
TURKEY (dark meat)	85	102	2600
HEART (beef)	85	221	2500
BUTTER	5	11	2500
LOBSTER	145	160	2400

FOOD	WEIGHT of Portion grams	CHOLESTEROL milligrams	SATURATED FAT milligrams
TURKEY (breast roasted)	85	63	1800
LIVER (chicken)	85	298	1600
EGG (yolk)	17	190	1600
SWORDFISH	106	55	1500
LIVER (beef)	85	204	1360
LIVER (pig)	54	157	1350
OYSTERS	70	73	1100
ANCHOVY (in oil)	85	54	1100
KIDNEY (beef)	85	391	900
SALMON (pink/baked)	150	90	849
SARDINES (in oil)	50	33	833
MUSSEL	85	49	700
OCTOPUS	85	123	636
HALIBUT	150	62	613
PRAWN	50	140	500
SOLE	127	93	500
TUNA	150	76	400
COD	180	101	300
CRAB (steamed)	118	85	300
HADDOCK	150	57	300
SHRIMP	50	65	227
WHELK	85	89	0

Table 6

Trans-Fat & Cholesterol in Food
Ranked in descending order of trans-fat content

Note: I gram = one thirtieth of an ounce. One milligram = one thousandth of one gram
100 MILLIGRAMS = ONE THREE HUNDREDTHS OF AN OUNCE

FOOD	WEIGHT of Portion grams	CHOLESTEROL milligrams	TRANS-FAT milligrams
HAMBURGER	250	188	1400
CHEESEBURGER (triple meat)	400	128	1200
LAMB (leg roasted)	85	85	595
ICE CREAM	66	16	528
SAUSAGES (pork)	100	55	410
CHEDDAR	28	27	392
MAGARINE	5	0	335

FOOD	WEIGHT of Portion grams	CHOLESTEROL milligrams	TRANS-FAT milligrams
PEANUT BUTTER	32	0	**300**
BEEF (rump) COOKED	100	76	**200**
CHOCOLATE: WHITE	44	10	**176**
CHOCOLATE: MILK	44	10	**176**
BUTTER	5	11	**150**
CHICKEN (dark meat)	114	93	**114**
DUCK (roasted)	85	98	**85**
TURKEY (dark meat)	85	102	**85**
KIDNEY (beef)	85	391	**85**
PARMESAN	6	5	**66**
SARDINES (in oil)	50	33	**50**
CHOCOLATE: PLAIN	44	3	**44**
CRISPS (potato)	30	0	**30**
FLORA PRO-ACTIVE	5	0	**25**
PORK (leg roasted)	85	85	**1**
CHICKEN BREAST (roasted)	196	184	**1**
HERRING	143	61	**1**
EEL	136	107	**1**
OIL (cod liver)	14	80	**1**
HEART (beef)	85	221	**1**
TURKEY (breast roasted)	85	63	**1**
LIVER (chicken)	85	298	**1**
EGG (yolk)	17	190	**1**
LIVER (beef)	85	204	**1**
LIVER (pig)	54	157	**1**
ANCHOVY (in oil)	85	54	**1**
HALIBUT	150	62	1
SOLE	127	93	1
HADDOCK	150	57	1
MILK (1% fat)	245	7	1
COTTAGE CHEESE	100	5	1
MUESLI	100	0	1
EGG (white)	33	0	1
BEVERAGES: COFFEE	200	0	1
TEA	200	0	1
BREAD (white average)	30	0	1
BREAD (wholewheat)	28	0	1
BREAKFAST CEREAL: BRAN FLAKES	50	0	1
CORNFLAKES	100	0	1
RICE KRISPIES	25	0	1
SHREDDED WHEAT	50	0	1
WEETABIX	50	0	1
OIL (corn)	14	0	1
OIL (hazelnut)	14	0	1

FOOD	WEIGHT of Portion grams	CHOLESTEROL milligrams	TRANS-FAT milligrams
OIL (olive)	14	0	1
OIL (palm)	14	0	1
OIL (sunflower)	14	0	1
OIL (walnut)	14	0	1
OIL (wheatgerm)	14	0	1
PASTA	57	0	1
YOGURT	100	0	1
CAMEMBERT	62	45	0
PANCREAS	85	223	0
MACKEREL	88	48	0
LOBSTER	145	160	0
SWORDFISH	106	55	0
OYSTERS	70	73	0
SALMON (pink/baked)	150	90	0
MUSSEL	85	49	0
OCTOPUS	85	123	0
PRAWN	50	140	0

Table 7

Arginine to Lysine Ratio of Foods
(ie plant to animal amino-acid ratios)
The higher the score – the better for your arteries

Food	More arginine than lysine	A/L Ratio
RED WINE		221.50
WHITE WINE		139.00
SHRIMP		10.00
PINE NUTS		5.25
HAZELNUTS		5.20
BRAZIL NUTS		5.05
WALNUTS		5.00
SESAME SEEDS		4.64
ORANGE JUICE		4.00
ALMONDS		3.77
COCONUT		3.33
PEANUTS		3.29
PEANUT BUTTER		3.21
ONION		3.00
SUNFLOWER FLOUR		2.72
RICE (long-grain white)		2.33
PUMPKIN SEEDS		2.22

Food	More arginine than lysine	A/L Ratio
SUNFLOWER SEEDS		2.17
RICE KRISPIES		2.00
RICE (brown)		2.00
PASTA		1.92
RICE (wild/dry)		1.84
BREAKFAST BRAN FLAKES		1.81
OATMEAL		1.72
WHELK		1.69
SHREDDED WHEAT		1.63
BREAD (white average)		1.60
PEAS (garden)		1.50
PEAS (processed)		1.50
ALCOHOL: BEER (average)		1.50
PEPPER (green)		1.36
CORNFLAKES		1.33
BRUSSEL SPROUTS		1.33
BREAD (wholewheat)		1.22
SOYBEANS (dry-roasted)		1.17
LENTILS		1.11
TOFU		1.08
BLACKEYED PEAS		1.02
LOBSTER		1.01
CRAB (steamed)		1.00

Food	Lysine = Arginine	A/L Ratio
ASPARAGUS		1.00
BANANA		1.00
BROCCOLI		1.00
CABBAGE		1.00
CARROTS		1.00
CAULIFLOWER		1.00
CORN		1.00
STRAWBERRY		1.00

Food	More lysine than arginine	A/L Ratio
OYSTERS		0.99
POTATO (sweet)		0.98
EGG (yolk)		0.98
MUSSEL		0.98
OCTOPUS		0.97
SCOLLOP		0.97
CUTTLE FISH		0.97
POTATO (flesh)		0.92
EGG (white)		0.92
LIMA BEANS		0.91
LIVER (beef)		0.91
BEANS (baked)		0.91

Food	More lysine than arginine	A/L Ratio
LETTUCE		0.89
KIDNEY (beef)		0.88
HAMBURGER		0.86
DUCK (roasted)		0.86
SAUSAGES (pork)		0.83
HEART		0.82
LIVER (chicken)		0.81
SPINACH		0.81
CHEESEBURGER (triple meat)		0.79
LIVER (pig)		0.79
PANCREAS		0.78
CRISPS (potato)		0.77
TURKEY (breast roasted)		0.76
TURKEY (dark meat)		0.76
BEEF (sirloin) COOKED		0.76
POTATO (flesh & skin)		0.75
CHICKEN BREAST (roast)		0.75
CHICKEN (dark meat)		0.74
PORK (leg roasted)		0.72
LAMB (leg roasted)		0.67
SARDINES		0.67
EEL		0.66
ANCHOVY		0.65
COD		0.65
HALIBUT		0.65
MACKEREL		0.65
SOLE		0.65
SWORDFISH		0.65
HADDOCK		0.65
TUNA		0.65
HERRING		0.65
SALMON (pink/baked)		0.65
MONKFISH		0.65
TOMATO		0.62
COTTAGE CHEESE		0.56
APPLE		0.50
CHOCOLATE (milk)		0.50
WHOLE MILK		0.50
MANGO		0.50
ICE CREAM		0.47
BUTTER		0.46
MILKSHAKE (Vanilla)		0.45
OVALTINE		0.45
CHEDDAR		0.45
MILK (1% fat)		0.45

Food	More lysine than arginine	A/L Ratio
AVOCADO		0.39
PARMESAN		0.38
PAPAYA		0.38
CREAM (25% fat)		0.33
YOGURT		0.33
CAMEMBERT		0.04

Index

Q10, 117
questions, 5, 43, 77, 87, 119, 128, 176, 186, 208, 209, 240, 252, 253

raison d'être, 273
ratio, 68, 112, 133, 264
reality, 27, 159, 192, 232, 257, 259
recommended daily amount, 108
Recommended Nutritional Intake (RNI), 118
reconnaissance, 8, 54,176, 177, 243
red wine, 68, 99, 113, 182, 192, 193, 231
Red Wine Polyphenolic Extracts, 99
relaxation, 164, 180, 181
re-modelling, 19
research trials, 209
resentment, 175, 179, 182
reservatrol, 99, 193
resourcefulness, 176
resuscitation, 24, 32
reversing the 'furring', 221
rhythm, 40, 197, 281
rhythm disturbances, 38
rich and the poor, 37, 221, 240, 241
risk, 15, 16, 17, 30, 35, 37, 39, 42, 43, 47, 49, 52, 53, 78, 82, 83, 85, 89, 90, 91, 92, 94, 98, 113, 119, 144, 150, 161, 162, 163, 164, 168, 172, 177, 178, 180, 182, 190, 192, 206, 207, 210, 220, 221, 244, 249, 250, 253, 254, 262, 264, 265, 266, 269, 280, 281, 287, 288
risk factors, 39, 82, 144, 190, 250, 264
RNI, 118, 119, 124, 139, 140, 141, 142, 143, 145, 149, 230, 244, 247
Rock n' Roll, 183
Romania, 238

roughage, 87
rowing, 183, 187
ruler, 128
Russia, 89
rusting, 64, 100, 266
RWPE, 99

salmon, 92, 277
salt, 89, 110, 112, 122, 124, 126, 129, 131, 132, 133, 138, 141, 142, 144, 148, 151, 223, 226, 227, 277, 302, 305
sardines, 89, 92
sartan, 43
SAS, 187, 203, 276
saturated fat, 4, 5, 57, 61, 62, 64, 68, 72, 117, 224, 228, 229, 237, 238, 327
sauces, 93, 128, 230
science, 30, 66, 67, 84, 233, 234, 242, 258, 265, 273
scientific consensus, 222
score, 57, 66, 71, 72, 74, 102, 105, 107, 108, 109, 112, 116, 119, 130, 132, 133, 134, 135, 139, 140, 141, 142, 193, 289, 293, 330
Scots, 98
screening, 17, 27, 54, 157, 160, 206, 243, 249, 253, 254, 265
Second World War, 178, 179
sedentary, 189, 190
selenium, 68, 69, 81, 86, 89, 90, 94, 117, 118, 124, 125, 145, 239, 317
self-esteem, 175
self-examination, 17, 160
sense of humour, 183, 203, 277
sense of value, 175
sesame seeds, 69, 133
sex, 185, 260
sexual activity, 113
shellfish, 61, 66, 86, 106, 107, 110, 116, 120, 145, 224
shortness of breath, 23, 31, 37, 50, 85, 254